Physiotherapy in Medical Conditions

Physiotherapy in Medical Conditions

Suraj Kumar BPT MPT PhD
SRF-ICMR, BEd (LI and CP)
MIAP, MDCP, Vice-President POSA
Lecturer and Incharge, Physiotherapy Department
Paramedical Vigyan Mahavidyalaya, RIMS and R
Saifai, Etawah, Uttar Pradesh, India

Anoop Aggarwal BPT MPT
MIAP, MDCP
Physiotherapist
Pt Deendayal Upadhyaya Institute for the Physically Handicapped
New Delhi, India

Foreword
Dharmendra Kumar

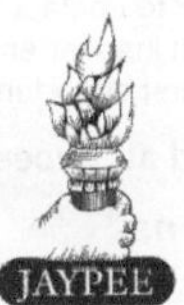

JAYPEE BROTHERS MEDICAL PUBLISHERS
The Health Sciences Publisher
New Delhi | London

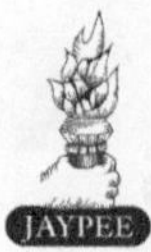

Jaypee Brothers Medical Publishers (P) Ltd

Headquarters
EMCA House
23/23-B, Ansari Road, Daryaganj
New Delhi 110 002, India
Landline: +91-11-23272143, +91-11-23272703
+91-11-23282021, +91-11-23245672
E-mail: jaypee@jaypeebrothers.com

Corporate Office
4838/24, Ansari Road, Daryaganj
New Delhi 110 002, India
Phone: +91-11-43574357
Fax: +91-11-43574314
E-mail: jaypee@jaypeebrothers.com

Overseas Office
J.P. Medical Ltd.
83, Victoria Street, London
SW1H 0HW (UK)
Phone: +44-2031708910
E-mail: info@jpmedpub.com

EU GPSR Authorised Representative
Logos Europe, 9 rue Nicolas Poussin
17000, La Rochelle, France
Phone: +33 (0) 6 67 93 73 78
E-mail: contact@logoseurope.eu

Website: www.jaypeebrothers.com
Website: www.jaypeedigital.com

Inquiries for bulk sales may be solicited at: jaypee@jaypeebrothers.com

Physiotherapy in Medical Conditions

First Edition: 2014

Reprint: **2025**

ISBN: 978-93-5152-165-5

Printed in India

Dedicated to

Our parents
Parents of Suraj Kumar:
Sri Raj Kumar Sinha
and
Smt Manorma Sinha
Parents of Anoop Aggarwal:
Sri Ashok Kumar Aggarwal
Smt Sudha Aggarwal
and
Badi Maa (Grandmother)
For always encouraging us with the prestigious guidance in the limited resources.

FOREWORD

Dear readers, congratulations on acquiring a book which has an immense potential to enhance your knowledge, improve professional capability and increase understanding about various medical conditions and their physiotherapeutic management.

This book contains meticulously designed and appropriately explained details of various topics including inflammation, edema, arthritis, skin diseases, deficiency diseases, psychiatric disorders, respiratory problems, cardiovascular diseases, neurological conditions, etc. This book will be very helpful to the physiotherapists and the other professionals who are working in the area of the rehabilitation management of disabling conditions.

The authors of the book, Suraj Kumar and Anoop Aggarwal, are innovative physiotherapists, scholars and good clinicians. They interact with the students with an open mind and facilitate the exchange of clinical and academic information based on their wide experience of the subject.

I wish all the readers very good luck in the quest of gaining and absorbing the knowledge provided in this book.

Dharmendra Kumar
Director
Pt Deendayal Upadhyaya Institute for
the Physically Handicapped
New Delhi, India

PREFACE

We are pleased to write the book *Physiotherapy in Medical Conditions.* The goal behind writing this book is to explain, in the language easily understood by the students, the ability to perform a good clinical examination, and we have no doubt, that the basic techniques are best learned by performance under the supervision. This task has been challenging and exciting because our rapidly increasing knowledge of physiotherapy continues to be growing. It is hoped that this book may help to fill some of these inevitable gaps until sound practice, based on experience, is achieved.

As with any product, there is always a scope for improvement; however, improvements are best made based on feedback from all the professionals.

- The book covers the basic as well as advanced details warranted for the clinical understanding, theoretical and practical knowledge with applied aspects.
- The book has been thoroughly updated by the subject experts.
- This book contains the bibliography to augment the authenticity of the facts related to various clinical conditions and their management.
- The book contains 9 topics including various subtopics.
- Illustrated throughout with photographs that support the explanations of the therapeutic application.

The language of the book is very reader-friendly and facilitates the learning process in an easy-to-understand manner. This book is designed for the physiotherapy students, who wish to acquire knowledge about different medical conditions. This book contains appropriately well-explained details of the medical topics which include inflammation, edema, arthritis, skin diseases, deficiency disorders, psychiatric, respiratory, cardiovascular and neurological conditions. This book is also very helpful for the physiotherapists and other professionals working in the area of rehabilitation management.

Suraj Kumar
Anoop Aggarwal

ACKNOWLEDGMENTS

Many friends have helped me along the path of framing the material and shared their highly valuable knowledge for this book. My grateful thanks to everyone who directly or indirectly helped and motivated me to write this book.

Special thanks to all those who have taught me—Dr Manda Chauhan, Dr Rajni Kalra, Dr Ramprabhu, Dr Ajay Bahl, Dr VP Sharma, Dr HK Tripathi, Dr Roshan Lal Meena, and Dr Tripta Ghai. I am grateful to my students for giving me the opportunity and privilege to understand various aspects of the clinical conditions and helped me to write this book. I express my special thanks to all those thousands of patients, treating and managing whom during the last ten years, I have received innumerable opportunities to enhance the clinical and academic knowledge.

The co-author of this book, Anoop Aggarwal, has really enlightened the clinical applicability of the book using his vast knowledge and clinical experiences. We wish to express true-hearted thanks to Dr Praerna Bhatnagar for her valuable suggestions during the various phases of book writing, and for arranging the various extremely-needed articles/journals for the completion of the book.

Finally, I would express my sincere thanks to my mother, father, my son (Tejasvi) and my wife (Rina Ranjana) who have listened to and supported me throughout the period of preparing and formulating the book.

I, along with my co-author, also thankfully acknowledge the suggestions of the following professionals:

- Akhilesh Shukla
- Arvind Kumar
- G Venu Vendhan
- Jaya Talwar
- Manda Chauhan
- NK Sinha
- Sandeep Babbar
- Shohrab A Khan

CONTENTS

Plate 1

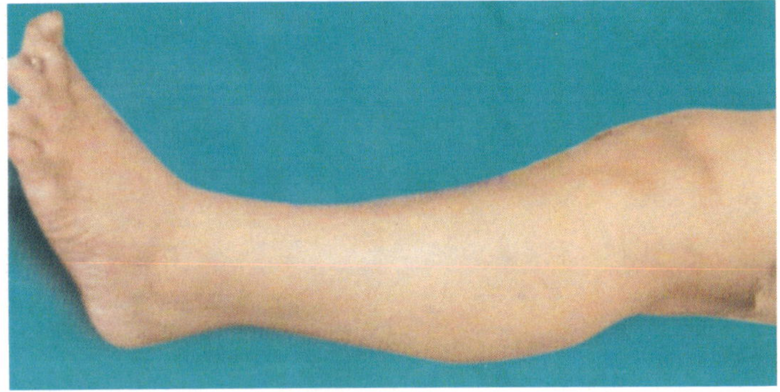

Fig. 2.1: The edema involving lower leg

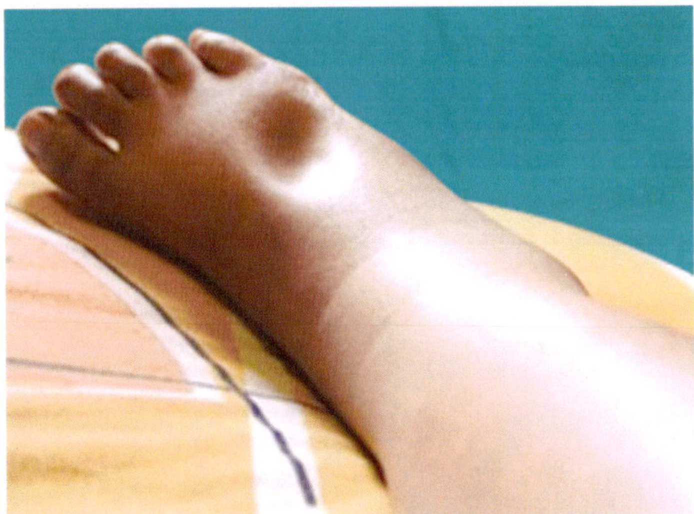

Fig. 2.2: Pitting edema of leg

Plate 2

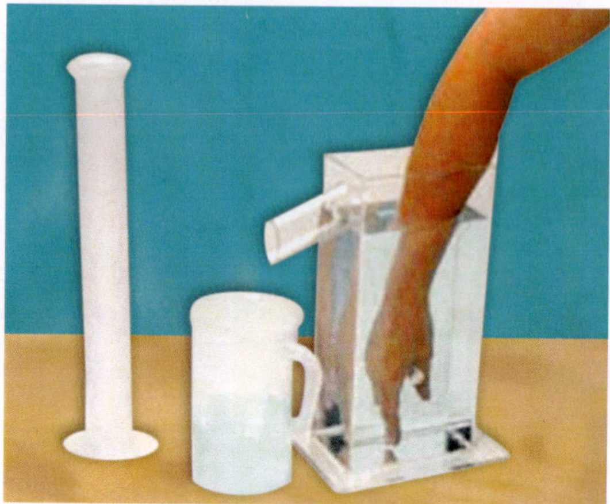

Fig. 2.4: Edema water-displacement volumetry

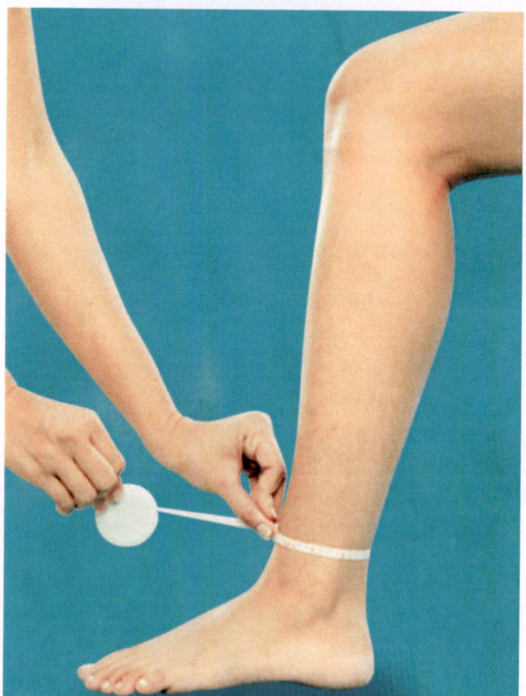

Fig. 2.5: Measurement of ankle edema by measuring tape

Plate 3

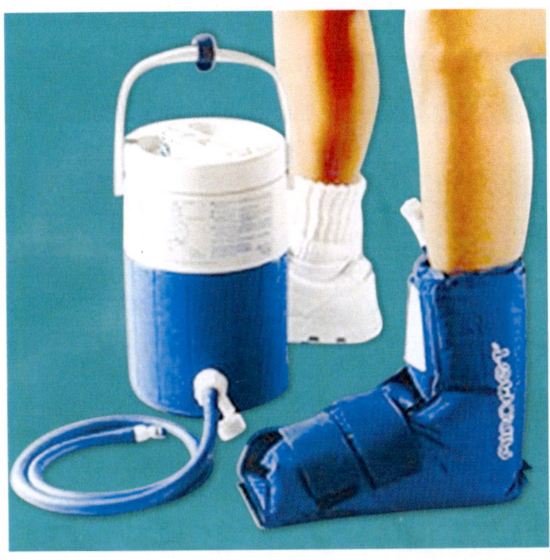

Fig. 2.6: Application of cryo-cuff for acute edema around ankle

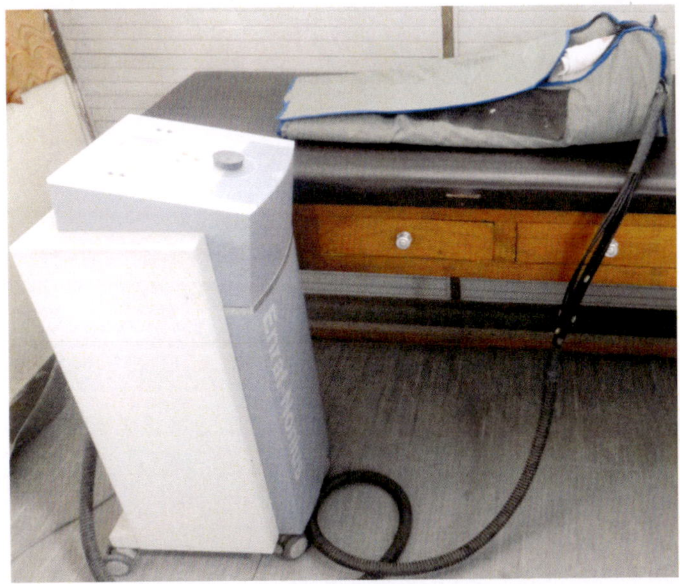

Fig. 2.7: The application of pneumatic compression pumps to manage the edema around ankle

Plate 4

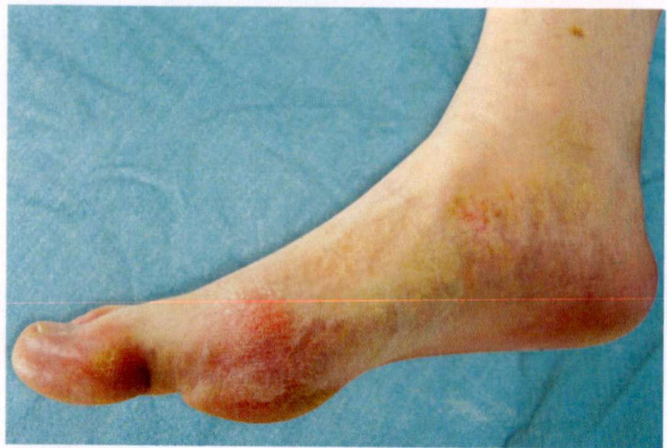

Fig. 3.5: MTP joint of foot, hot, swollen and tender

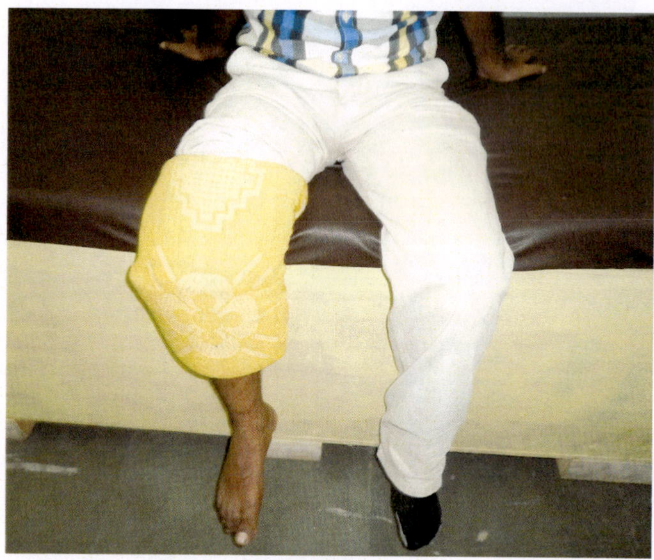

Fig. 3.9: Application of hot pack for the knee joint pain

Plate 5

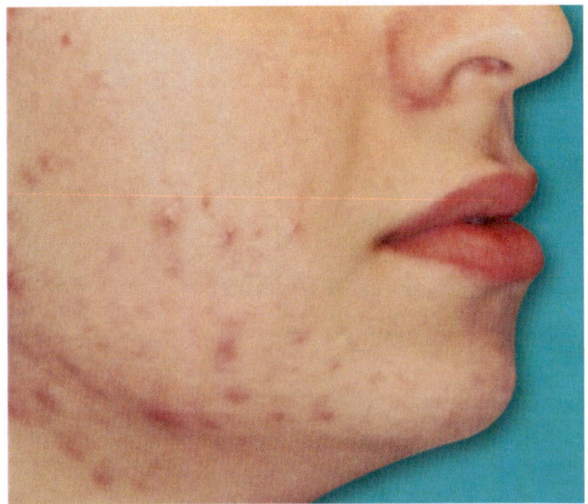

Fig. 4.1: Pimples in acne

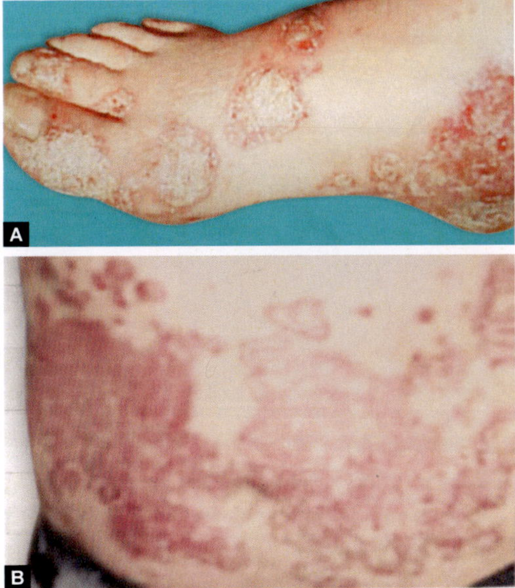

Figs 4.2A and B: (A) Clearly defined plaques on foot; (B) Red color patches on abdominal region

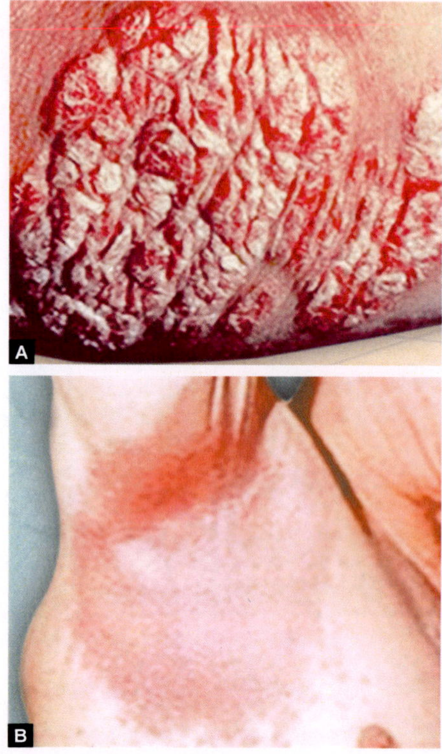

Figs 4.4A and B: (A) Plaque Psoriasis; (B) Inverse psoriasis in axilla region

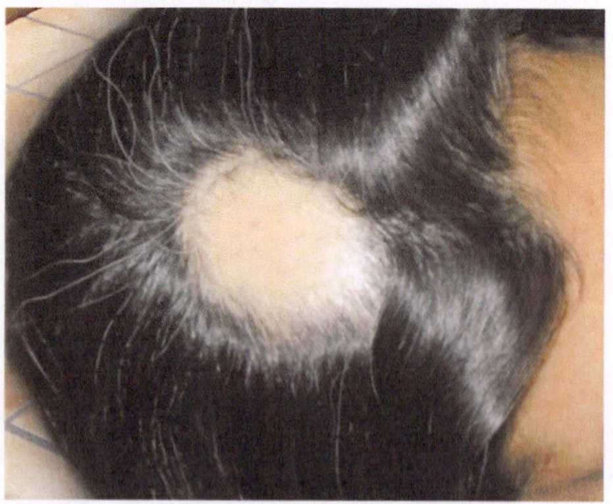

Fig. 4.5: Alopecia areata

Plate 7

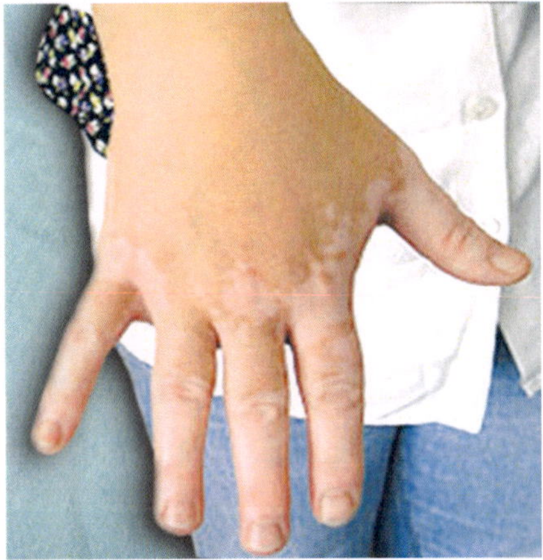

Fig. 4.6: White/light colored skin patch on hand

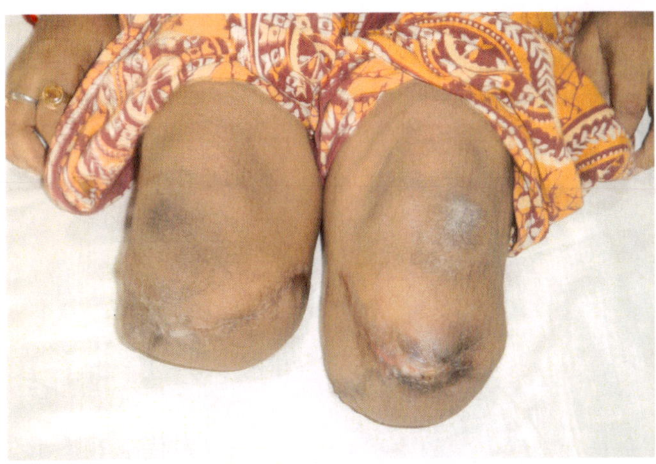

Fig. 4.9: Below knee amputation secondary to leprosy

Plate 8

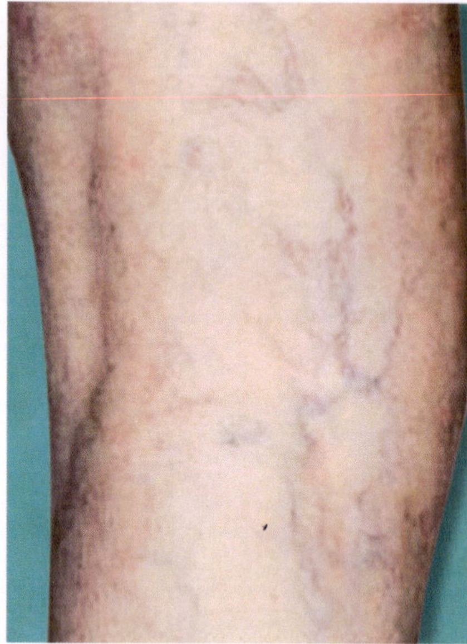

Fig. 8.4: Spider vein in the posterior aspect of knee

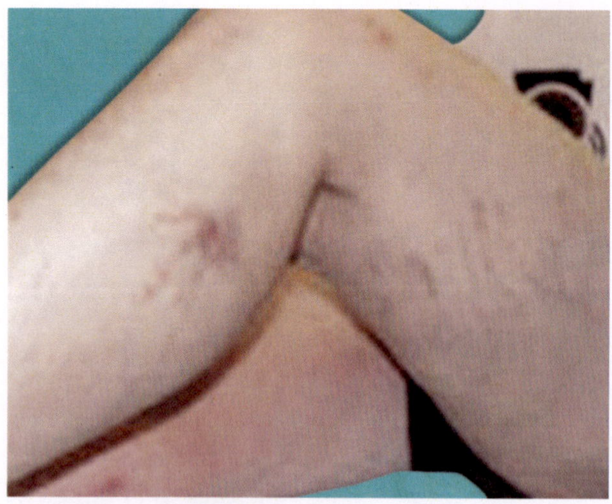

Fig. 8.5: Telangiectasias

Plate 9

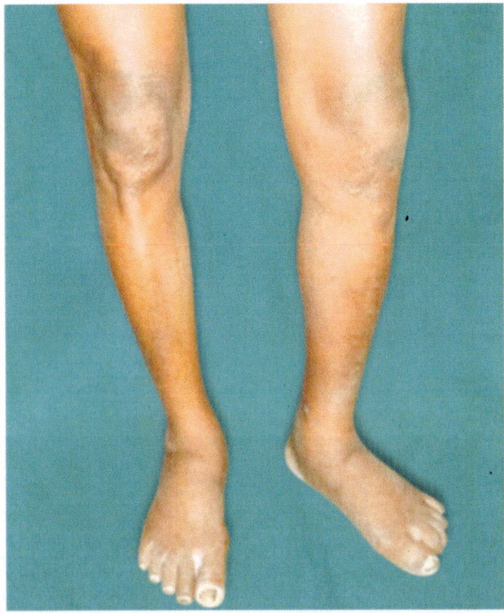

Fig. 8.6: Deep vein thrombosis of right leg with redness and swelling

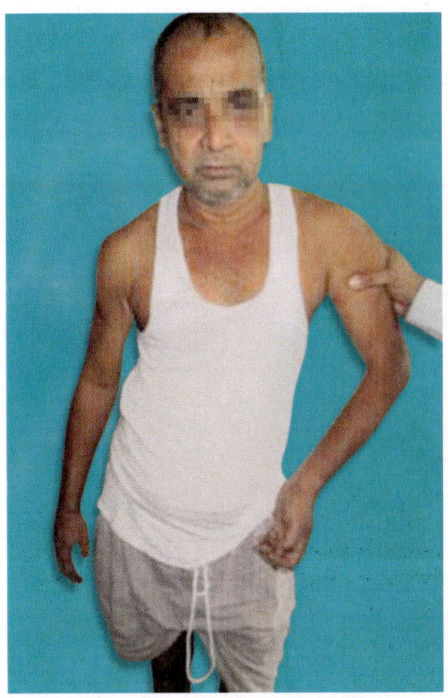

Fig. 9.2.1: The attitude of the joints in a typical hemiplegic patient

CHAPTER

1

Inflammation

DEFINITION

Inflammation is the sequence of changes which take place in living tissue in response to damage. It is natural reaction of the body towards any event or any foreign material (chemical, mechanical, geometrical, and others) which tends to irritate the environment of the body (Coleman et al, 1973).

Inflammation is the protective or defensive mechanism (Ferrero-Miliani et al, 2007) that occurs in the living tissue as a result of injury. It involves a series of changes affecting vessels and cells surrounding the affected area. If the injury is severe enough to cause destruction of tissue (necrosis) then the inflammatory reaction will occur in the surrounding area which was injured.

If there was no process of inflammation then wounds and infections would never heal. There would occur the progressive destruction of the tissue. Yet the chronic inflammation can lead to variety of pathological conditions like arterial hardening (atherosclerosis) and rheumatoid process.

Importance of the Inflammation

The inflammation is an important process which serves following two-fold purpose:

- Removal of the irritant, debris and dead cells. Increased blood cells engulf and often digest bacteria, dead cells, or other debris that might cause or continue the inflammation.
- Preparation of the way for repair by increasing the blood supply and the fresh healing factors to the place.
- Macrophages may play a more direct role in muscle repair and remodeling than merely removing tissue debris. Role for macrophages has been identified in muscle repair and regeneration *in vivo* (Lesaudron et al, 1999).

- Due to the increased blood supply the fluid content in the region increases and this dilutes the irritant which was leading to the irritation in the region.
- Antibodies, which are also present in the edema fluid, neutralize toxic substances.

This is an important event in case of injury of the cell or body parts however in some cases it may be required to suppress this process. In some cases these inflammatory reactions may be fatal or harmful to body. It occurs when some organ transplantation procedure has been done and there is risk that this foreign organ may be damaged if inflammatory process takes place. This requires the suppression of immunity or inflammatory process which can be achieved by cytotoxic drugs or immunosuppressors drugs.

Inflammation sometime can also lead to the injury and damage to the tissue of the body (Flow chart 1.1). During inflammation the neutrophils can cause direct lysis of muscle cell membranes through a superoxide-dependent mechanism (Nguyen and Tidball, 2003).

Stages of Inflammation

Over the next few weeks, *resolution* occurs, and the normal tissue architecture is restored. Blood clots are removed by fibrinolysis, and if it is not possible to return the tissue to its original form, *scarring* results from in-filling with fibroblasts, collagen, and new endothelial cells.

Inflammation may occur rapidly as "acute inflammation" or it may persist for prolonged period and chronically long duration when it is called as "chronic inflammation". Both of these inflammations present different pictures. The inflammation is considered acute for the first 24 hours, when there is primarily neutrophil infiltration (Yager and Nwomeh, 1999). By 1 week, the inflammation converts to chronic, as identified histologically by macrophage infiltration (Radhkrishna et al, 2003).

Acute inflammation is earlier response of the body to the irritant stimulus and during this the increased migration of plasma and WBCs occur into the injured region (Fig. 1.1.). Also the activation of local vascular and immune system causes the appearance of cardinal features of the inflammation (Rubor, tumor, dolor, color, and loss of functions) occurs. In chronic inflammation, the inflammation persists for prolonged time and this is due to the destruction of the damaged cells and the formation of new healed tissue.

Flow chart 1.1: Sequence of events occuring during inflammation

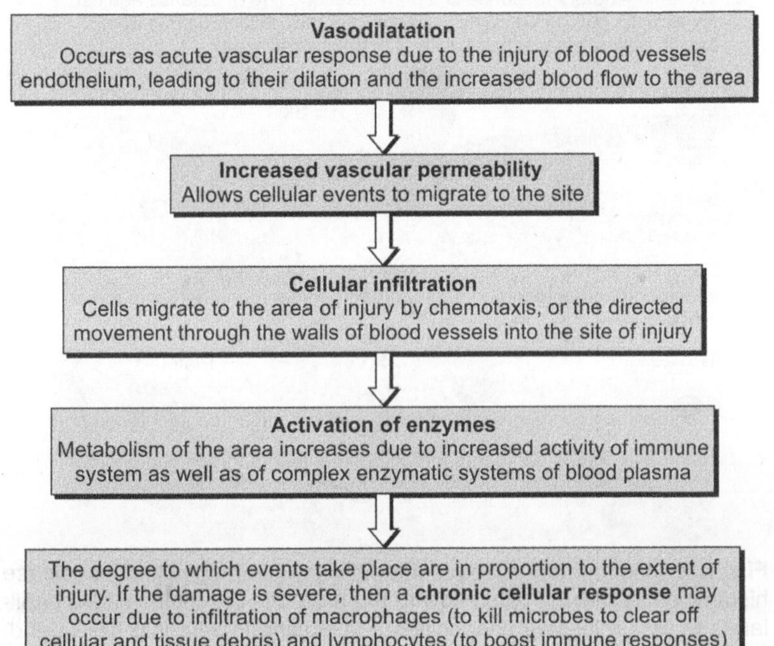

ACUTE INFLAMMATION

Causes

There are a large number of factors which can cause the inflammatory reaction and they can be listed under the following headings:

- Physical—thermal, mechanical, irradiation
- Chemical—acids and alkalis, body fluids which escape into tissues (bile, urine), metabolic products of bacteria (toxins)
- Intra-cellular replication viruses
- Hypersensitivity reactions such as reaction of antibody to antigenic material
- Necrosis of tissue result in inflammation in surrounding area.

Changes of Acute Inflammation

Whatever the causes of inflammation, the reaction follows a basic pattern. However, the appearance of the tissue will depend on the type of tissue affected, the nature of the irritant and the duration.

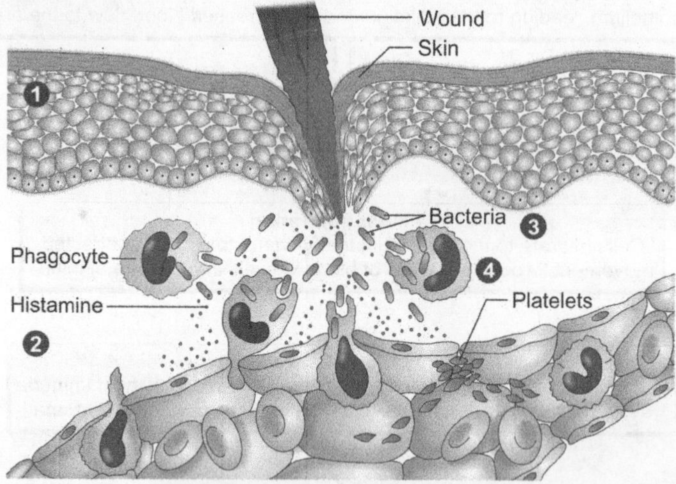

Fig. 1.1: Inflammatory changes after injury: 1. Damaged tissues release histamines increasing blood flow to the area; 2. Histamines cause capillaries to leak releasing phagocytes and clotting factors into the wound; 3. Phagocytes engulf bacteria, dead cells and cellular debris; 4. Platelets move out of the capillary to seal the wounded area

The basic pattern of changes concern:

- Vascular
- Surrounding tissues
- The lymph flow.

Vascular Changes in Acute Inflammation

The initial change may be observed in relation to superficial vessels, as a whitening of the skin. This is a momentary vasoconstriction caused by the irritant and is quickly followed by the main inflammatory changes designed to deal with the injury. The first of these changes is a relaxation of the circular muscle of the arterioles which may be brought about by chemical mediator and possibly by the axon reflex. This is believed to be regulated by the chemical mediator released in direct relation to the irritant. However, it may be that the axon reflex produces the more widespread flare noticed by Lewis is the 'triple response'.

Accompanying the relaxation of the arterioles there is an engorgement of the capillaries and post-capillary venules as the result of the increased blood flow (active hyperemia). This active hyperemia is followed by a slowing of the blood flow which results from a number of factors. There is inflammatory exudate into the surrounding tissues which increases the viscosity of the blood in the area and thus offers more resistance to flow. The viscosity is also increased by the red cells clinging together (rouleaux). The leucocytes tend to adhere to the walls of the post-capillary venules and further hinder blood flow. In some instances there may be a temporary stasis and clotting may occur.

The inflammatory exudate is composed of protein-rich plasma which differs from the normal passage of fluid into the tissues due to hydrostatic pressure which is called transudation. The passage of proteins is accompanied by a relatively greater quantity of fluid than in normal plasma and this further increases the viscosity of the blood. There is usually an axial flow in the blood vessels with the cells and plasma lying centrally land only plasma peripherally. However, as the flow of blood slows down, the larger white cells tend to fall towards the periphery (margination) while the red cells maintain an axial flow and form rouleaux. The leucocytes (Polymorph nuclear leucocytes and monocytes) which have adhered to the endothelial wall tend to pass out into the tissue space by an active process of emigration. This process occurs mainly in the venules, and the leucocytes thrust pseudopodia through the gaps in the endothelial cells and then squeeze through into the tissues. It is thought that this may be the result of chemical attraction due to a chemical mediator produced at the site of injury (chemotaxis). Some of the red cells may also pass into the tissue spaces (diapedesis).

Surrounding Tissues Changes

As already stated, there is an exudation of fluid from the vessels into the tissues and this may serve a number of purposes. The increase of fluid to the infected tissue dilutes the toxins and may prevent or diminish further tissue damage. It helps to carry bacteria and toxins to lymph vessels and nodes where the antigenic effect may further assist the defense mechanisms by producing an immune response. If the inflammatory exudates bring plasma proteins into contact with bacteria these antigens lead to production of antibodies. If the plasma contains antibodies which will react with the infecting organisms they may be destroyed and removed by phagocytosis. If the ground substance of the tissues is a gel, this changes to a fluid thus preventing an early rise in tissue tension. There is a proliferation of connective tissue cells.

Lymph Flow Changes

The tissues become swollen with the increased quantity of fluid in inflammation and this causes a dilation of the lymph vessels and some of the fluid escapes from the site of the lesion. The antigenic effect has been mentioned in the previous paragraph.

Although the basic changes are similar for all tissues, there are differences according to the type of tissue. For example, in mucous membrane there is an increased production of mucus which may become mucopurulent depending on the causative factor. Similar reactions will occur with serous secreting membranes.

Signs and Symptoms of Acute Inflammation

Inflammation is characterized locally by redness, heat, pain, swelling and loss of function. In some circumstances, such as bacterial or viral infection, there may be general signs depend upon the type and degree of injury to the tissues and the efficiency of the body's defense mechanism in that area.

The acute inflammation is characterized by five cardinal features (Rubor, tumor, dolor, color and loss of function) (Parakrama and Taylor, 2005).

- *Rubor/Redness*: This is due to the local vasodilatation and the increased blood supply to the region.
- *Color/Heat*: The increased flow of blood resulting from the dilatation of vessels may cause a local increase of temperature. This can occur in superficial tissue where the temperature may be lower than the blood because contact with the external environment.
- *Dolor/Pain*: This is partly due to the tension created in the tissues by the exudates. If the space is small the pressure on the nerve endings will be greater. Pain may also be due to an increased concentration of hydrogen ions or the chemical substances released by the damaged tissue. This irritates the local nerve endings and lead to the pain sensation.

- *Tumor/Swelling*: The inflammatory exudates accumulate in the area resulting in swelling. This occurs due to increased permeability of capillary walls thus fluid passes into the tissue spaces. The amount of swelling depends on the severity of the inflammation, the tensions of the particular tissues land the extent to which the fluid can drain away. It may also depend on the type of tissue involved.
- *'Functio laesa'/Loss of Function*: Inflammation will upset the normal function of the tissues, and the extent of this malfunction will depend on several factors. Pain, particularly in relation to muscle and joints, will limit movement and there may be reflex inhibition of muscle action. Swelling around a joint will limit movement apart from the resulting pain. Depending on the tissues involved, the inflammation may either alter or impede the function. If mucus secreting epithelium is inflamed the secretion of mucus is increased as in the common cold.

These features of the inflammation are apparent mostly on the superficial skin while are almost inconsistently found in the cases where the deeper sited areas are inflamed like deeper visceral organs involvement, where the nerve endings are almost absent.

Further stages following acute inflammation.

RESOLUTION

If the inflammatory agent is very mild the damaged cells and the exudate will be quickly removed and the area will rapidly return to normal. This is known as resolution. A more severe injury, provided it is not accompanied by tissue destruction, should also resolve but the process will take a little longer, possibly up to several weeks.

This return to normal occurs in the following way:

- Removal of excess fluid. Most of the excess fluid drains away via the lymphatics. Some of the fluid will flow back into the capillaries as the vessels return to their normal permeability and the balance of hydrostatic pressure and osmotic pressure between the tissue fluid and plasma is restored.
- Removal of cellular debris and damaged phagocytes. Debris may be digested by phagocytes or enzymes in the exudate. Some debris is carried in the lymph stream to the nodes where it is dealt with by the cells lining the sinuses.

- Undamaged polymorphs. These pass back into the blood and lymph streams and macrophages wander back into the surrounding connective tissues.

SUPPURATION

This occurs as a result of a pyogenic bacterial infection which leads to necrosis of tissue and formation of pus. It can also occur in body cavities such as the pleural space, peritoneum or joint without involving necrosis of tissue, the toxins produced by the bacteria cause necrosis of tissue which is then digested by the polymorph enzymes leaving a space filled with pus (abscess). Pus comprises an inflammatory exudate containing living and dead polymorphs, bacteria, necrotic tissue, and fibrin. This is creamy in color and consistency and sticky due to DNA released from the dead polymorphs.

The formation of an abscess tends to lead to an increase of bacteria and spread of infection for the following reasons: exudate from the inflammatory reaction flows into lymphatic vessels but in an abscess there is inadequate drainage and exudate tends to become stagnant. There is an increase of polymorphs into the cavity and with the exudate this increases the pressure. The exudate in the cavity is an ideal medium for the growth of bacteria and liberation of toxins which then cause necrosis of surrounding tissue, because of the increased pressure, pus from the abscess tends to extend into surrounding tissues where there is least resistance.

CHRONIC INFLAMMATION

This type of inflammation is characterized by the proliferation of tissue cells to give fibrous-tissue; this contrasts with the exudative changes of acute inflammation: Chronic inflammation may be secondary to acute inflammation when the body's defense is not sufficient to allow resolution and there is persistent low grade irritation.

Primary chronic inflammation may be produced by the same factors which produce acute inflammation but the injury or irritant produces a mild reaction. This may be due to the nature of the irritant, the dosage, the state of the body's defense and part of the body affected. Certain bacterial and fungal infections produce a chronic inflammation, e.g. tubercle bacillus and syphilis. Some dusts or chemicals produce irritation of the lungs resulting in chronic bronchitis, asbestosis or similar conditions. Repetitive minor trauma may result in chronic inflammation as in a sprained ankle.

Changes of Chronic Inflammation

The changes are a mixture of the vascular and proliferative changes of acute inflammation—the attempt to clear the debris and the microorganisrns and the processes of healing. This is the state in which inflammation and healing are going on at the same time.

In many cases of chronic inflammation there is extensive exudation of protein-rich fluid leading to the production of considerable quantities of fibrin. This is particularly seen in chronic, suppurative inflammation and inflammation of serous sacs. Many cells are present in the area including large quantities of macrophages which may have fused to form giant cells. These cells soften and remove the dead cells and debris.

Lymphocytes and plasma cells are also found in great numbers.

The function of the later cells is uncertain but they are a feature of the granulation tissue in chronic inflammation. Endothelial cells are also present forming the new capillaries. These are especially noticeable in the lining of chronic abscess cavities and they break down readily leading to hemorrhage.

Fibroblasts are present in large numbers and lay down the collagen which produces a large quantity of fibrous tissue. If the cells of the chronically inflamed tissue can divide, then regeneration occurs. Quite often there is excessive production of new cells, which is particularly noticeable in epithelial tissues.

Signs and Symptoms of Chronic Inflammation

These will depend on the area involved but generally lead to impaired function as a result of the formation and shrinkage of fibrous tissue. Adhesions may form in relation to ligaments around joints and will restrict movement; tubes and orifices may be affected leading to stenosis, e.g. the mitral valve in chronic endocarditis or the small intestine in regional ileitis. It can lead to reduction of elasticity in tubes as in chronic bronchitis.

Healing

In the floor of any open and healing wound tiny raised red dots can be clearly seen. To this tissue the term granulation tissue has been applied. The name originates from the Latin 'granum', a seed or granule. Each do or granule consists of new blood vessels, macrophages, fibroblasts and other cells.

No matter what body tissue is damaged, healing begins with the formation of granulation tissue. The final result may differ depending upon whether the parenchymal cells are capable of mitotic division or not. The cells of some tissues such as epithelium, bone marrow, lymph glands and the spleen continue to divide throughout life. Such tissues have great power of regeneration. Some cells, e.g. the cells of the liver, have the power to divide but only do so if the need arises. On the other hand, nerve and muscle cells have no power to reproduce themselves and in this case granulation tissue will eventually be converted into scar tissue.

Regeneration is the replacement of lost tissue by similar tissue. Repair is replacement by scar tissue when the cells of the damaged organ or tissue are unable to divide.

Healing of Skin Wounds

A wound where there is little tissue loss and no infection may heal by first intention (primary union). If there is a greater degree of tissue destruction then healing may occur by second intension (secondary union).

Healing by First Intention

This should occur following a clean cut or surgical incision and follows a basic pattern.

Blood Clot: Blood escaping from cut vessels clots on the surface and fills the gap between the edges of the wound. This serves as an adhesive and protective cover.

Inflammatory reaction is mild and occurs during the first twenty-four hours resulting in exudation of fluid and invasion of the site by macrophages which ingest and digest fibrin, red cells and cellular debris.

Epithelial Cells: Within twenty-four hours the squamous epithelium bridges the gap and is followed by hypertrophy of all the layers of the skin adjacent to the wound. The epithelial cells may extend down into the dermis but are later removed.

Dermis and Subcutaneous Tissue: There is a proliferation of net blood vessels and fibroblasts leading to the formation of granulation tissue. Vascular sprouts extend into the wound and unite to form vascular network and at the same time the lymphatic channels are re-established.

Fibrous Tissue Proliferation: Fibroblasts proliferate and move into the area and within four to five days mature collagen fibers are produced and probably unite the cut edges of the incision from about the end of the first week.

The strength of the newly formed skin is nearly normal by about fourteen days and continues to develop slowly over the next few weeks. The normal skin formed in this manner is devoid of hair follicles, sweat and sebaceous glands which cannot reproduce.

Healing by Second Intention

There is no real difference in the healing process except that there is necrotic tissue and debris to be removed and a gap to be filled. The process of healing therefore takes longer, more granulation tissue is formed and more scar tissue results. The gap is filled by clotted exudate and blood. Then phagocytic cells invade the clot. Capillaries and fibroblasts grow in from the sides and floor of the wound, filling it with granulation tissue.

If the cells of the damaged tissue can divide, new cells infiltrate the granulation tissue, but if they cannot, the tissue becomes increasingly fibrous. The collagen fibers thicken and new layers are laid down at right angles to each other, so that eventually a tough bundle or membrane of collagen fiber is formed. Tension on these fibers seems to determine the direction in which they lie. Epithelial cells at the edges of the wound multiply and migrate down the sides into the wound between the connective tissue and the clot, forcing the latter up. As the granulation tissue grows up from the floor and sides, the tongues of epithelial cells growing down on the edges of the gap are forced up until they cover the surface. Should there be much loss of epitheliurn, cells are obtained from the bases of the hair follicles and sweat glands.

While all this is going on some of the new blood vessels begin to atrophy while others show such proliferation of the endothelium that their lumen is obliterated. As revascularization and thickening increase, pale, vascular scar tissue is formed. This has a great tendency to contract, thereby deforming the surrounding tissues.

Local Factors Which may Affect Wound Healing

One of the most important of these is the vascularity of the damaged tissue. A good blood supply is necessary both for inflammatory reaction and to support the processes of repair. Circulation varies in different tissues. Some, such as bone and muscle, are highly vascular; others, such as cartilage and ligaments, have very poor nutrition and heat less readily.

- When the circulation is impaired by disease, healing can be seriously affected, as can be readily seen in peripheral vascular disease. The blood supply can also be reduced by:
  - Prolonged pressure
  - Edema
  - Chronic inflammation since this is accompanied by thickening of the intima and obliteration of the lumen of the blood vessels.
- Infection will delay healing since the toxins produced by microorganisms destroy tissue.
- Persistent irritation will cause healing to be slowed, e.g. the presence of foreign bodies.
- Continual breakdown of granulation tissue due to rough handling will delay healing.
- Repeated dressing of a wound will have a similar effect.
- Too early movement will sometimes delay healing if it causes further damage or destruction of granulation tissue.
- The speed of healing is increased by physical measures which stimulate the circulation. Thus heat, ultraviolet light, ultrasound, and moderate exercise may all help the healing process if applied correctly.

Healing of Other Soft Tissues

Healing of damaged tendons takes place in an identical way to that of other soft tissues except that tendon cells are found in the granulation tissue and very slowly regeneration will occur. If the ends of the tendon are not joined, however, union will be by fibrous issue and the danger then is that repeated stretching due to movement will elongate the fibrous tissue, lengthening the tendon and reducing power.

In a minor injury of a muscle with rupture of individual fibers, regeneration can occur but in more severe injuries scar tissue forms.

Cardiac muscle fibres have no ability to divide, consequently damage to the heart muscle is healed by fibrous tissue thus an infarct is converted into fibrous tissue. Nerve tissue within the brain and spinal cord has no power of regeneration since nerve cells cannot reproduce, and axons can only grow if there is a neurlemma. Nerve fibres in the central nervous system do not have a neurilemmal sheath. Peripheral nerves on the other hand can regenerate if the cells of origin of the axons are still intact.

PHYSICAL THERAPY INTERVENTION

Acute Phase Management

Aims during acute phase of inflammation are:

- Prevention of excessive exudates and bleeding
- Rest of the inflamed part to reduce the muscle spam and prevent the irritation of tissue
- Maintenance of normal circulation to the affected part
- Maintenance of normal muscle bulk and tone.

In order to fulfill these aims the various physical therapy interventions are used. To prevent excessive exudates or bleeding, the ice, pressure bandages or evaporating lotions can be used. During initial acute stages (about up to 3 days) during pain the cryotherapy along with rest, is recommended to decrease pain and swelling. The application of cryotherapy along with compression and the elevation further aid to reduce the signs of inflammation.

PRICE (Pressure, Rest, Ice, Compression, and Elevation) are the preferred principles during acute phase management (Ivins, 2006). The relaxation exercises and the rest further reduce the inflammatory response. Rest may be given in various ways according to the site of the injury. Patient may be confined to bed; the upper limb/lower limb may be splinted or supported in a sling.

Electric currents are used to decrease the pain, by the mechanism of pain-pathway blocking, and activating the local mechanoreceptors to decrease the perception of pain (Abram and Stephen, 1993).

TENS is found to be ineffective in reducing hyperalgesia in the early, acute phase of inflammation, and 4 hours after induction. However, it helps to reduce secondary hyperalgesia which appears approximately 24 hours to 2 weeks later. Thus, clinically, after the early, acute phase of inflammation. TENS may be more effective in reducingpain and hyperalgesia (Carol Vance et al, 2007).

The ultrasound therapy in pulsed mode and low intensity laser therapy are used due to their non-thermal and pain reduction effects. They also augment the healing process.

The prolonged rest must be discouraged as it reduces the circulation to the region due to diminished muscle activity. It might prevent the organization of the healing tissue and may cause the muscle disused atrophy (Stein and Wade, 2005) and diminished muscle tone/bulk. In cases where the rest is still necessary then the active exercises of the proximal and distal portion may help to maintain the circulation to the affected region. When the dynamic movement of the body part is not possible then isometric contractions, passive movements and massage are the suitable means.

Chronic Phase Management

Aims during chronic phase of inflammation are:

- To revascularize the area
- Deliberate attempt to stretch the tissues in appropriate fashion so as to break the adhesions
- To increase the healing tissue strength.

Revascularization can be increased in many ways. Sometime an injection of a local anesthesia, to overcome vasospasm by temporarily paralyzing the vasoconstrictor fibers and thus it will promote the hyperemia. The deep massage can be used to increase the revascularization further.

In order to reduce the adhesions the ultrasound therapy, deep transverse friction massage and vigorous exercises are suitable. The ultrasonic therapy helps to increase the fibroblast activity and thus helps to increase the collagen tissue formation. The deep transverse friction massage helps to break the haphazard linking of the collagen fibers so that the haphazard collagen cross-link now does not restrict the tissue mobility or impair the revascularization process. The vigorous exercises are used to increase the strength of the healing tissues.

Functional re-education of the injured muscles are used. In initial stages when the muscle contraction is absent or is too weak, then the faradic muscle stimulation helps to preserve the movement pattern and tissue excitability. As condition improves, the faradic stimulation may be combined with the active muscle contraction. Further progression can be done to attempt the muscle contraction independently without the aid of electrical stimulation.

The low power laser therapy helps to improve the collagen fiber quality and thus helps to lay down the collagen fiber of high tensile strength (Dicky et al, 2002). The thermal dosage of ultrasonic therapy may be used now.

The cryotherapy can be replaced by thermotherapy to improve the blood circulation to the region, to improve its metabolic activity, to wash out the metabolite waste products and to bring more fresh nutrients to the region to boost up healing processes. Thermotherapy can reduce the muscle spasm and improve collagen tissue extensibility, thus it can be employed before range of motion exercises and the stretching exercises.

The external pressure via intermittent pneumatic compression pump may be used to improve the lymphatic return from the region.

Management of Suppurative Inflammation

Aims of management in case of suppurative inflammation:

- To destroy the micro-organisms and prevent their manipulations
- Encourage rapid healing, and to prevent contracture of fibrous tissue
- To prevent the restriction of movement in joints
- Restoration of normal muscle functions (common aim in all types of inflammations).

The therapeutic modalities are mostly avoided, still whenever necessary they should be used with caution.

In case of deep sited infections, if the infected tissue communicates with the exterior (Such as in case of PID, pelvic inflammatory diseases) then the SWD (short wave diathermy) will help to drain out the pus by improving the blood flow and along with this the drainage of pus from deeper tissue to the superficial openings.

The ultraviolet therapy or infrared radiations are used to promote of a good blood supply and to promote rapid healing.

Gentle active movements taking aseptic precautions in the necessary handling of the area can be used for improving circulation.

BIBLIOGRAPHY

1. Abram, Stephen E. Advances in Chronic Pain Management since gate control. Regional Anesthesia and Pain Medicine 1993;18;2.
2. Carol GT Vance, Radhakrishnan R, Skyba DA, Sluka KA. Transcutaneous Electrical Nerve Stimulation at Both High and Low Frequencies Reduces Primary Hyperalgesia in Rats with Joint Inflammation in a Time-Dependent Manner. Physical Therapy 2007;87(1):44-51.
3. Chandrasoma P, Taylor CR. "Part A. General Pathology, Section II. The Host Response to Injury, Chapter 3. The Acute Inflammatory Response, sub-section Cardinal Clinical Signs". Concise Pathology (3rd edition (Computer file) ed.). New York, NY. McGraw-Hill 2005.
4. Coleman DL, King NR, Andrade JD. The foreign body reaction: A chronic inflammatory response Journal of Biomedical Materials Research 1973;8(5):199-211.
5. Dicky TC Fung, Gabriel YF Ng, Mason CP Leung, David KC Tay. Therapeutic Low Energy Laser Improves the Mechanical Strength of Repairing Medial Collateral Ligament. Lasers in Surgery and Medicine 2002;31:91-6.
6. Ferrero-Miliani L, Nielsen OH, Andersen PS, Girardin SE. "Chronic inflammation: Importance of NOD2 and NALP3 in interleukin-1beta generation". Clin Exp Immunol 2007;147(2):227-35.
7. Ivins D. "Acute ankle sprain: An update". American family physician 2006;74(10):1714-20.
8. Lescaudron L, Peltekian E, Fontaine-Perus J, Paulin D, Zampieri M, Garcia L, Parrish E. Blood borne macrophages are essential for the triggering of muscle regeneration following muscle transplant. Neuromuscul Disord 1999;9:72-80.
9. Nguyen HX, Tidball JG. Interactions between neutrophils and macrophages promote macrophage killing of muscle cells *in vitro*. J Physiol 2003;547:125-32.
10. Radhakrishnan R, Moore SA, Sluka KA. Unilateral carrageenan injection into muscle or joint induces chronic bilateral hyperalgesia in rats. Pain 2003;104:567-77.
11. Stein TP, Wade CE. Metabolic Consequences of Muscle Disuse Atrophy. J Nutr 2005;135:1824S-8S.
12. Yager D, Nwomeh B. The proteolytic environment of chronic wounds. Wound Repair Regeneration 1999;7:433.

CHAPTER

2

Edema

DEFINITION

Edema is an abnormal accumulation of fluid under the skin or in intercellular spaces or in cavities of the body or in the body tissues. Edema most commonly occurs in the feet and legs, where it is referred to as peripheral edema. The swelling is the result of the accumulation of excess fluid under the skin in the spaces within the tissues. All tissues of the body are made up of cells and connective tissues that hold the cells together. This connective tissue around the cells and blood vessels is known as the interstitium. Most of the body's extracellular fluids that are found outside of the cells are normally stored in two spaces; the blood vessels (as the "liquid" or serum portion of your blood) and the interstitial spaces (not within the cells). In various diseases, excess fluid can accumulate in either one or both of these compartments (Fig. 2.1).

The body's organs have interstitial spaces where fluid can accumulate. An accumulation of fluid in the interstitial air spaces (alveoli) in the lungs occurs in a disorder called pulmonary edema.

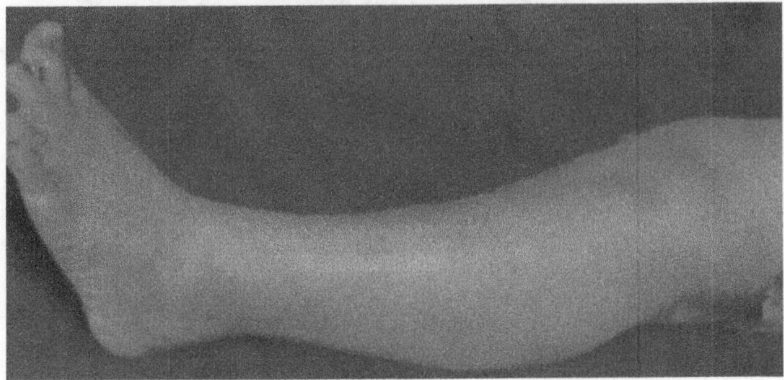

Fig. 2.1: The edema involving lower leg
(*For color version, see Plate 1*)

In addition, excess fluid sometimes collects in the abdomen (abdominal or peritoneal cavity - called "ascites") or in the chest (lung or pleural cavity - called "pleural effusion"). Anasarca refers to the severe, widespread accumulation of fluid in the all of the tissues and cavities of the body at the same time.

PITTING EDEMA AND NON-PITTING EDEMA

Pitting edema (Fig. 2.2) can be demonstrated by applying pressure to the swollen area by depressing the skin with a finger. If the pressing causes an indentation that persists for some time after the release of the pressure, the edema is referred to as pitting edema. Any form of pressure, such as from the elastic in socks, can induce pitting with this type of edema (Table 2.1).

In non-pitting edema, which usually affects the legs or arms, pressure that is applied to the skin does not result in a persistent indentation. Non-pitting edema can occur in certain disorders of the lymphatic system such as lymphedema, which is a disturbance of the lymphatic circulation that may occur after a mastectomy, lymph node surgery, or congenitally. Another cause of non-pitting edema of the legs is called pretibial myxedema, which is a swelling over the shin that occurs in some patients with hyperthyroidism. Non-pitting edema of the legs is difficult to treat. Diuretic medications are generally not effective, although elevation of the legs periodically during the day and compressive devices may reduce the swelling.

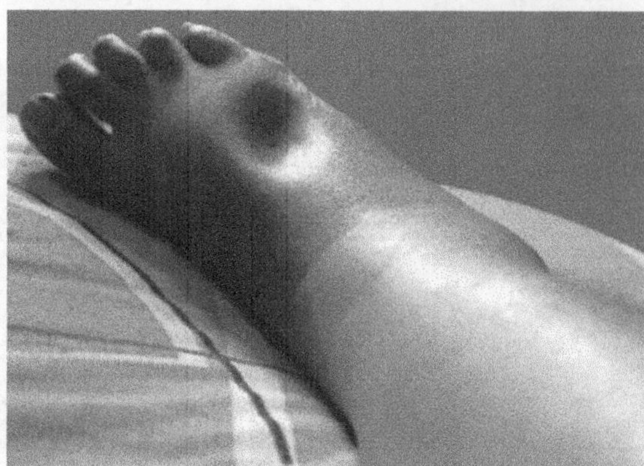

Fig. 2.2: Pitting edema of leg (*For color version, see Plate 1*)

TABLE 2.1 Grading for the assessment of pitting edema (Seidel et al, 1995)

Grade 1 + edema (Pit depth ≤ 2 mm)	*Grade 2 + edema (Pit depth 2-4 mm)*	*Grade 3 + edema (Pit depth 4-6 mm)*	*Grade 4 + edema (Pit depth 6-8 mm)*
Slight pitting No visible distortion Pit disappears rapidly	More deeper pit No easily detectable distortion Pit disappears 10-15 seconds	Pit noticeably deep Pit lasts more than 1 minute The affected extremity is fuller and swollen	Pit is very deep Pit lasts 2-5 minutes Dependent extremity is grossly distorted due to swelling

Causes

Edema is caused by either systemic diseases, that is, diseases that affect the various organ systems of the body, or by local conditions involving just the affected extremities. The most common systemic diseases associated with edema involve the heart, liver, and kidneys. In these diseases, edema occurs primarily because of the body's retention of too much salt (sodium chloride). The excess salt causes the body to retain water. This water then leaks into the interstitial tissue spaces, where it appears as edema.

The most common local conditions that cause edema are varicose veins and thrombophlebitis (inflammation of the veins) of the deep veins of the legs. These conditions can cause inadequate pumping of the blood by the veins (venous insufficiency). The resulting increased back-pressure in the veins forces fluid stay in the extremities (especially the ankles and feet). The excess fluid then leaks into the interstitial tissue spaces, causing edema.

Mechanism

Edema can result from (Fig. 2.3) the interaction of about five factors:

- Increased hydrostatic pressure (The pressure exerted by the fluid at equilibrium due to force of gravity) tends to exert higher radially directed pressure on the blood vessel wall thus tends to push fluid out of the vascular tubes.
- Reduced oncotic pressure within blood vessels (Oncotic pressure is the osmotic pressure due to proteins in blood plasma. It tends to retain and attract water in the circulatory system) tends to

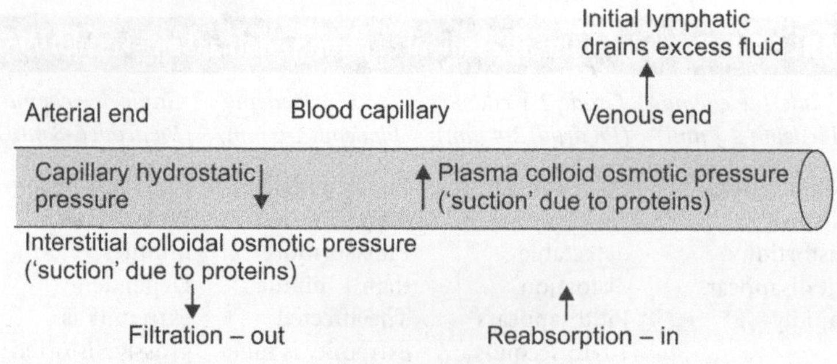

Fig. 2.3: The mechanism of edema production

loose the tendency to keep the water retained with in the vascular channels thus fluid tends to gush out of vessels.

- Increased blood vessel wall permeability occurs due to variety of conditions or early stages of inflammation. The increased vessel wall permeability provides reduced impedance to the outflow of fluid.
- Obstruction of lymphatic impaired fluid clearance it tends to cause accumulation of fluid with in lymphatic channels and also tends to augment the hydrostatic pressure.
- Alteration of the water retaining properties of the tissues may provide reduced space available for fluid accumulation or this may cause reduction of the oncotic pressure.

Rate of outflow of the fluid is primarily dependent on the force balance between hydrostatic pressure and the oncotic pressure (Starling Equation). The capillaries and post capillary venules provide the common interface for the leakage of water due to its semi-permeable nature.

Formation of edema can occur either by an increase in hydrostatic pressure within the blood vessel, a decrease in the oncotic pressure within the blood vessel or an increase in vessel wall permeability. The latter has two effects. It allows water to flow more freely and it reduces the oncotic pressure difference by allowing protein to leave the vessel more easily.

Classification (Based on Region Affected)

Edema may be called as generalized or as localized/tissue specific depending on the area of its involvement.

- *Generalized edema*: This type of edema involves whole body and multiple organs. It commonly occurs in case of the malfunctioning of the heart, lungs, kidneys or liver. In cardiac failure the peripheral fluid stagnation occurs and this causes increased hydrostatic pressure. In case of kidney or liver pathology the clearance of the metabolites from blood stream fails thus increased in oncotic pressure occurs in the widespread body tissues.
- *Organ-specific edema*: Edema will occur in specific organs as part of inflammation, as in pharyngitis, tendonitis or pancreatitis, for instance. Certain organs develop edema through tissue specific mechanisms.

Cerebral edema is extracellular fluid accumulation in the brain. It may lead to drowsiness, altered sensorium or loss of consciousness. *Pulmonary* edema occurs when hydrostatic pressure in the pulmonary vasculature rises high or obstruction of pulmonary veins (common in left ventricle failure) impairs the removal of blood from lungs. In *lymphedema* abnormal removal of interstitial fluid is caused by failure of the lymphatic system. This may be due to obstruction from pressure from a cancer or enlarged lymph nodes, destruction of lymph vessels by radiotherapy, or infiltration of the lymphatics by infection (such as elephantiasis). Most common cause of the same is the failure of the pumping action of muscles due to immobility, or paralysis. Some medicines like indomethacin (NSAID) reduce plasma rennin activity and aldosterone level thus increases sodium and potassium retention thus it may impair the lymphatic action and may lead to edema (Akbarpour, 1985).

ADVERSE EFFECTS OF EDEMA

- Edema is closely related to disturbances in circulation
- Persistently the fluid is present in the tissue spaces it interferes with nutrition of cells because fresh gases and nutrients are not available and waste products are not removed metabolism and tissue functioning may be seriously impaired the severity of impairment varies with the amount of edema, duration of edema or the nature of edematous fluid.
- The prolonged impairment may lead to atrophy, loss of muscle contractile nature, impaired healing process, impaired immunity mechanisms.

- If fluid present in the interstitial space for prolonged time fluid tends to organize into fibrous tissues and area gets hardened the organized fibrous content is foreign to body it is acted upon by immune mechanisms cells and blood vessels proliferate in this its size may increase and may obliterate blood vessels causing impaired circulation or disturbance of local nutrition.
- Excessive edema around joint impairs joint ROM (Range of motion)
- Accumulated fluid irritates nerve endings and causes pain.

ASSESSMENT OF EDEMA

Edema is often an early sign of significant fluid retention, which could eventually result in significant cardiac overload and conditions such as heart failure. Although many physicians are aware of the importance of monitoring edema, accuracy and consistency in assessing edema has been a challenge (Kimberly et al, 2009).

A variety of methods (periphery circumference, volume displacement, patient's self report) have been available to assess edema, however each has own set of advantages and disadvantages.

The most widely-used technique is a subjective clinical assessment where an examiner applies pressure with his/her index finger to a single location on the patient's ankle (Raju et al, 2002). This technique captures pit depth and the time needed (see Table 2.1) for the skin to return to its original appearance (recovery time) as a single edema score ranging from 0 to 4 (Seidel et al, 1995).

Water-displacement volumetry (Fig. 2.4) is widely considered to be the quick and common method of edema assessment, can be used for irregular ends of extremity (Thulesius et al, 1973); however, it is time consuming, needs space, difficulty to perform and not possible in case of ICU or wards of hospitals.

Ankle circumference; for consistent ankle circumference (Fig. 2.5) measurements (in cm), each ankle is marked with a marker at approximately 7 cm proximal to the midpoint of the medial malleolus. The circumference of the extremity is measured using a tension-controlled measuring tape, rather than a standard measuring tape, to minimize measurement error due to differences in the amount of tension applied. The measure of circumference is compared over days to see the progress or reduction of the edema.

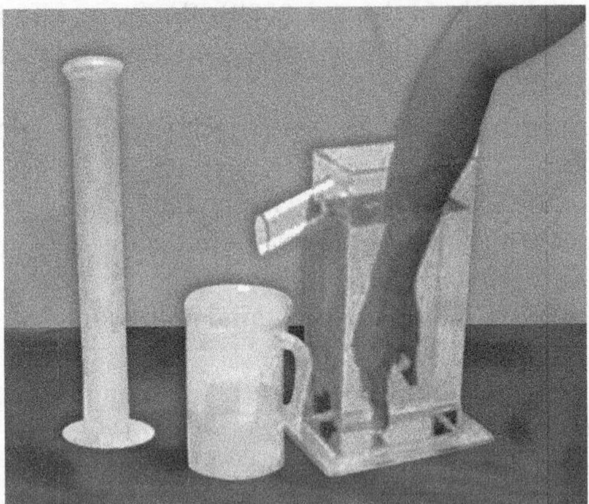

Fig. 2.4: Edema water-displacement volumetry
(*For color version, see Plate 2*)

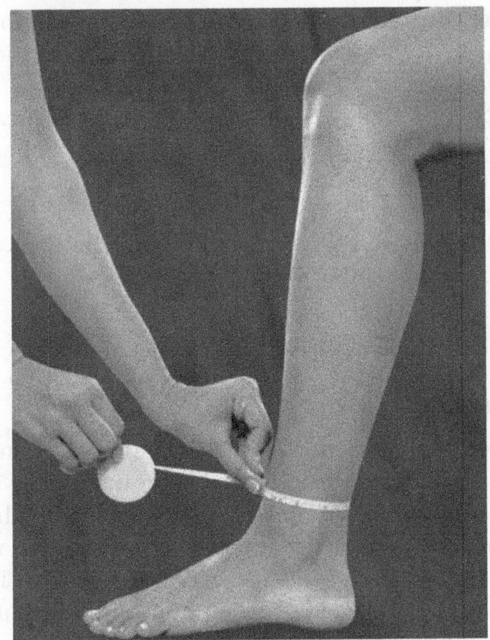

Fig. 2.5: Measurement of ankle edema by measuring tape
(*For color version, see Plate 2*)

Figure-of-Eight (Kimberly et al, 2009). The figure-of-eight method uses eight landmarks on the ankle and foot to measure ankle circumference in centimeters:

1. Midway between the tibialis anterior tendon and the lateral malleolus
2. Distal to the tuberosity of the navicular
3. Proximal to the base of the 5th metatarsal
4. Tibialis anterior tendon
5. Distal to the distal tip of the medial malleolus
6. Achilles tendon
7. Distal to the distal tip of the lateral malleolus
8. Back to origin.

All these landmarks are marked and the measuring tape is wrapped to link them and the sum total of all the distances between points is used to record the circumference of the periphery.

The *other non-invasive methods of edema assessment* (Stanton and Badger, 2000) include:

1. *Optoelectronic volumetry*: The use of perometer device which measures the interruption of infrared light by limb
2. Tonometry to measure the physical characteristics of edema tissue
3. Harpenden skinfold calipers to measure the truncal edema
4. MRI, CT scan less used to measure the extent of edema in the corss-section of the body deeper layers
5. Ultrasound to evaluate the depth of the edema involvement.

Classification (based on underlying mechanism along with physiotherapy management).

INCREASED VENOUS PRESSURE

General Edema

Chronic venous insufficiency is one of the most common causes of the edema involving distal lower extremities. It is a condition where the veins fail to pump the blood back into the heart for reoxygenation, due to dilated/damaged valves, reduced venous tone or increased tortuosity of veins. The venous pressure is increased in *cardiac failure*. The veins do not get emptied and thus the amount of blood in them increases leading to the raised pressure at the venous end of the capillary which now counteracts the osmotic pressure of the plasma proteins, thus impeding the reabsorption of tissue fluid.

Management

Treatment involves the appropriate management of cardiac failure, or venous insufficiency including the use of drugs such as digoxin and diuretics.

■ LOCAL EDEMA

Gravity

An important factor in determining the site of edema. Even in healthy people edema of the feet and legs can occur if the limbs remain dependent for too long, as on a long flight.

Management

Change of posture can be of great importance in controlling edema. Example is the prevention of edema of the lungs in a patient with left ventricular failure by sleeping propped-up in bed against pillows.

Inactivity

The venous return, especially from the legs under normal condition depends on compression of the veins by muscular activity in conjunction with competent valves in the veins which prevent reverse flow. If the muscles are inactive the venous return is poor, the venous capillary pressure is raised and so edema occurs. An extreme example is paralytic edema and the edema due to poor muscle tone.

Management

- *Poor muscle tone*: Physiotherapist can help to restore the strength and tone of the muscles by teaching graded exercises.
- *Laxity of the fascia*: Limb is elevated and a firm (but not tight) elastic bandage may be used.
- *Paralytic edema*: Passive measures to promote venous return will be required. These include:
  - Elevation of the affected limb
  - Passive movement of joints
  - Artificial exercise of the paralysed muscles by interrupted direct current (now rare)
  - Light massage which is sometimes effective in dispersing the fluid into regions not affected by the paralysis. Care must be

taken neither to increase the paralytic vasodilation nor to bruise or stretch the atonic muscle fibres.

Varicose Veins

These greatly impair venous return from the legs. The dilatation of the veins causes valves to become incompetent so that even with muscular activity the venous return is poor.

Management

Venous return can be improved by raising the legs or by providing support, e.g. with an elastic stocking. Surgical treatment of varicose veins is often effective.

PHYSICAL THERAPY MANAGEMENT OF EDEMA

The management of edema greatly underlies on the cause of the edema, thus accurate diagnosis to reveal its cause must be done.

Acute Inflammation

During this phase the movement or stress will aggravate the problem rest is needed. The cryotherapy is helpful as it reduces the metabolic activity and thus reduce the blood flow to the region.

Patient may need bed rest or at least the rest of the affected part by help of splint.

Once the symptoms of acute inflammation phase start getting over, the movement or activity in controlled environment is important to avoid the organization in the fibrous tissues.

The circulation of the affected part has to be maintained to allow healing procedures to function optimally and also to avoid fluid stagnation and organization in to fibrous lumps.

To improve the circulation:

- Active exercise
- Rhythmic contraction of muscle
- Isometrics of the affected extremity.

Reduced Plasma Proteins

The plasma proteins may be reduced by inadequate intake as in starvation, or excessive loss as in Protein-losing nephritis.

Management

Management includes raising the level of plasma proteins, particularly, albumin by intravenous infusion and treatment of the cause.

Increased Capillary Permeability

The sluggish circulation associated with raised venous pressure tends to cause anoxia of the endothelial cells. The resulting increased capillary permeability is thus a factor in circulatory edema. Damage to the capillary endothelium is also a factor in the edema occurring in nephritis, e.g. periorbital edema. Allergy, e.g. wasp sting may also damage the endothelium of capillaries and produce local edema which can be a hazard to life if the sting involves the tongue. The edema of nettle-rash is similar and may be controlled by antihistamine drugs, histamine being one of the main substances causing damage to the capillary endothelium in allergic states.

Rums are an important cause or increased capillary permeability. The resulting edema fluid has a high protein content so that it clots and organises readily. This may result in permanent disfiguration if appropriate steps are not taken to promote its reabsorption. The underlying principles and practical measures have already been described but unfortunately their application may be impeded by the extent of injury caused by the burns.

Management

An over-riding consideration is the maintenance of blood pressure by the infusion of plasma or plasma substitute to replace the fluid and protein lost from the circulation into the tissue spaces as edema fluid.

Obstruction to Lymphatic Drainage

Raised venous pressure, which obstruct both veins and lymphatics, there may also be selective lymphatic obstruction. This occurs after repeated attacks of lymphadenitis and lymphangitis following radical surgery, e.g. for carcinoma of the breast and as a long-term effect of filarial infection (elephantiasis). The edema produced by lymphatic obstruction is usually of the non-pitting variety due to fibrosis.

Management

Unless treated early it rarely responds to physiotherapy.

- Physiotherapy modalities for edema
  - Cryotherapy in acute edema the application of cryotherapy under pressure is helpful to reduce the edema. This can be easily done by the cryo-cuff (Fig. 2.6).
- Manual lymphatic drainage (massage)
  - Direct intervention by a therapist (Kathrin et al, 2000). The effleurage method is most promising and the direction of the massage stroke must be directed towards the lymph nodes so as to facilitate the lymphatic drainage and venous return.
  - Self-massage by the patient
  - Sometimes the self-massage may be done in aquatic environment to combine the effect of aqua therapy, and active efforts to achieve lymphedema reduction (Dorit et al, 2007)
- Compression
  - Nonelastic or low-stretch bandages or custom-fitted garments
  - Intermittent, sequential pneumatic compression pump
  - Elastic bandages and inelastic bandages also provide a good mean to reduce the swelling and edema. Previous researches have proved a lesser efficacy of the elastic bandages while

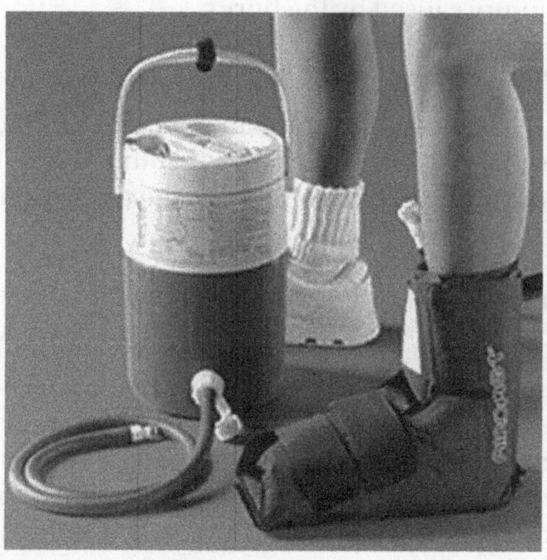

Fig. 2.6: Application of cryo-cuff for acute edema around ankle
(*For color version, see Plate 3*)

compared to the inelastic bandages (Partch et al, 1999). The elastic bandages are not useful to reduce edema if less than four layers are used (Partch et al, 1999). Even the efficacy of the elastic bandages to prevent edema is less while compared to the semi rigid dressings for the management of pre-prosthetic stage amputee patients (Michael Muller, 1982).
  - Other possible alternatives for the compression therapies include elastic stockings, elastic bandages, Unna boots.
- Individualized exercise program
  - Active ROM (pumping exercises)
  - Flexibility exercises
  - Low-intensity resistance exercises
  - Cardiovascular conditioning
  - Rest of the limb in antigravity position—sometimes it is believed that the positioning of limb in antigravity position helps to increase the venous return from the periphery towards center. The 20 to 30 minute resting periods daily with the legs at an angle of 30° are sufficient to reduce the edema that affects the elderly (Perrin and Guex, 2000).
  - However this method of edema reduction by rest is found to be appropriate only for those patients who cannot ambulate. In fact this method is found to be much lesser effective while compared to the muscle exercises (Belczak et al, 2009).
  - Skin care and daily living precautions.

Prevention of Lymphedema

- Avoid static, dependent positioning of the lower extremities, such as prolonged sitting or standing. Avoid sitting with legs crossed.
- When traveling long distances by car, stop periodically and walk around or support an involved upper extremity on the car's window ledge or seat back.
- Elevate involved limb(s) and perform repetitive pumping exercises frequently during the day.
- Avoid vigorous, repetitive activities with the involved limb. Avoid carrying heavy loads, such as a suitcase, a heavy backpack, or shoulder bag. Avoid use of heavyweights when exercising.
- Wear compressive garments while exercising.
- Avoid wearing clothing that restricts circulation, such as sleeves or socks with tight elastic bands. Do not wear tight jewelry such as rings or watches.

- Monitor diet to maintain an ideal weight and minimize sodium intake.
- Avoid hot environments or use of local heat.
- If possible, avoid having blood pressure taken on an involved upper extremity or injections in either an involved upper or lower extremity.

Skin Care

- Keep the skin clean and supple; use moisturizers but avoid perfumed lotions.
- Avoid infections; pay immediate attention to a skin abrasion or cut, an insect bite, a blister, or a burn.
- Protect hands and feet; wear socks or hose, properly fitting shoes, rubber gloves, oven mitts, etc.
- Avoid contact with harsh detergents and chemicals.
- Use caution when cutting nails. Women need to use an electric razor when shaving legs or underarm area.
- Avoid hot baths, whirlpools, and saunas that elevate the body's core temperature.

PNEUMATIC COMPRESSION THERAPY (PCT)

Vascular compression from PCDs (pressure compression device) may stimulate the release of endothelial mediators that modulate symptoms. Additionally, PCDs may improve local perfusion by enhancing venous and lymphatic drainage with consequent relief of mild, otherwise subclinical ischemia (Christopher et al, 2008).

Pneumatic compression device has inflatable garment (Fig. 2.7) for the leg/arm and an electrical pump that fills the garment with compressed air. The garment can be inflated and deflated in various cyclic modes. This therapy is used to provide the external pressure so as to counteract the venous hypertension by facilitating venous return toward the heart, improving venous return and lymphatic drainage. It reduces edema by increasing local hydrostatic pressure and lowering superficial venous pressure, preventing the leakage of fluids and macromolecules, improving cutaneous blood flow, and aiding fibronolysis (Montori et al, 2002).

External pneumatic compression (EPC) therapy involves the application of pressure from the external source, the pneumatic (Air) assisted pressure generating device. It is used to reduce venous stasis

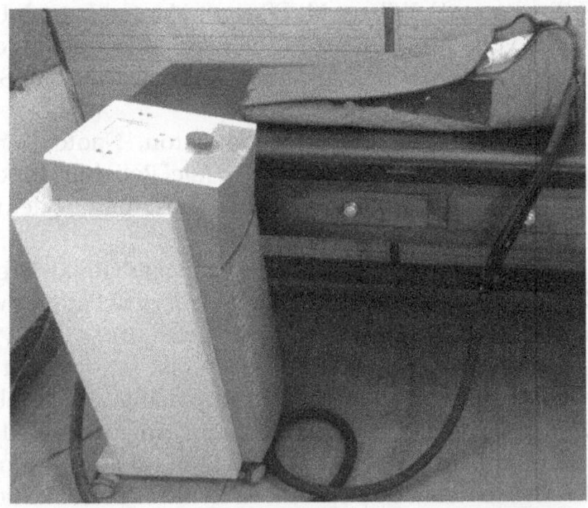

Fig. 2.7: The application of pneumatic compression pumps to manage the edema around ankle (*For color version, see Plate 3*)

by compressing the superficial veins and forcing blood into the deep veins, which then return it to the heart. EPC uses air as a compression medium. EPC devices are sleeve- or boot-shaped chambers that fill with air and electrical pumps with gauges that provide intermittent compression to the lower extremities. EPC therapy is also known as intermittent pneumatic compression (IPC) therapy.

Other possible alternatives for the compression therapies include elastic stockings, elastic bandages, Unna boots.

BIBLIOGRAPHY

1. Akbarpour F, Afrasiabi A, Vaziri N. "Severe hyperkalemia caused by indomethacin and potassium supplementation". South Med J 1985;78(6):756-7.
2. Belczak Cleusa Ema Quilici, Cavalheri Gildo, Jose Maria Pereira de Godoy, Belczak Sergio Quilici, Caffaro Roberto Augusto. Comparison of reduction of edema after rest and after muscle exercises in treatment of chronic venous insufficiency. Int Arch Med 2009;2:18.
3. Christopher J, Lettieri, Arn H Eliasson. Pneumatic Compression Devices Are an Effective Therapy for Restless Legs Syndrome. Chest. 2009;135(1):74-80.
4. Dorit Tidhar, Jacqueline Drouin, Avi Shimony. Aqua Lymphatic Therapy in Managing Lower Extremity Lymphedema. J Support Oncol 2007;5:179-83.

5. Härén K, Backman C, Wiberg M. Effect of Manual Lymph Drainage As described by vodder on edema of the hand after fracture of the distal Radius: A Prospective Clinical Study. Journal of Plastic Surgery and Hand Surgery. 2000;34(4):367-72.
6. Kimberly G Brodovicz, Kristin McNaughton, Naoto Uemura, Gary Meininger, Cynthia J. Girman, Steven H Yale. Reliability and Feasibility of Methods to Quantitatively Assess Peripheral Edema. Clinical Medicine & Research 2009;7(1/2):21-31.
7. Michael J Mueller. Comparison of Removable Rigid Dressings and Elastic Bandages in Preprosthetic Management of Patients with Below-Knee Amputations. Physical Therapy. 1982;62(10):1438-41.
8. Montori VM, Kavros SJ, Walsh EE, Rooke TW. Intermittent pneumatic compression for nonhealing wounds in patients with limb ischemia: the Mayo Clinic experience (1998-2000). Int Angiol. 2002;21(4):60-6.
9. Partsch H, Menzinger G, A Mostbeck. Inelastic Leg Compression Is More Effective to Reduce Deep Venous Refluxes than Elastic Bandages. Dermatologic Surgery 1999;25(9):695-700.
10. Perrin M, Guex JJ. Edema and leg volume: methods of assessment. Angiology 2000;51(1):9-12.
11. Raju S, Owen S Jr, Neglen P. The clinical impact of iliac venous stents in the management of chronic venous insufficiency. J Vasc Surg 2002;35:8-15.
12. Seidel HM, Ball JW, Dains JE, Benedict GW. Heart and blood vessels. In: Schrefer S, ed. Mosby's Guide to Physical Examination, 3rd ed. St. Louis, MO: Mosby. 1995;419.
13. Stanton AWB, Badger C, Sitzia J. Non-invasive assessment of the lymphedematous limb. Lymphology 2000;122-35.
14. Thulesius O, Norgren L, Gjöres JE. Foot-volumetry, a new method for objective assessment of edema and venous function. Vasa 1973;2(4): 325-9.

CHAPTER

3

Arthritis

INTRODUCTION

The term arthritis is derived from the Greek: "arthron" meaning "joint" and "itis" meaning inflammation. In specific the inflammation involves synovial membrane, articular cartilage disruption and the peri-articular structures (Reeves et al, 2010). The term "Arthritis" is an umbrella term which includes more than 100 different types of joint related conditions such as rheumatoid arthritis, osteoarthritis, gout, pseudogout, psoriatic arthritis, and fibromyalgia to name a few.

The degree of the inflammation varies in each of these conditions, and it also varies from one stage to other stage of same pathology. Each of the arthritic conditions has specific pathology and the presentation. Complications, including infection, delays in wound healing, malunion, nonunion, implant failure, and degeneration of adjacent joints soon after primary fusion, have been described in the literature (Reeves et al, 2010).

Most types of arthritis involve joint inflammation. Inflammation is the body's natural response to injury or infection. For an example of inflammation, take a simple scratch of your body automatically releases chemicals that cause fluids to accumulate and white blood cells to gather around the area of the scratch. As your body fights foreign substances and bacteria, inflammation, redness, heat, swelling and pain occur at the sight of the injury (Peter Brookes, 2003).

In some forms of arthritis, unfortunately, the self-defence mechanism of body starts irreversibly attacking the joint structures and leads to initially temporary (and then irreversible) damage to the joint.

In arthritic conditions mere the symptomatic treatment to alleviate pain may not be sufficient. Early detection and the correct treatment strategy is important because it can help to protect joint structure and leads more active and comfortable lives.

COMMON TYPES OF ARTHRITIS

Rheumatoid arthritis (RA) is a chronic, degenerative, systemic disease that leads to the destruction of articular cartilage of the joints (Reeves et al, 2010). It is the most common and serious inflammatory form of arthritis which adversely affects the peripheral joints of hand (Fig. 3.1) and foot. It is the prototypical autoimmune form of arthritis (Gary, 2003). Because it may cause most of its damage in the first year, early diagnosis and aggressive therapy is critical. Left untreated RA may shorten life-expectancy by as much as 18 years as it may lead to other complications such as rheumatoid fever, rheumatoid heart disease, etc.

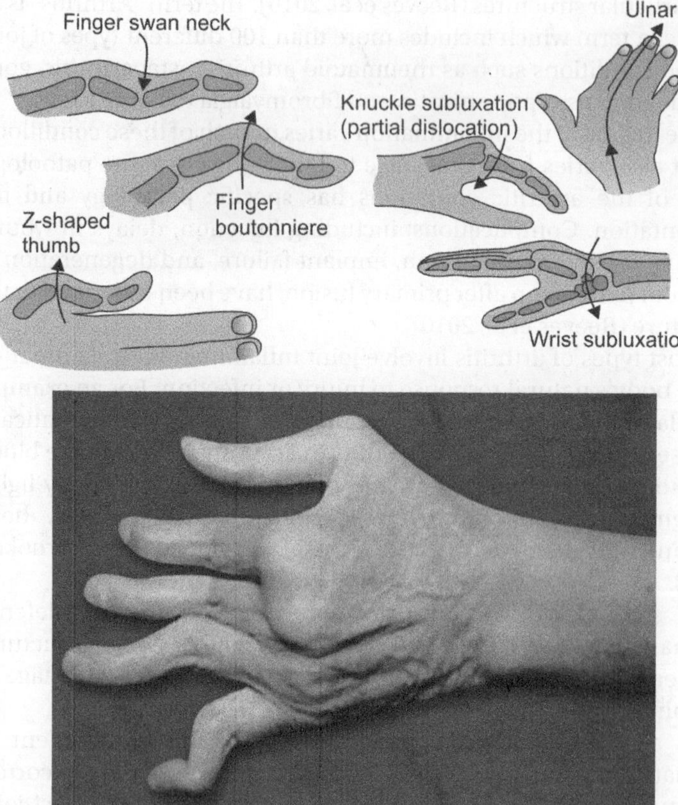

Fig. 3.1: Typical hand deformities in rheumatoid arthritis

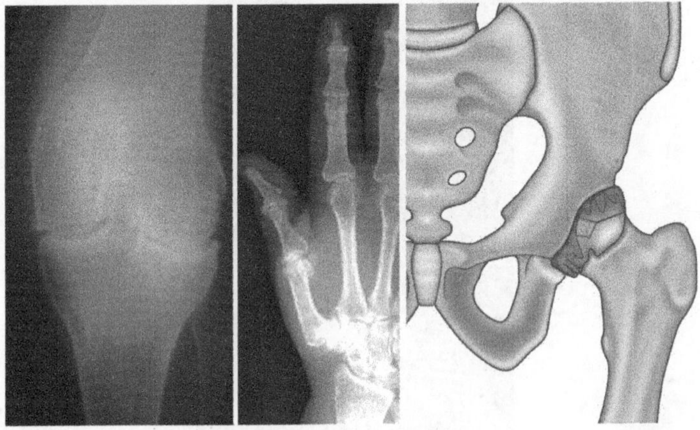

Fig. 3.2: Involvement of weight-bearing areas in osteoarthritis. (Knee and thumb CMC and hip joint)

Osteoarthritis

This type of arthritis is thought to be associated with aging (James et al, 2002). Osteoarthritis affects weight-bearing areas (Thomas P et al, 2004) such as the spine, hips, knees (Fig. 3.2), base of the thumbs, and feet. Genetics and mechanical factors (Thomas P et al, 2004) also play a big role. Research is being done on medications that will slow down the progression of this disease.

Ankylosing Spondylitis

This inflammatory form of arthritis affects the spine and the sacroiliac joints. Since it often presents with low back pain, it is often misdiagnosed. In most cases of the AS the involvement of the Sacroiliac joint (SI) and the bony fusion (Fig. 3.3) of the vertebral bodies occurs in form of "bamboo spine" like appearance on X-ray due to calcification of the longitudinal ligaments of the spine. AS is very treatable however accurate diagnosis and aggressive therapy are advisable.

Fibromyalgia

Fibromyalgia is a soft tissue form of arthritis that is due to defective neurotransmitter function in the brain. Because these neurotransmitters are responsible for many sensory functions,

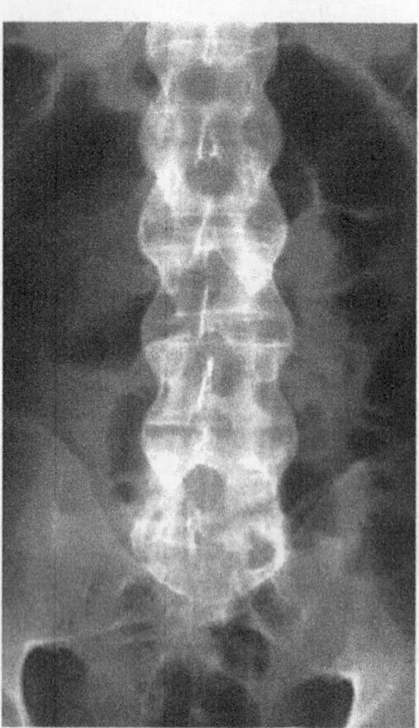

Fig. 3.3: Ankylosing spondylitis: The reduction of the joint space of sacroiliac joint and the bony fusion of the vertebral bodies

patients with fibromyalgia present with bizarre symptoms. It is imperative that other forms of arthritis be ruled out first. During this disease the multiple trigger points occur along the skeletal muscles. Some of the regions in the body are more prone to develop such trigger points. The common areas (Fig. 3.4) are depicted in the diagram.

Polymyalgia Rheumatica

Polymyalgia rheumatica occurs after the age of 50 and presents with severe stiffness and aching in the neck, shoulders, and hips. Because it is very treatable, accurate diagnosis is needed. Because so many other conditions look like it, an accurate diagnosis is not always easy.

Psoriatic Arthritis

Psoriatic arthritis is a potentially serious inflammatory form of arthritis that is often found in association with psoriasis. Because it may begin and progress insidiously, it can cause serious problems. Early diagnosis and aggressive intervention are recommended.

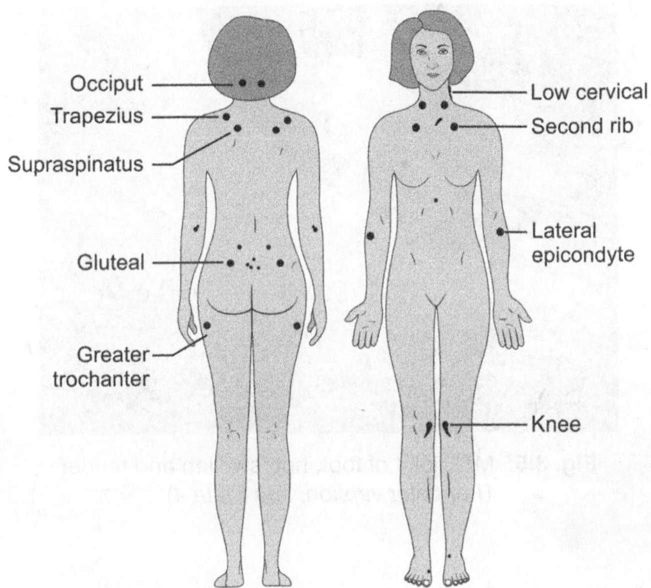

Fig. 3.4: Trigger points location in fibromyalgia

Reactive Arthritis

Reactive arthritis is a form of arthritis that comes on after infections. Also known as Reiter's syndrome, arthritis urethritica, venereal arthritis and polyarteritis enterica, is an autoimmune condition (Ruddy and Shaun, 2001) that develops in response to an infection in another part of the body. The most common being types of infections being intestinal or genitourinary. Young adults are often affected. Appropriate medical treatment is very effective.

Gout

This common form of arthritis is due to deposition of monosodium urate (MSU) crystals. In addition to joints such as first metatarsophalangeal joint of foot (Fig. 3.5), heel, wrist and fingers (Schlesinger, 2010), the kidneys are a big target of this disease (Terkeltaub, 2010). Dietary changes and medicines are very effective in treating this disorder.

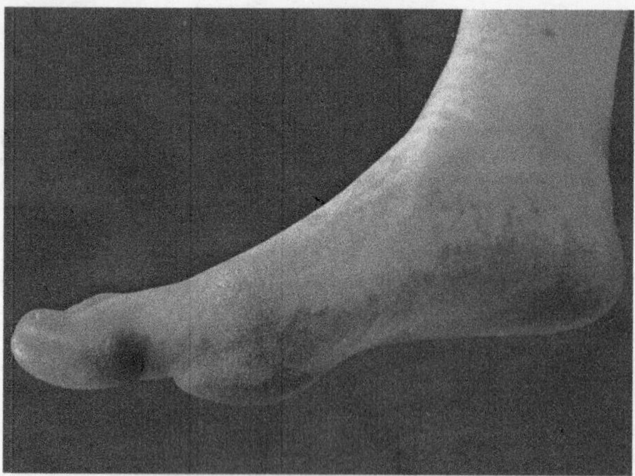

Fig. 3.5: MTP joint of foot, hot, swollen and tender (*For color version, see Plate 4*)

Pseudogout

This form of arthritis is also due to crystals—deposits of calcium pyrophosphate or hydroxyapatite in most instances. Pseudogout may mimic other types of arthritis such as gout and rheumatoid arthritis. Further, it may coexist with other types of arthritis making it very difficult to diagnose.

Systemic Lupus Erythematosus

This relatively common autoimmune disease is systemic in nature and capable of affecting many internal organ systems. SLE most often affects women in the child-bearing years. Early diagnosis and management are necessary since this disorder is potentially life-threatening.

Polymyositis

This inflammatory form of muscle disease is often associated with arthritis. Because it is a systemic condition that affects all muscles—including those that are responsible for the functioning of the heart, lungs, etc., careful examination and appropriate aggressive medical therapy are necessary.

Lyme Disease

Lyme disease occurs as a result of infection with Borrelia burgdorferi (Ryan and Ray, 2004). The organism is transmitted by a deer tick bite. Early recognition and antibiotic therapy is effective in most cases.

OSTEOARTHRITIS

Osteoarthritis (OA), is degenerative joint disease (DJD) or osteoarthrosis, which occurs when the cartilage in the joints begins to break down. The cartilage serves as a cushion between bones, allowing the joint to move without pain. Therefore, individuals with osteoarthritis experience pain and reduced mobility in their joints where cartilage is degrading (Fig. 3.6) because in such joints the amount of forces between joint forming bones could be very high. Osteoarthritis may affect any joint in the body, however it is more common in the weight bearing joints like knee, hip and the spinal joints (Jordan et al, 2000). In initial stages it may be difficult to identify the difference between osteoarthritis and rheumatoid arthritis, however few comparative points may be kept in mind to identify these differences (Table 3.1).

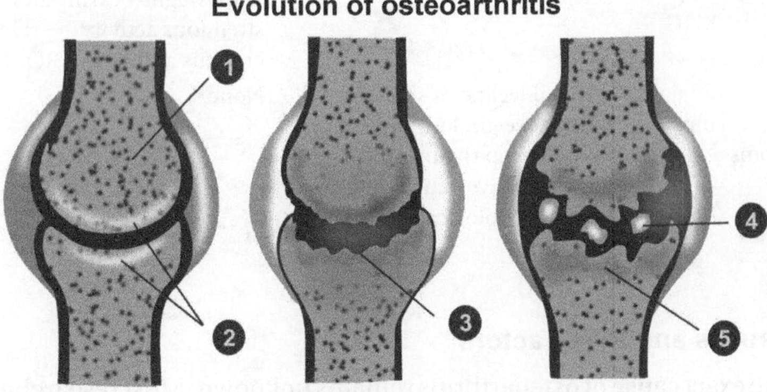

Fig. 3.6: Cartilage degradation in the weight-bearing joints

TABLE 3.1 Comparison between RA and OA

Characteristics	*Rheumatoid arthritis*	*Osteoarthritis*
Joint affected	It affects many joints simultaneously and bilateral; typically • Smaller joints such as MCP and PIP of hands, wrists, elbows, shoulders • Cervical spine may be involved • MTP, talonavicular and ankle	Affects a few joints (usually asymmetrical) typically • DIP, PIP, 1st CMC of hands • Cervical and lumbar spine • Hips, knees, 1st MTP of feet
Progression	May develop suddenly, and may progress during weeks or months	Develops slowly over many years in response to mechanical stress
Manifestations	Inflammatory synovitis and irreversible structural damage to cartilage occurs due to pannus formation and it leads to bone and articular cartilage erosion	Cartilage degradation, altered joint architecture, osteophyte formation
Age of onset	Between age 15 and 50	After age of 40
Joint signs and symptoms	Redness, warmth, swelling, and prolonged morning stiffness increased joint pain with activity	Morning stiffness (usually less than 30 min), increased joint pain with weight-bearing and strenuous activity crepitus and loss of ROM
Systemic signs and symptoms	General feeling of sickness and fatigue, weight loss and fever may develop rheumatoid nodules, may have ocular, respiratory, hematological, and cardiac symptoms	None

Causes and Risk Factors

The exact cause of osteoarthritis remains unknown. Most researchers believe that several factors, including obesity, age, joint injury or stress, genetics, and muscle weakness, may contribute to the development of osteoarthritis.

Aging: Osteoarthritis may develop at any age however the individuals older than 45 years show higher incidences of the joint degeneration. The major risk factor for developing osteoarthritis is aging. Approximately 70% of people over the age of 65 (Sharma et al, 2007) show some degree of osteoarthritis upon X-ray examination.

Congenital or developmental disorders: Such as hip displacement, Legg-Calve-Perthes disease (an infection of the hip bone), and bone dysplasias (group of disorders characterized by abnormalities of cartilage and bone growth). Such joints may increase the stresses on the joint forming bones thus increase risk of OA.

Endocrine disorders: The exact mechanism of relation between endocrineal disorder and the OA remains uncleared yet the individuals with diabetes may be prone to osteoarthritis. Other endocrine problems which may also promote the OA development, include acromegaly (overproduction of growth hormone), hypothyroidism (low thyroid hormone levels), hyperparathyroidism (high parathyroid hormone levels), and obesity.

Enzymes: Some researchers believe that cartilage damage may occur when cartilage releases too many enzymes (including collagenase and hyaluronidase) involved in the natural breakdown and regeneration of cartilage. If the body releases too many of these enzymes, the cartilage will be destroyed faster than it can be regenerated. This may occur when the cartilage damaging cells work faster than the cartilage forming cells.

Ethnicity: The rate of osteoarthritis varies by ethnic group. In the United States, Caucasians and African-Americans have higher rates of arthritis than Latinos or other ethnic groups. Osteoarthritis also tends to favor specific joints over others in certain ethnic groups. Older African-American men are about 33% more likely than Caucasian men to have hip osteoarthritis. Asians appear to have a higher incidence of osteoarthritis in the knee, an equal risk for osteoarthritis in the spine, and a lower risk for osteoarthritis in the hips than Caucasians.

Gender: Before age 45 (Schouten et al, 1992), osteoarthritis occurs more frequently in males (although it is not common in younger adults). After age 55, it develops more often in females. Some research suggests that women may also experience greater muscle and joint pain, in general, than men. After 55, the females may be at higher risk of OA development due to the hormonal factors.

Genetic disorders: A genetic defect may promote the breakdown of the protective architecture of cartilage. Examples include collagen disturbances such as Ehlers-Danlos syndrome.

Neuropathic: Diseases, such as diabetes, can cause nerve problems. The loss/defect of sensation may affect how the joint position is sensed and condition of the joints or limbs is sensed. In such cases joints may move in abnormal way and again the risk of OA is high.

Trauma: Traumatic events to the body may lead to osteoarthritis. If a broken bone does not line up and heal properly, the bone may lose stability or damage cartilage (Darryl D'lima et al, 2001). Other trauma may be repetitive movements that damage bone and cartilage over time, such as in occupations including athletics.

Other risk factors include: Wilson's disease (a genetic condition causing copper deficiency) and obesity. Obesity increases joint weight bearing and joint loading.

Signs and Symptoms

Because osteoarthritis develops slowly, many individuals do not experience symptoms until several years after cartilage breakdown begins. Common symptoms include joint pain, swelling and/or stiffness in a joint (especially after joint use), joint discomfort before or during a change in the weather, bony lumps on the fingers, and loss of joint flexibility (Fujiwara et al, 2000).

The joints that are most often affected by osteoarthritis include the fingers, spine, and weight-bearing joints (Thomas P et al, 2004), such as the hips, ankles, feet, and knees (Fig. 3.2). Stiffness in the joint may occur after inactivity, such as upon rising in the morning or after a long car ride. Stiffness may indicate the possibility of inflammation in the joint (Mulherin et al, 1996).

Once symptoms develop, they are generally the worst during the first year of the disease. Pain often is described as a deep ache and is confined to the affected joint, called localized pain. In most cases, pain increases with use of the joint and subsides with rest. However, as the disease progresses, pain may become persistent. Osteoarthritis may cause pain at night that interferes with sleep.

If individuals overuse the affected joints and do not receive treatment, the cartilage in the joints may further wear down completely. When this happens, the bone may rub against bone, causing severe pain and joint damage.

Complications

Pain: In OA the intensity of pain depends on the extent of joint involvement. In some cases, the medication or dosage may need to be taken for pain relief.

Joint damage: In some cases, osteoarthritis can lead to severe joint damage. In such cases, surgery, such as a joint replacement, may be necessary. Individuals should have annual checkups to check the progression of the joint damage and to take appropriate means to prevent this progression.

Cosmetic concerns: Due to joint degeneration the bones may put abnormal stresses on the surrounding skin and this may cause formation of the pressure bumps called as nodules. These bumps can occur on any joint, but they are most common in the hands. These nodules may be disfiguring and painful in some individuals.

Limited mobility: Patients with arthritis may have limited mobility in the joints, such as limited movement of the knee or shoulder. Joint mobility decreases as the joint becomes more damaged. Advanced cases of OA might have difficulty in coping with daily life activities and functioning.

Depression: Some osteoarthritis patients may suffer from depression. This is because the associated disability and, pain may interfere significantly with the patient's lifestyle. Such individuals should consult their healthcare providers if they experience feelings of sadness, low self-esteem, loss of pleasure, apathy, and sometimes, difficulty functioning for two weeks or longer, with no known underlying cause. These may be signs of depression.

Diagnosis

General: Once individuals are diagnosed with osteoarthritis, they should visit their healthcare providers regularly, at least once a year. Individuals should stay in close contact with their doctors to ensure that their symptoms are managed and joint damage is monitored.

X-ray: X-rays are often the first test performed if a patient has symptoms of osteoarthritis. If the patient has osteoarthritis, the X-ray images will often show loss of cartilage in the affected joints, narrowing of the space between bones, and bumps called nodules. X-ray based classification is now accepted to classify the grade of OA (Table 3.2).

TABLE 3.2 Kellgren and Lawrence key for radiological assessment of osteoarthritis (Kellgren and Lawrence JS; 1957)

Grade	*Classification*	*Description*
0	Normal joint	No characteristic symptoms of osteoarthritis
1	Doubtful OA	Indications of osteophytes Significance doubtful
2	Minimal OA	Definite osteophytes
3	Moderate OA	Moderate narrowing of joint space
4	Severe OA	Joint space very narrow, with subchondral-bone sclerosis

Arthrocentesis: In arthrocentesis, a needle is inserted into the affected joint, and a small sample of fluid is removed and analyzed to rule out other conditions, such as gout or infection. This test may also temporarily relieve some pain and inflammation in the joint.

Arthroscopy: A surgical procedure called arthroscopy may also be performed. During the surgery, a small incision is made into the affected joint. Then a tube called an arthroscope is inserted into the joint. This tube has a small light and camera, which allows the healthcare provider to see the inside of the joint. If abnormalities, including cartilage or ligament damage are seen, the individual is diagnosed with osteoarthritis.

Treatment

General: Osteoarthritis is managed with medications that reduce pain and inflammation. In severe cases, surgery may be necessary to repair damage.

The initial treatment of the OA consists of non-steroidal anti-inflammatory drugs (NSAIDs) for pain relief and the carefully designed exercise therapy regime for reducing the stresses on the joints. If this is not implemented appropriately then damage to joint may warrant surgery.

Antidepressants: Some individuals with arthritis may also suffer from depression.

Arthroscopic lavage and/or debridement: In some cases, individuals with osteoarthritis may suffer from severe joint damage. In such cases, surgical procedures called arthroscopic lavage and/or arthroscopic debridement may be recommended, in which a tubular instrument called arthroscope is inserted into joint via small incision and saline is squirted through joint. This allows to see the inside of joint and helps to remove any blood, fluid or loose body inside joint.

If any loose fragments of bone/cartilage is found in joint then arthroscopic debridement can be performed simultaneously.

Both of these procedures may provide temporary pain relief and improved joint function. However, they may not be effective in advance cases of osteoarthritis. Therefore, individuals should discuss the potential risks and health benefits of the procedure with their healthcare providers.

Corticosteroids: Corticosteroids, such as prednisone and methylprednisolone, are occasionally used to reduce inflammation and pain and slow joint damage caused by osteoarthritis. These drugs are generally very effective when used short-term (weeks to a few months). However, if these drugs are used for six months or longer, they may become less effective and serious side effects may develop. Side effects may include easy bruising, thinning of bones, cataracts, weight gain, a round face, and diabetes.

Fusing bones: If there is serious joint damage, the bones of a joint, such as the ankle, may be surgically fused together in a procedure called arthrodesis. This surgery helps increase stability and reduces pain. Although the joint may be pain-free after bone fusing, the joint no longer has any flexibility and cannot bend or move, which may limit an individual's ability to move around easily. This is performed in cases where the muscle optimal joint control by muscle actions cannot be achieved and where the fusion of joint is less painful than the unfused joint.

Joint replacement surgery: In some cases, individuals with osteoarthritis suffer from permanent joint damage. In such instances, joint replacement surgery may be necessary. During the procedure, the damaged joint is surgically removed, and it is replaced with a plastic or metal device called prosthesis. The most commonly replaced joints are the hip and knee, but other joints, including the elbow, shoulder, finger, or ankle joints, can be replaced.

Joint replacement surgeries (Fig. 3.7) are generally most successful for large joints, such as the hip or knee. Researchers estimate that hip or knee replacements last at least 20 years in 80% of patients. After a successful surgery and several months of rehabilitation,

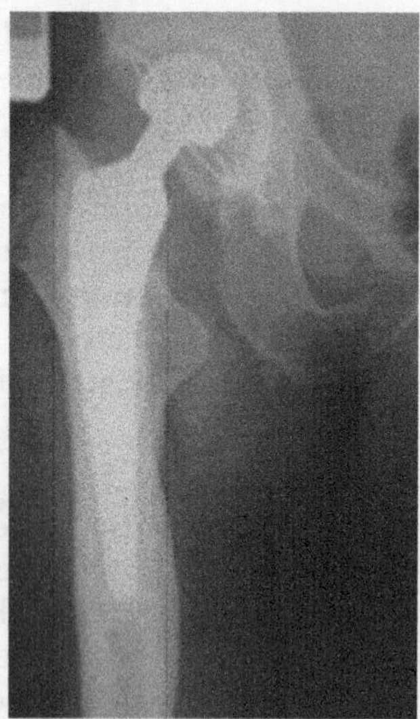

Fig. 3.7: Total hip joint replacement

individuals are able to use their new joints without pain (Ackerman and B ennell, 2004).

Medication

Non-selective: Nonsteroidal anti-inflammatory drugs (NSAIDs) like ibuprofen have been used to relieve pain and inflammation caused by osteoarthritis. These medications are generally taken long-term to manage symptoms.

The frequency and severity of side effects vary with NSAIDs. The most serious side effects include kidney failure, liver failure, ulcers, heart-related problems, and prolonged bleeding after an injury or surgery. About 15% of patients who receive long-term NSAID treatment develop ulcers in the stomach or duodenum.

Narcotic analgesics like acetaminophen/codeine may be prescribed to treat severe arthritis pain. These just reduce pain during short-term flare-ups and do not reduce swelling.

Topical pain relievers are creams, ointments, gels, and sprays that are applied to the skin.

Physiotherapy Management

Cool compress or ice pack: Applying a cool compress (cooling with pressure) or ice pack to the affected joint (Figs 3.8A and B) helps to reduce swelling and pain. This is more in cases where pain is high and the patient's pain tolerance is less.

Heat: During chronic cases the Application of a hot pack to affected joints (Fig. 3.9) may help reduce pain, relax muscles, and increase

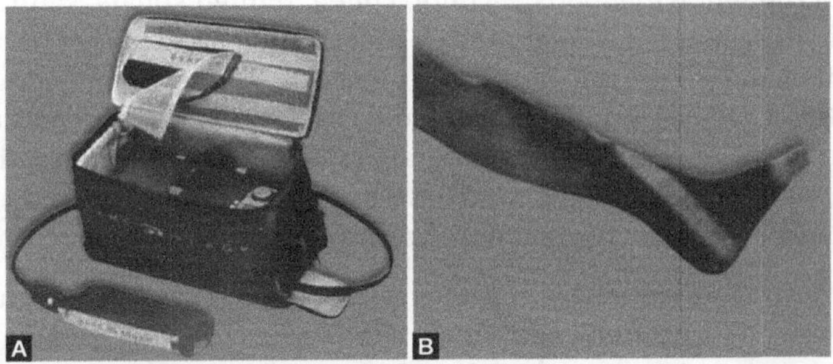

Figs 3.8A and B: Application of ice pack with compression at ankle joint

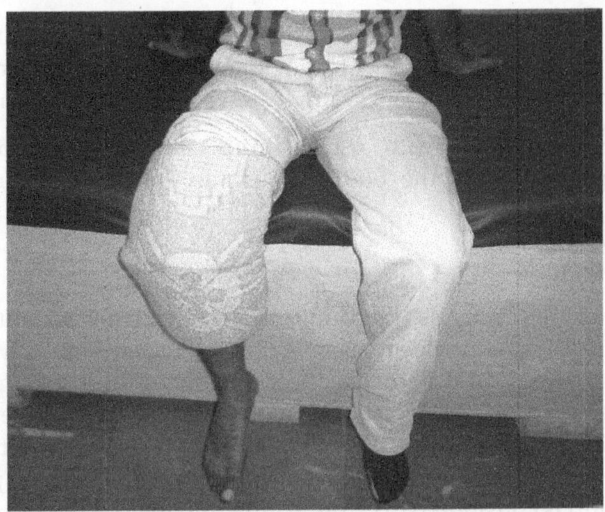

Fig. 3.9: Application of hot pack for the knee joint pain
(*For color version, see Plate 4*)

blood flow to the joint. It may also be an effective treatment before exercise. Alternatively, individuals may take a hot shower or bath before exercise to help reduce pain.

Lifestyle adjustments: Many lifestyle changes, including regular exercise, weight management, and healthy diet, may help reduce symptoms of osteoarthritis.

A dietary opinion from nutritionist may help to remove inflammatory foods from the diet, including dairy products, wheat, potatoes, peppers, eggplant, tomatoes, and tobacco. It is best to avoid the following foods: alcohol, coffee, refined sugars, saturated fat, hydrogenated fat (margarine), excess salt, spinach, cranberries, plums, buckwheat, and nuts.

Green vegetables, diet may include: carrots, avocado, sea weeds, spirulina, soy products, whole grains (such as brown rice, millet, oats, wheat, and barley), seeds (sesame, flax, and pumpkin), and cold-water fish (such as salmon, herring, and tuna).

Footwear: Individuals with osteoarthritis should wear comfortable footwear that properly supports their weight. This may reduce the amount of strain put on the joints during walking.

Walking aids: Individuals with osteoarthritis may require canes (Fig. 3.10),.walkers, or other assistive devices during ambulation.

Braces: If the joints are severely affected, braces may be beneficial to prevent the progression of joint deformities and to avoid the imbalance between different groups of muscles working around joint.

Posture: Individuals with osteoarthritis should maintain good posture. This allows the body's weight to be evenly distributed among joints.

Prevention

Regular exercise may also help individuals control their weight. There are many ways for people to exercise including: gardening, walking, sports activities, and dancing. Individuals who are beginning an exercise program should choose activities that fit their levels of strength and endurance. The type of exercise is not as important as a consistent exercise schedule. Exercise that causes extreme pain or discomfort is considered to be unhealthy, and may cause permanent damage to the joints.

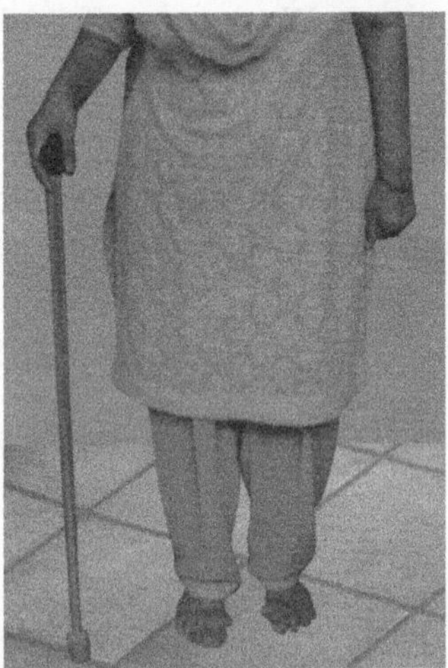

Fig. 3.10: Use of cane by arthritic patient during ambulation to reduce joint load and joint pain. Figure also shows the hallux valgus deformity with bunion (Swelling deformity of great toe)

Individuals who maintain a healthy body weight have a decreased risk of developing osteoarthritis. Eating a healthy and well-balanced diet may help individuals control their weight. Daily calorie needs of individuals range from the 1,000-calorie diets for toddlers to 3,200-calorie diets for teenage boys.

RHEUMATOID ARTHRITIS

Rheumatoid arthritis (RA) is a long-term disease that leads to inflammation of the joints and surrounding tissues. It can also affect other organs.

Causes, Incidence, and Risk Factors

The RA is considered to be an autoimmune disease (Gary, 2003; Thomas DJ et al, 1983). The body's immune system normally fights off foreign substances, like viruses. But in an autoimmune disease, the immune system confuses healthy tissue for foreign substances. As a result, the body attacks itself.

RA can occur at any age. Women are affected 3 times more often than men (Areskoug JK & Oberg, 2009).

RA usually affects joints on both sides of the body in variable amount. Wrists, fingers, knees, feet, and ankles are the most commonly affected. The course and the severity of the illness can vary considerably. Infection, genes, and hormones may contribute to the disease.

Symptoms

The disease usually begins gradually with constitutional symptoms such as:

- Fatigue
- Loss of appetite
- Morning stiffness (lasting more than 1 hour)
- Widespread muscle aches
- Weakness

Eventually, joint pain appears. During acute phase the joint can become warm, tender, and stiff. When the synovial lining of the joint becomes inflamed, it gives off more synovial fluid (this is called synovitis) and the joint becomes swollen. Joint pain is often felt on both sides of the body, and may affect the fingers, wrists, elbows, shoulders, hips, knees, ankles, toes, and neck (Allaire et al, 2009).

Additional symptoms include:

- Anemia due to failure of the bone marrow to produce enough new red blood cells
- Eye burning, itching, and discharge
- Hand (see Fig. 3.1) and feet deformities (Figs 3.11A and B)
- Limited range of motion
- Low-grade fever
- Lung inflammation
- Nodules under the skin (usually a sign of more severe disease)
- Numbness or tingling
- Paleness
- Skin redness or inflammation
- Swollen glands.

Joint destruction may occur within 1-2 years after the appearance of the disease.

Hallux Valgus

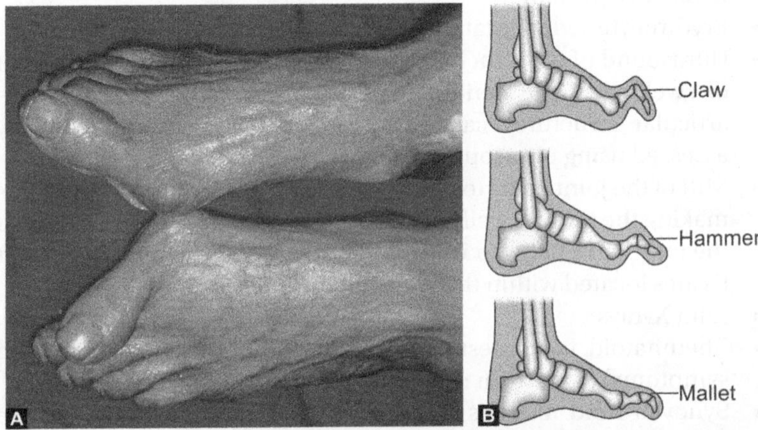

Figs 3.11A and B: Foot deformities in RA

Investigations

The criterias to diagnose RA were laid by American Rheumatology association in 1987. These are as follows:

- Morning stiffness in and around joints lasting at least 1 hour before maximal improvement
- Soft tissue swelling (arthritis) of 3 or more joint areas observed by a physician
- Swelling (arthritis) of the proximal interphalangeal, metacarpophalangeal, or wrist joints
- Symmetric swelling (arthritis)
- Rheumatoid nodules
- The presence of rheumatoid factor
- Radiographic erosions and/or periarticular osteopenia in hand and/or wrist joints.

Criteria 1 through 4 must have been present for at least 6 weeks. Rheumatoid arthritis is defined by the presence of 4 or more criteria, and no further qualifications (classic, definite, or probable) or list of exclusions are required.

A specific blood test is available for diagnosing RA and distinguishing it from other types of arthritis. It is called the anti-CCP antibody test (Pooja et al, 2004). Other tests that may be done include:

- Complete blood count
- C-reactive protein
- Erythrocyte sedimentation rate
- Ultrasound of the joint helps to identify the location and amount of swelling in the periarticular structures. However, the intra-articular structures cannot be adequately and appropriately assessed using ultrasound alone.
- MRI of the joint helps to have a detailed overview of the structures making the joint as well as the structures located in the vicinity of the joint. MRI helps to identify the status and the integrity of soft tissues located within the joints or around the joint.
- Joint X-rays
- Rheumatoid factor test (positive in about 75% of people with symptoms) (American rheumatology association criteria, 1987).
- Synovial fluid analysis helps to analyse the constituent of the synovial fluid and helps to identify various possible factors which might lead to arthritis or the articular pathology.

Deformities

In RA, bones and cartilage get damaged which causes inappropriate orientation of articular surfaces with respect to each other thus tendons may slip towards a wrong direction of action; due to repeated joint swelling ligaments get "slacken in wrong" action of muscles combined with the compromised joint stability causes joints to deform or subluxate.

In hand the Rheumatoid arthritis can cause the wrist or knuckle subluxation, ulnar drift of hand (the fingers get drifted towards ulnar border of hand), 'neck' or 'boutonniere' finger or 'z-shaped thumb' deformities, Heberden's nodes and Bouchard's nodes.

In feet the deformities may involve flat foot, hammer toe, hallux valgus, and bunions.

Treatment

RA usually requires lifelong treatment, including medications, physical therapy, exercise, education, and possibly surgery. Early, aggressive treatment for RA can delay joint destruction, however simultaneously it must be kept in mind that excessive stresses on the joint must also be avoided.

Medications

Diseases modifying antirheumatic drugs (DMARDs) are the current standard of care for RA, in addition to rest, strengthening exercises, and anti-inflammatory drugs. Methotrexate is the most commonly used DMARD for rheumatoid arthritis.

Anti-inflammatory medications: These include aspirin and nonsteroidal anti-inflammatory drugs (NSAIDs), such as ibuprofen. Although NSAIDs work well, long-term use can cause stomach problems, such as ulcers and bleeding, and possible heart problems.

Corticosteroids: These medications work very well to reduce joint swelling and inflammation. Because of potential long-term side effects, however, corticosteroids should be taken only for a short time and in low doses when possible.

Prognosis

Regular blood or urine tests should be done to determine how well medications are working and if drugs are causing any side effects.

RA differs from person to person. People with rheumatoid factor, the anti-CCP antibody, or subcutaneous nodules seem to have a more severe form of the disease. People who develop RA at younger ages also seem to get worse more quickly.

Many people with RA work full-time. However, after many years, about 10% of those with RA are severely disabled, and unable to do simple daily living tasks such as washing, dressing, and eating.

In the past, the average life expectancy for a patient with RA could be shortened by 3-7 years. Those with severe forms of RA would often die 10-15 years earlier than expected. However, as treatment for rheumatoid arthritis has improved, severe disability and life-threatening complications have decreased considerably and many people live relatively normal lives.

Complications

Rheumatoid arthritis is not solely restricted to joint destruction, rather it can involve almost all organs of body. Rupture of muscle tendons may occur due to chronic inflammation which occludes the small blood vessels supplying the muscles.

In rheumatoid arthritis the necrosis and erosion of transverse and the alar ligament of cervical spine may occur. Thus, now the odontoid process of axis cannot be contained in the ring of atlas. This may injure spinal cord and may prove to be life-threatening.

Disruption of long spinal ligaments may lead to increased motion between C1 and C2 vertebral bodies. Thus, during flexion atlas subluxates on axis and may impinge on spinal cord impingement or may cause vertebral arteries injury.

Rheumatoid vasculitis (inflammation of the blood vessels) may occur and lead to skin ulcerations and infections, bleeding stomach ulcers. It may also impair blood supply to nerves and may cause pain, numbness, or tingling. Vasculitis may also affect the brain, nerves, and heart (Rheumatic heart disease), which can cause stroke, heart attack, or heart failure.

The medicines used for the treatments of RA may also cause serious side effects.

Surgery

Surgical treatment may be needed for highly resistant cases who fail to respond to conservative management and develop high level of disability.

Main indications of surgery are: Refractory cases who do not respond to conservative care; when the associated disability causes significant reduction in the functional status of the patient; when the pain and deformity cause irreversible injury to the anatomical or physiological systems of the patient.

Unlike OA the RA may need multiple joint surgeries and must be careful because the disease will continue to progress even after the joint surgeries.

Common used surgical procedures are:

Synovectomy: It is helpful in early stage and helps to control the inflammation.

Synovectomy—lymphocytes of the synovial layer fail to attack in presence of IgM now; no antigen-antibody reaction now; no release of lysozyme enzyme; no pannus formation; no cartilage destruction further (Wynn Parry and Stanley, 1993).

Synovectomy is done in cases where synovitis persists for > 6 months and not responds to medical treatment.

Debridement: Of the damaged cartilage fragments. Removal of the loose body or joint fragments from the joint.

Arthroplasty: May involve the partial or complete joint replacement.

Corrective surgeries for fingers. Resection of the metatarsal heads to reduce the deformity.

Osteotomy: To recorrect the joint surfaces alignment and to optimize the weight transferring and load bearing. Osteotomy involves the cutting portion of bone to gain appropriate limb alignment and also helps to optimize force distribution so as to delay the abnormal joint/bone stresses.

Osteotomy also delays the need of joint replacement and simultaneously improves functional status of the patient.

It is treatment of choice in case of young adults where extensive synovectomy cannot be performed as it would lead to excessive cartilage destruction (Coventry, Ilstrup and Wallrich, 1993).

Arthrodesis: Performed to stabilize the joints when the other procedures cannot gain the joint stability. In case of spine the severe arthritis causes instability and ligament necrosis or excessive bone loss which cannot allow joint replacement, then arthrodesis or joint fusion are important to get stability.

Decompression surgeries: In cases where the spinal stenosis causes the spinal cord compression, the decompression surgeries are important and thus laminectomy may be needed.

Physiotherapy Management of RA

Most of RA patients suffer depression and psychological distresses due to the chronic nature of the disease. Social support groups may be helpful.

In RA the chronic inflammation causes blood circulation of tendons and muscles to get adversely affected, the rotator cuff muscles may rupture, need rotator cuff muscles strengthening.

In RA if excessively increase in the motion occurs between spinal segments, orthotic support is important.

The management of the deformities and associated pain/disability also needs therapeutic interventions.

In order to manage bunions the cryotherapy, ultrasound therapy, shoe wear modifications are important.

The Ottawa Panel found evidence to recommend and support the use of therapeutic exercises, especially knee functional strengthening, whole-body functional strengthening, general physical activity, and whole-body, low-intensity exercises, for the management of RA. (Ottawa Panel guidelines, 2004).

Range-of-motion exercises and individualized exercise programs prescribed by a physical therapist can delay the loss of joint function.

Joint protection techniques, heat and cold treatments, and splints or orthotic devices to support and align joints may be very helpful.

Sometimes therapists will use special machines to apply deep heat or electrical stimulation to reduce pain and improve joint mobility.

Occupational therapists can construct splints for the hand and wrist, and teach how to best protect and use joints when they are affected by arthritis. They also show people how to better cope with day-to-day tasks at work and at home, despite limitations caused by RA.

Frequent rest periods between activities, as well as 8 to 10 hours of sleep per night, are recommended.

Life style modifications and energy conservation strategies:

- Avoid stressful life and fatiguing exercises
- Manage/avoid fatigue
- Teach proper mechanics of the body
- Avoid joint strains
- Control body weight.

Orthotic Devices

Splints help to support a joint and improve its function thus reduce pain and prevent deformity.

Wrist hand synovitis—the static wrist hand orthosis are important. Night resting splints help to control the signs of inflammation. Resting position for splinting is 5-10 degree extension and MCP flexion of 10-20 degrees with corrected ulnar drift.

Ulnar drift splints help to keep fingers in neutral position with the finger separators and thus help to prevent ulnar drift contracture (Figs 3.12A and B).

To correct swan-neck deformity: PIP double-ring flexion splints are used.

To correct Boutonniere deformity: PIP double-ring extension splints are used.

Assistive aids may be useful. May use book stand instead of holding a book while reading; may use levered taps to reduce effort needed to use them; long handle equipments; light weight equipments.

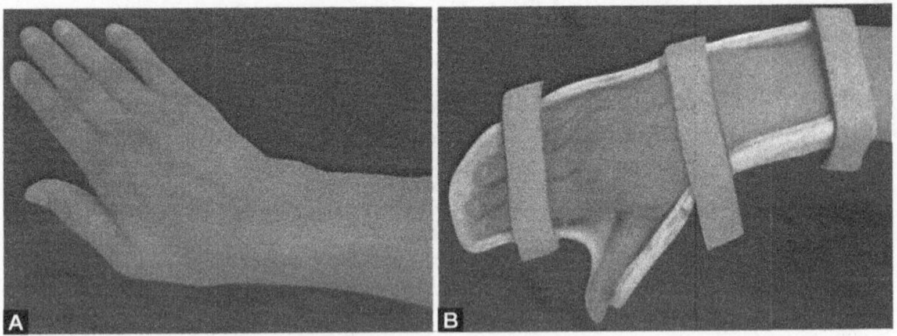

Figs 3.12A and B: Ulnar drift of hand: Splint to prevent ulnar drift in rheumatoid hand

Precautions with exercises: Must avoid forceful griping exercises. Should do light intensity relatively long-term exercises to improve endurance without causing fatigue.

During increased inflammatory stage may use cryotherapy to reduce the inflammation.

During chronic inflammation the hot packs are helpful to improve the circulation and to reduce the swelling.

Preoperative physical therapy care for arthrodesis involves: Maintaining an improving mobility, Range of motion (ROM) at proximal and distal joints; getting pain free movement of proximal and distal joints; normal strength of proximal and distal joints and the contra lateral side joints. This is important to do appropriate preoperative physiotherapy treatment because if proximal and distal joints are not normal then surgeries may not help to improvise function of the operated joint.

Prior to surgery the correction of all possible tightness and contractures is important.

After the *postoperative surgeries* the proper physical therapy is need to rehabilitated the patients back to normal life.

ANKYLOSING SPONDYLITIS

Ankylosing spondylitis is a long-term disease that causes inflammation of the joints between the spinal bones, and the joints between the spine and pelvis. It eventually causes the affected spinal bones to fuse together.

Causes, Incidence, and Risk Factors

Ankylosing spondylitis (AS) is a seronegative spondyloarthropathy that predilects young men. It is difficult to diagnose in its early stages and challenging to manage, once detected (Cameron and Silvano, 2000).

The cause of ankylosing spondylitis is unknown, but genes seem to play a role.

Strong correlation is found between Human Leukocyte Antigen (HLA-B27) and the AS.

The disease most often begins between ages 20 and 40, but may begin before age 10. It affects more males than females. Risk factors include:

- Family history of ankylosing spondylitis
- Male gender

Symptoms

The disease starts with low back pain that comes and goes.

- Pain and stiffness are worse at night, in the morning, after the period of inactivity during sleep.
- The pain typically gets better with activity or exercise.
- Back pain may begin in the sacroiliac joints (between the pelvis and the spine). Over time, it may involve all or part of the spine.
- Patients do have the typically flexed posture where neck has forward head attitude and the whole spine has flexed appearance (Fig. 3.13).

There may be a progressive loss motion or mobility in the lower spine. You may not be able to fully expand your chest because the joints between the ribs are involved.

Patient may have pain while doing deep breathing. This is due to the inflammation at the site of attachments of the intercostals ligaments (this inflammation is known as enthesis) which get stretched up during deep breathing.

Fatigue is also a common symptom.

Other, less common symptoms include:

- Eye inflammation or uveitis
- Heel pain
- Hip pain and stiffness
- Joint pain and joint swelling in the shoulders, knees, and ankles
- Loss of appetite

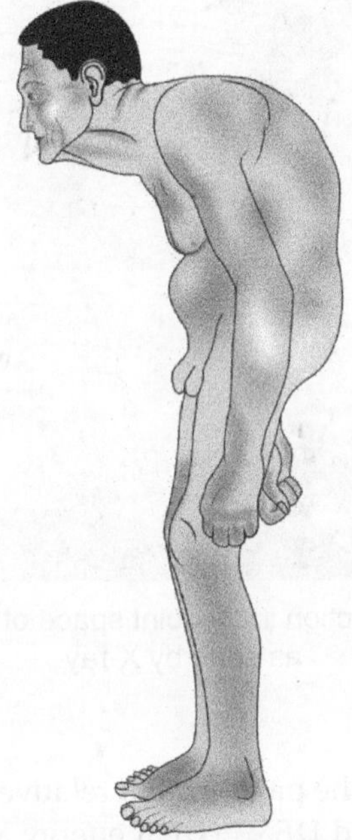

Fig. 3.13: Typical flexed posture of spine in AS patients

- Slight fever
- Weight loss.

Signs and Tests

Laboratory tests may include:

- CBC
- ESR may be increased in about 75% cases (Vander IE et al, 2002)
- HLA-B27 antigen
- X-rays of the spine and pelvis.

Investigations

X-rays reveals sacroilitis, however this visible appearance on X-ray is possible only after significant reduction in the joint gap has occurred. The earlier X-rays may reveal the reduction in the joint space of sacroiliac joint (Fig. 3.14).

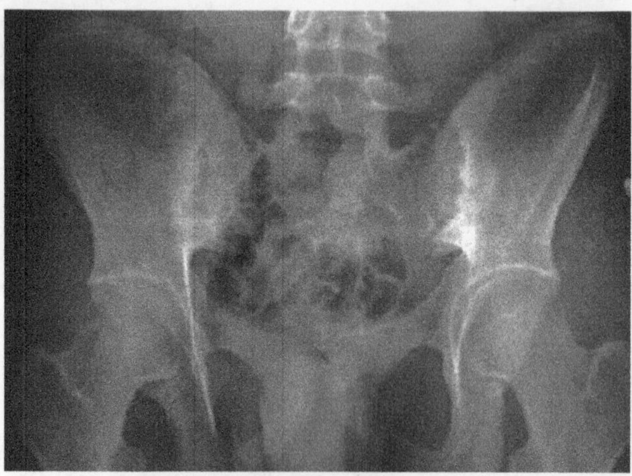

Fig. 3.14: The reduction in the joint space of the sacroiliac joint, as seen by X-ray

CT scan can reveal the pathology in relatively earlier stages.

MRI, ultrasound and DEXA (Dual energy X-ray absorptiometry) are other important investigations.

The diagnosis of the AS is made on the basis of the criteria laid by New York (Table 3.3).

Assessment of the AS patients (Zochling and Braun, 2005)

Back pain intensity assessment is important to be documented. This assessment may be recorded by VAS (visual analogue scale).

Spinal Stiffness: Assessment of the spinal stiffness in morning and its duration reflects disease activity and its impact on physical function. When syndesmophytes and ankylosis are present then stiffness does not change over the course of the day (Zochling and Braun, 2005). Change in the duration of morning stiffness can be interpreted as a change in inflammation, as structural damage does not change over this time frame.

Cervical region mobility can be assessed by occiput to wall distance, tragus to wall distance and cervical rotation range of motion.

Thoracic mobility can be assessed by recording the measurement of chest expansion between maximum expiration and maximum inspiration at level of nipple.

TABLE 3.3 Modified New York Criteria for ankylosing spondylitis (Linden et al, 1984; Cameron and Silvano, 2000)

- Diagnosis
  - Clinical criteria
    - Low back pain and stiffness for more than 3 months which improves with exercise, but is not relieved by rest
    - Limitation of motion of the lumbar spine in both the sagittal and frontal planes
    - Limitation of chest expansion relative to normatl values corrected for age and sex
  - Radiological criterion sacroiliitis grade 2 bilaterally or sacroilitis grade 3–4 unilaterally
- Grading
  - Definite ankylosing spondylitis if the radiologic criterion is associated with at least 1 clinical criterion
  - Probably ankylosing spondylitis if:
    - Three clinical criteria are present
    - The radiologic criterion is present without any signs or symptoms satisfying the clinical criteria. (Other causes of sacroiliitis should be considered)

Lumbar spine mobility is assessed by lumbar spine Range of motion, spinal lateral flexion ranges, finger to floor distance during forward bending.

Course of the AS

The course of the AS is highly variable as there may be periods of acute exacerbations and the remission.

Treatment

Nonsteroidal anti-inflammatory drugs (NSAIDs) to reduce inflammation and pain.

Corticosteroid therapy or medications to suppress the immune system may also be prescribed. Drugs called TNF-inhibitors (etanercept, adalimumab, infliximab), which block an inflammatory protein, have been shown to improve the symptoms of ankylosing spondylitis.

Drugs that block cell growth (cytotoxic drugs) are used in people who do not respond well to corticosteroids or who are dependent on high doses of corticosteroids.

Surgery may be done if pain or joint damage is severe.

Exercises can help improve posture and breathing. Lying flat on the back at night can help maintain normal posture.

Prognosis

The course of the disease is unpredictable. Symptoms may come and go at any time. Most people are able to function unless the hips are severely involved.

Complications

Rarely, people may have problems with the aortic heart valve (aortic insufficiency) and heart rhythm problems.

Some patients may have pulmonary fibrosis or restrictive lung disease.

Prevention

Prevention is unknown. Awareness of risk factors may allow early detection and treatment.

Physical Therapy Management of AS

To relieve pain the cryotherapy or hot fomentation may be helpful to relieve spasm and the muscle tightness.

Pool therapy and hydrotherapy (Fig. 3.15) are very useful in these patients as buoyancy supports body weight and reduces the joint loading and stresses.

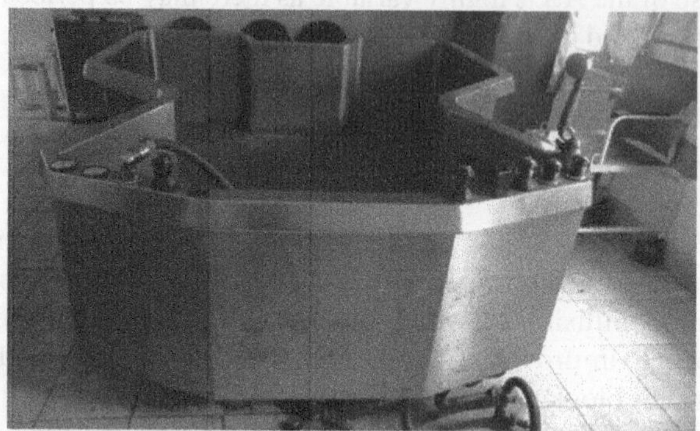

Fig. 3.15: Hydrotherapy application for the AS patients

Spinal and pelvic mobility exercises are important to prevent the progressive restriction in the ranges at joints.

Thoracic mobility exercises help to maintain the chest expansion, the pulmonary capacity and the breathing stamina.

Proper postural care is important, to prevent the deterioration in the posture of the body.

Cervical retraction exercises are important to prevent the development of the forward head posture.

The development of upper and lower crossed syndromes should be avoided. The stretching of the pectorals, hip flexors and lumbar extensors are important. The endurance of lumbar extensors is important to prevent the forward deviation of the spine.

Deep breathing exercises (Figs 3.16A and B) are helpful to maintain lung expansion and the thorax region.

Mobility exercise (Figs 3.17A to G) for the sacroiliac joints are important to preserve the pelvic joint mobility and to prevent the progressive loss of spinal range of motion.

ADHESIVE CAPSULITIS

Frozen shoulder is when the shoulder is painful and cannot move normally because of inflammation involving the shoulder joint capsule.

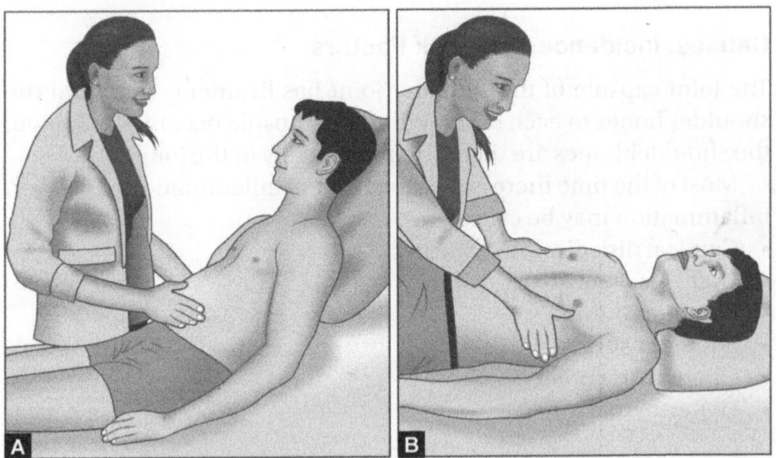

Figs 3.16A and B: Deep breathing exercises for AS patients: (A) Diaphragmatic breathing; (B) Inter-costal breathing facilitation (Adapted from Carolyn Kisner)

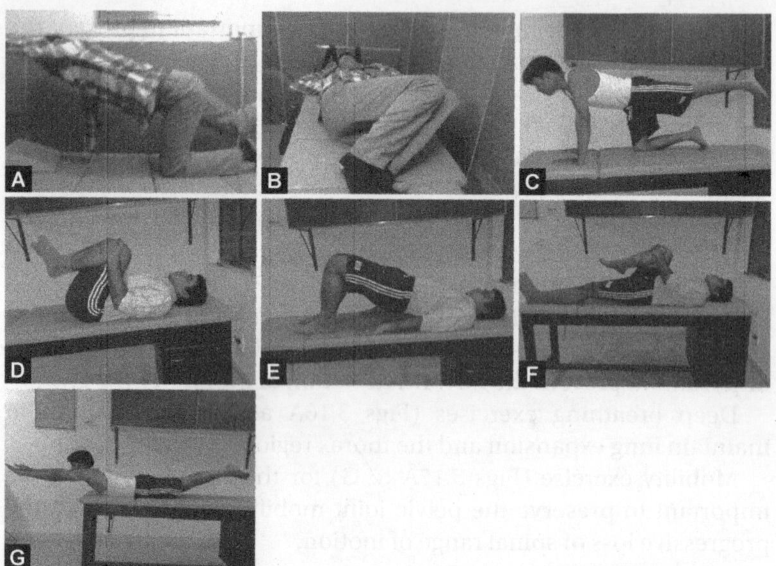

Figs 3.17A to G: Mobility exercises for the AS patient: (A) Prone hip and contralateral arm extension; (B) Trunk rolling; (C) Prone lying hip extension; (D) Bilateral hip knee flexion; (E) Bridging; (F) Unilateral knee to chest; (G) Upper and lower spine extension (Combined)

Causes, Incidence, and Risk Factors

The joint capsule of the shoulder joint has ligaments that hold the shoulder bones to each other. When the capsule becomes inflamed, the shoulder bones are unable to move freely in the joint.

Most of the time there is no cause for the inflammation. However, inflammation may be caused by:

- Cervical disk disease of the neck
- Diabetes
- Shoulder trauma
- Shoulder surgery
- Open heart surgery
- Hyperthyroidism

Symptoms

The main symptoms are:

- Decreased motion of the shoulder
- Pain
- Stiffness

Frozen shoulder without any known cause starts with pain. This pain prevents you from moving your arm. The lack of movement (Figs 3.18A to D) leads to stiffness and decreased motion. Eventually you cannot perform activities such as reaching over your head.

Signs and Tests

The healthcare provider will make the diagnosis based on your symptoms and an examination of your shoulder.

You may have X-rays of the shoulder to make sure there is no other problem, such as arthritis. Sometimes an MRI exam may show inflammation, but there are no specific findings that diagnose frozen shoulder.

Treatment

Pain is treated with nonsteroidal anti-inflammatory medications (NSAIDs) and steroid injections. Steroid injections along with physical therapy can significantly improve motion. It can take as long as 6 - 9 months to see improvement. The physical therapy is intense and needs to be done every day.

Any risk factors for frozen shoulder may also need to be treated.

Surgery is recommended if therapy is not successful. Your health care provider will release the scar tissue by bringing the shoulder through a full range of motion. This procedure is done under *anesthesia*.

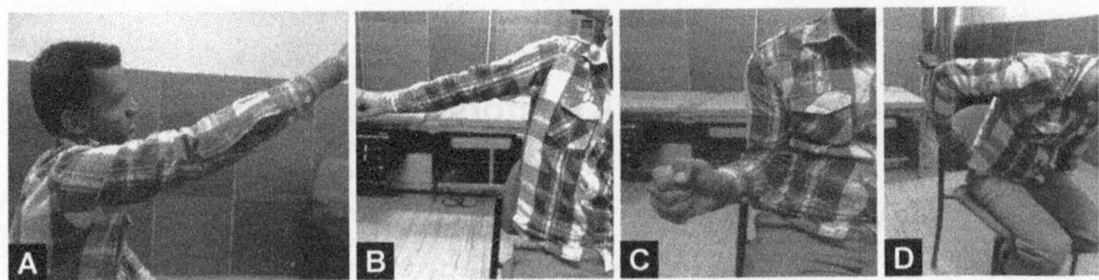

Figs 3.18A to D: The restricted movement of the shoulder joint in patients with adhesive capsulitis: (A) Restricted flexion; (B) Restricted abduction; (C) Restricted external rotation; (D) Restricted internal rotation

Arthroscopic surgery can be used to cut the tight ligaments and remove the scar tissue from the shoulder. Some surgeons may use repeated pain blocks after surgery so you can participate in physical therapy.

Prognosis

Treatment with therapy and NSAIDs will usually return the motion and function of the shoulder within a year. Even if left untreated, the frozen shoulder can get better by itself in 18–24 months.

Even if surgery restores motion, you must continue physical therapy for several weeks or months afterward to prevent the frozen shoulder from returning. Treatment may fail if you cannot tolerate physical therapy.

Complications

- Stiffness and pain continue even with therapy
- The arm can break if the shoulder is moved forcefully during surgery.

Prevention

The best way to prevent frozen shoulder is to contact your health care provider if you develop shoulder pain that limits your range of motion for an extended period of time. This will allow early treatment and help avoid stiffness.

People who have diabetes will be less likely to get frozen shoulder if they keep their condition under control.

BURSITIS

Bursitis is inflammation of the fluid-filled sac (bursa) that lies between a tendon and skin, or between a tendon and bone. The condition may be *acute* or *chronic*.

Causes, Incidence, and Risk Factors

Bursae are fluid-filled cavities near joints where tendons or muscles pass over bony projections. They assist movement and reduce friction between moving parts.

Bursitis can be caused by chronic overuse, trauma, rheumatoid arthritis, gout, or infection. Sometimes the cause cannot be determined. Bursitis commonly occurs in the shoulder, knee, elbow, and hip. Other areas that may be affected include the Achilles tendon and the foot.

Chronic inflammation can occur with repeated injuries or attacks of bursitis.

Symptoms

- Joint pain and tenderness
- Swelling
- Warmth over the joint.

Treatment

Temporary rest or immobilization of the affected part may be required to reduce the symptoms of the bursitis.

If the bursitis is due to gout or due to infective reasons, the concerned medical/orthopedic management might be required before starting any physiotherapy intervention.

Nonsteroidal anti-inflammatory drugs (NSAIDs) such as ibuprofen may relieve pain and inflammation. Formal physical therapy may be helpful as well.

If the inflammation does not respond to the initial treatment, it may be necessary to draw out fluid from the bursa and inject corticosteroids. Surgery is rarely required.

Exercises for the affected area should be started as the pain resolves. If *muscle atrophy* (weakness or decrease in size) has occurred. Your healthcare provider may suggest exercises to build strength and increase mobility.

Bursitis caused by infection is treated with antibiotics. Sometimes the infected bursa must be drained surgically.

Prognosis

The condition may respond well to treatment, or it may develop into a chronic condition if the underlying cause cannot be corrected.

Complications

- Chronic bursitis may occur
- Too many steroid injections over a short period of time can cause injury to the surrounding tendons.

Prevention

Avoid activities that include repetitive movements of any body parts whenever possible.

MYALGIA

Muscle aches and pains are common and can involve more than one muscle. Muscle pain also can involve ligaments, tendons, and fascia, the soft tissues that connect muscles, bones, and organs.

Alternative Names

Muscle pain; **Myalgia**; Pain - muscles.

Considerations

Muscle pain is most frequently related to tension, overuse, or muscle injury from exercise or physically-demanding work. In these situations, the pain tends to involve specific muscles and starts during or just after the activity. It is usually obvious which activity is causing the pain.

Muscle pain also can be a sign of conditions affecting your whole body, like some infections (including *the flu*) and disorders that affect *connective tissues* throughout the body (such as *lupus*).

One common cause of muscle aches and pain is *fibromyalgia*, a condition that includes tenderness in your muscles and surrounding soft tissue, sleep difficulties, fatigue, and headaches.

Common Causes

The most common causes are:
- Injury or trauma including sprains and strains
- Overuse: using a muscle too much, too soon, too often
- Tension or stress.

Muscle pain may also be due to:
- Certain drugs, including:
  - ACE inhibitors for lowering blood pressure
  - Cocaine
  - Statins for lowering cholesterol
- Dermatomyositis
- Electrolyte imbalances like too little potassium or calcium
- Fibromyalgia

- Infections, including:
  - Influenza (the flu)
  - Lyme disease
  - Malaria
  - Muscle abscess
  - Polio
  - Rocky mountain spotted fever
  - Trichinosis (roundworm)
- Lupus
- Polymyalgia rheumatica
- Polymyositis
- Rhabdomyolysis.

Physical Therapy Care

For muscle pain from overuse or injury, apply ice for the first 24–72 hours of an injury to reduce pain and inflammation. After that, heat often feels more soothing.

Muscle aches from overuse and fibromyalgia often respond well to massage. Gentle stretching exercises after a long rest period are also helpful.

Regular exercise can help restore proper muscle tone. Walking, cycling, and swimming are good aerobic activities to try. A physical therapist can teach you stretching, toning, and aerobic exercises to feel better and stay pain-free. Begin slowly and increase workouts gradually. Avoid high-impact aerobic activities and weight lifting when injured or while in pain.

Be sure to get plenty of sleep and try to reduce stress. Yoga and meditation are excellent ways to help you sleep and relax.

If home measures are not working, call your doctor, who will consider prescription medication, physical therapy referral, or referral to a specialized pain clinic.

If your muscle aches are due to a specific disease, follow the instructions of your doctor to treat the primary illness.

Prevention

- Warm up before exercising and cool down afterward
- Stretch before and after exercising
- Drink lots of fluids before, during, and after exercise
- If you work in the same position most of the day (like sitting at a computer), stretch at least every hour.

FIBROMYOSITIS

Fibromyalgia is a common condition characterized by long-term, body-wide pain and tender points in joints, muscles, tendons, and other soft tissues. Fibromyalgia has also been linked to fatigue, morning stiffness, sleep problems, headaches, numbness in hands and feet, depression, and anxiety.

Fibromyalgia can develop on its own or along with other musculoskeletal conditions such as rheumatoid arthritis or lupus.

Alternative Names

Fibromyositis; Fibrositis.

Causes, Incidence, and Risk Factors

The cause of this disorder is unknown. Physical or emotional trauma may play a role in development of the syndrome. Some evidence suggests that fibromyalgia patients have abnormal pain transmission responses.

It has been suggested that sleep disturbances, which are common in fibromyalgia patients, may actually cause the condition. Another theory suggests that the disorder may be associated with changes in skeletal muscle metabolism, possibly caused by decreased blood flow, which could cause chronic fatigue and weakness.

Others have suggested that an infectious microbe, such as a virus, triggers the illness. At this point, no such virus or microbe has been identified.

Pilot studies have shown a possible inherited tendency toward the disease, though evidence is very preliminary.

Men and women of all ages get fibromyalgia, but the disorder is most common among women aged 20 to 50.

Symptoms

The overwhelming characteristic of fibromyalgia is long-standing, body-wide pain with defined tender points. Tender points are distinct from trigger points seen in other pain syndromes. Unlike tender points, trigger points can occur in isolation and represent a source of radiating pain, even in the absence of direct pressure.

Fibromyalgia pain can mimic the pain that occurs with various types of arthritis. However, the significant swelling, destruction, and deformity of joints seen in diseases such as rheumatoid arthritis does not occur with fibromyalgia syndrome alone.

The soft-tissue pain of fibromyalgia is described as deep-aching, radiating, gnawing, shooting or burning, and ranges from mild to severe. Fibromyalgia sufferers tend to wake up with body aches and stiffness.

For some patients, pain improves during the day and increases again during the evening, though many patients with fibromyalgia have day-long, unrelenting pain. Pain can increase with activity, cold or damp weather, anxiety, and stress.

Specific symptoms:

- Body aches
- Chronic facial muscle pain or aching
- Fatigue
- Irritable bowel syndrome
- Memory difficulties and cognitive difficulties
- Multiple tender areas (muscle and joint pain) on the back of the neck, shoulders, sternum, lower back, hips, shins, elbows, knees
- Numbness and tingling
- Palpitations
- Reduced exercise tolerance
- Sleep disturbances
- Tension or migraine headaches.

Signs and Tests

Diagnosis of fibromyalgia requires a history of at least 3 months of widespread pain, and pain and tenderness in at least 11 of 18 tender-point sites (Fig. 3.4). These tender-point sites include fibrous tissue or muscles of the:

- Arms (elbows)
- Buttocks
- Chest
- Knees
- Lower back
- Neck
- Rib cage
- Shoulders
- Thighs.

Sometimes, laboratory and X-ray tests are done to help confirm the diagnosis by ruling out other conditions that may have similar symptoms. The following conditions have been associated with fibromyalgia or mimic its symptoms:

- Cancer
- Cervical and low-back degenerative disease
- Chronic fatigue syndrome
- Depression
- HIV infection
- Hypothyroidism
- Irritable bowel syndrome
- Lyme disease
- Rheumatoid arthritis
- Sleep disorders.

Management

In mild cases, symptoms may go away when stress is decreased or lifestyle changes are implemented. A combination of treatments including medications, patient education, physical therapy, and counseling are usually recommended. Many fibromyalgia sufferers have found support groups helpful.

Eating a well-balanced diet and avoiding caffeine may help with problems sleeping, and may help reduce the severity of the symptoms. Lifestyle measures to improve the quality of sleep can be effective for fibromyalgia.

Some reports indicate that fish oil, magnesium/malic acid combinations, or vitamins may be effective. Reducing stress and improving coping skills may also help reduce painful symptoms.

Improved fitness through exercise is recommended. Studies have shown that fibromyalgia symptoms can be relieved by aerobic exercise. The best way to begin a fitness program is to start with short sessions of just a few minutes of gentle, low-impact exercises such as walking and swimming. The length of each session can be increased slowly, as tolerated. Attempts at keeping to an exercise program often fail because they are begun too aggressively, with sessions that are too long or too intense. Starting out slowly and gently can help ease you into an effective program you can stick with.

Starting slowly helps stretch and mobilize tight, sore muscles. High-impact aerobics and weight lifting could cause increased discomfort. Symptoms may be relieved by gentle stretching and light massage, as well as acupressure, acupuncture, and relaxation techniques.

BIBLIOGRAPHY

1. Ackerman IN, Bennell KL. Does pre-operative physiotherapy improve outcomes from lower limb joint replacement surgery? A systematic review. Australian Journal of Physiotherapy 2004;50:25-30.
2. Allaire S,Wolfe F, Niu J, et al. Current risk factors for work disability associated with rheumatoid arthritis: recent data from a US national cohort. Arthritis Rheum 2009;61(3):321-8.
3. Andriacchi TP, Mündermann A, Smith RL, Eugene J. Alexander, Chris O Dyrby, Seungbum Koo. A Framework for the in vivo Pathomechanics of Osteoarthritis at the Knee. Annals of Biomedical Engineering 2004;32(3).
4. Areskoug JK, Oberg U. A literature review of the sexual health of women with rheumatoid arthritis. Musculoskeletal Care 2009;25.
5. Brooks P. Inflammation as an important feature of osteoarthritis. Bulletin of the World Health Organization 2003;81(9):689-90.
6. Cameron McDermaid, Silvano Mior. Ankylosing spondylitis presenting to a chiropractic office a report of two cases. Journal of Canadian Chiropractic Association 2000;44(2):87-97.
7. Coventry MB, ILstryp DM, Wallrichs SL. Proximal tibial osteotomy: A critical long-term study of 87 cases. Journal of bone and joint surgery, 1993;75:196-201.
8. D'Lima Darryl, Hashimoto Sanshiro, Chen Peter, Colwell Clifford W. Jr Lotz, Martin K. Impact of Mechanical Trauma on Matrix and Cells. Clinical Orthopedics and Related Research 2001;391:S90-S9.
9. DJ Thomas, A Young, AN Gorsuch, GF Bottazzo, AG Cudworth. Evidence for an association between rheumatoid arthritis and autoimmune endocrine disease. Ann Rheum Disease 1983;42:297-300.
10. Firestein S. Review article evolving concepts of rheumatoid arthritis. Nature 2003;423:356-61.
11. Fujiwara, Atsushi Lim, Tae-Hong An, Howard S Tanaka, Nobuhiro Jeon, Chang-Hoon Andersson, Gunnar BJ Haughton, Victor M. The Effect of Disc Degeneration and Facet Joint Osteoarthritis on the Segmental Flexibility of the Lumbar Spine. Spine 2000;25(23):3036-44.
12. IE van der Horst-Bruinsma, DO Clegg, BAC Dijkmans. Treatment of ankylosing spondylitis with disease modifying antirheumatic drugs. Clin Exp Rheumatol 2002;20(Suppl. 28):S67-S70.
13. Jordan JM, Kington RS, Lane NE, Nevitt MC, Zhang Y, Sowers MF. Systemic risk factors for osteoarthritis. In: Felson DT, conference chair. Osteoarthritis: new insights. Part 1: The disease and its risk factors. Ann Intern Med 2000;133:637-9.

14. Kellgren JH, Lawrence JS. Radiologic assessment of osteoarthrosis. Ann Rheum Dis 1957;16:494-501.
15. Khosla P, S Shankar, Duggal L. Anti CCP Antibodies in Rheumatoid Arthritis. J Indian Rheumatol Assoc 2004;12:143-6.
16. Linden S, Valkenburg HA, Cats A. Evaluation of diagnostic criteria for ankylosing spondylitis. A proposal for modification of the New York criteria. Arthritis Rheum 1984;27:361-8.
17. Mann RA, Schakel ME. 2nd. Surgical correction of rheumatoid forefoot deformities. Foot Ankle Int. 1995;16(1):1-6.
18. Martin JA, Joseph A. Buckwalter. Aging articular cartilage chondrocyte senescence and osteoarthritis. Biogerontology 2002;3(5).
19. Mulherin D, Fitzgerald O, Bresnihan B. Clinical improvement and radiological deterioration in rheumatoid arthritis: evidence that the pathogenesis of synovial inflammation and articular erosion may differ. Rheumatology 1996;35(12):1263-8.
20. Ottawa Panel Evidence-Based Clinical Practice Guidelines for Therapeutic Exercises in the Management of Rheumatoid Arthritis in Adults. Physical Therapy 2004;84(10).
21. Reeves CL, Peaden AJ, Shane. The complications encountered with the rheumatoid surgical foot and ankle. Clin Podiatr Med Surg 2010;27(2):313-25.
22. Ruddy, Shaun. Kelley's Textbook of Rheumatology, 6th Ed. WB Saunders. 2001.pp.1055-64.
23. Ryan KJ, Ray CG. Sherris Medical Microbiology (4th ed.). McGraw Hill. 2004.pp.434-7.
24. Schlesinger N. "Diagnosing and treating gout: A review to aid primary care physicians". Postgrad Med 2010;122(2):157-61.
25. Schouten JS, van den FA Ouweland, Valkenburg HA. A 12-year follow-up study in the general population on prognostic factors of cartilage loss in osteoarthritis of the knee. Ann Rheum Dis 1992;51:932-7.
26. Sharma MK, Swami HM, Bhatia V, Verma A, Bhatia SPS, Kaur G. An Epidemiological Study of Correlates of Osteoarthritis in Geriatric Population of UT Chandigarh, Indian Journal of Community Medicine 2007;32(1):1-3.
27. Terkeltaub R. "Update on gout: new therapeutic strategies and options". Nat Rev Rheumatol 2010;6(1):30-8.
28. The american rheumatism association revised criteria for the classification of rheumatoid arthritis. Arthritis and Rheumatism. 1987(31)3:315-24.
29. Wynn Parry CB, Stanley JK. Synovectomy of hand. British Journal of Rheumatology 1993;32:1089-95.
30. Zochling, Braun. Assessment of ankylosing spondylitis. Clin Exp Rheumatol 2005;23(Suppl. 39):S133-S41.

CHAPTER

4

Skin Diseases

ACNE

Acne is a very common skin disorder of the pilosebaceous units of skin. Pilosebaceous units of skin consist of sebaceous glands that connect to hair follicles (canals) lined with keratinocytes. The sebaceous glands are responsible for production of sebum (skin oil). Acne is very common inflammatory skin disorder of these pilosebaceous unit and is characterized by comedones (clogged pores) and pimples (papules and pustules), due in part to the excessive production of sebum (Flow chart 4.1). When excessive amounts of sebum and dead keratinocytes accumulate in the hair follicle, they often solidify as a soft plug. The plug may be complete and form a whitehead (closed comedone) or may be incomplete and form a blackhead (open comedone). These plugged, sebum-filled follicles allow overgrowth of *Propionibacterium acnes* (*P. acnes*), which are skin bacteria that are normally present in hair follicles. *P. acnes* break the sebum down into substances that irritate the skin and cause inflammation. This inflammation may lead to eruptions called as pimples, cysts or nodules. Acne can occur anywhere on the body, but it is most common in areas with high concentrations of sebaceous glands (e.g., face, neck, chest, shoulders, upper back).

Presentation

Presentation of acne varies from person to person. In few cases it may not be more than just a simple and short lasting cosmetic concern, while for others few it might involve extensive spread over large area, and may lead to high degree of discomfort along with cosmetic concern. However for most sufferers, acne is not a serious medical condition, and can usually be kept under control with treatment. Although scarring is common, treatment during and after an outbreak can help.

Flow chart 4.1: Events leading to acne

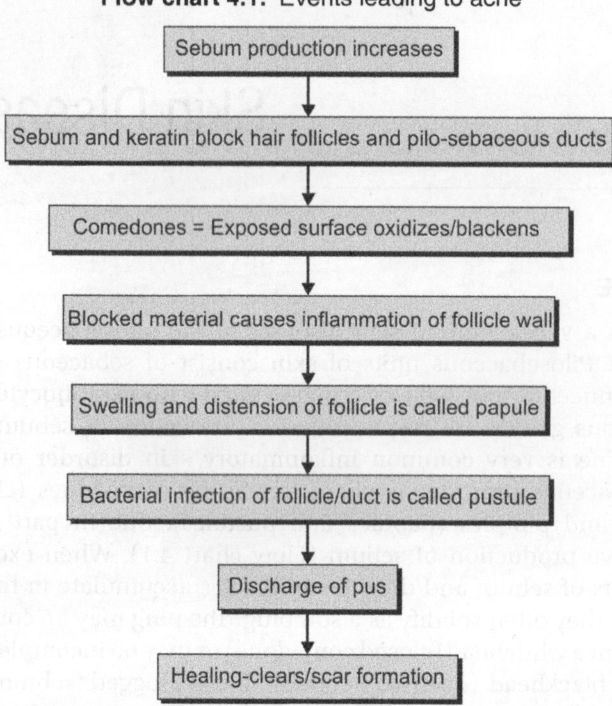

Associated Problems

Serious medical complications not occur, however emotional problems are more common in acne suffers.

- Scars form after lesions clear
- Emotional distress
- Poor social relationships, self-esteem or a person's outlook on life
- Social withdrawal (Zaenglein and Thiboutot, 2006)
- Poor body image
- Feelings of depression (Zaenglein and Thiboutot, 2006)
- Anger and frustration.

Acne myths, such as the belief that acne is linked to poor hygiene, may contribute to this poor social regard.

Acne is the most common skin condition affecting people worldwide as nearly 85 percent of all people between the ages of 11 and 30 develop acne (Van et al, 2009). Acne can affect people of all ages, but is most common in teenagers. It usually occurs in puberty (typically between the ages of 10 and 13), when androgens (male sex hormones) increase in both males and females. Most cases of acne last between 5 to 10 years. Typically, the severity of acne decreases by the age of 30, but this is not always the case.

Classification

There are many different types of acne. "Common" acne (acne vulgaris) can be divided into four categories according to severity:

- Type 1: Predominantly comedones (whiteheads and blackheads) with an occasional small pimple (papule or pustule). This is the mild form and does not involve scarring.
- Type 2: Comedones and more numerous pimples, mainly facial. This form involves mild scarring.
- Type 3: Numerous comedones and pimples, spreading to the back, chest and shoulders. It may lead to formation of cyst or nodule and moderate scarring.
- Type 4: Numerous large cysts and nodules on face, neck and upper trunk. This is severe form and causes significant scarring.

Another common form of acne is acne rosacea (rosacea), which includes facial discoloration (reddening). Other types of less common acne may be characterized by severity and symptoms or by causes.

Acne fulminans. Rare type of acne marked by inflamed, tender, crusting lesions on the upper trunk and face. Acne fulminans occurs suddenly and typically affects adolescent males. It is often accompanied by fever, high levels of white blood cells and an elevated sedimentation rate. It is occasionally accompanied by inflammation in several joints.

Causing Factors of Acne

- Chlorinated agents or chlorinated chemicals, such as the chlorine used to treat pool water
- Excessive use of make-up, lotions and oil based creams
- Petroleum products and oils. Direct skin exposure to greasy or oily substances (e.g., from scalp or hair, mineral or cooking oils) and certain cosmetics may cause acne
- Systemic or topical use of steroids, including corticosteroids and anabolic steroids. Often occurs predominantly on the upper back and shoulders
- Halogen acne (Zouboulis and Xia, 2009)

- Summer acne or tropical acne occurs in hot, humid weather or is made worse by such weather. It predominantly affects the neck, chest, back and legs, and often occurs in individuals unaccustomed to such climates
- Acne neonatorum is form of acne which is common among newborns and infants.

Risk Factors

There are many factors that influence these contributing factors and outbreaks after onset, including:

- Hormonal changes. These may include changes due to:
  - Puberty—increased secretion of androgens (male sex hormones) results in increased size and activity of sebaceous glands
  - Menstruation
  - Pregnancy
  - Oral contraceptives. Women starting or stopping birth control pills may experience an improvement or worsening of acne (Thiboutot and Chen, 2003)
  - Stress—may have an affect on hormones, causing individuals undergoing high levels of stress to experience an outbreak or worsening of acne
  - Corticosteroids, anabolic steroids (such as those used by athletes) and barbiturates may lead to acne outbreaks.
- Heredity—severe acne may have a genetic component (Bataille et al, 2002)
- Allergies and sensitivities—some individuals due to their lower immunity are more sensitive to the bacteria that cause acne
- Friction or pressure on skin—friction and pressure, such as that caused by telephones, helmets, tight collars and backpacks, may lead to acne outbreaks
- Environmental factors—humidity, pollution, changes in the season and other environmental factors may lead to an outbreak of acne
- Junk foods such as chocolate and greasy foods (e.g., French fries, pizza) are often blamed for acne
- Smoking habits (Capitanio et al, 2009)
- Poor hygiene.

Signs and Symptoms

Acne is characterized by an outbreak of lesions on the skin. These lesions include:

- Whiteheads (closed comedones). The openings of the hair follicles become clogged and completely blocked. The soft plug is a white color. These are noninflammatory.
- Blackheads (open comedones). The openings of the hair follicles become clogged and partially blocked. The plug darkens and is open to the surface of the skin. These are noninflammatory.
- Pimples (papules and pustules). Raised, reddish spots with white centers that signal inflammation or infection in the follicle (Fig. 4.1). These may be without pus (papules) or may contain pus (pustules). They may be tender or painful.
- Nodules—solid, raised reddish bumps.
- Cysts-thick lumps beneath the skin formed by the build-up of secretions deep in the hair follicle.

Diagnosis and Treatment

Acne is typically managed by a dermatologist (skin specialist). The diagnosis of acne relies upon the patient's medical history and a physical examination. In most cases, acne is obvious and does not require any additional testing.

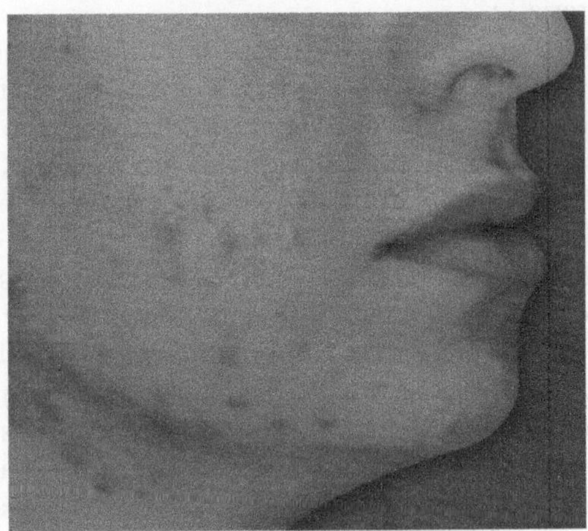

Fig. 4.1: Pimples in acne
(*For color version, see Plate 5*)

The goal of acne treatment is to minimize scarring, prevent further eruptions of blemishes and improve those that are already present. Individualized treatment depends upon the followings:

- Acne severity
- Types of lesions present
- Patient's age
- Patient's skin type
- Patient's overall health and medical history
- Patient's tolerance for specific medications, procedures or therapies
- Patient and physician's expectations for the course of the condition
- Patient's opinion or preference.

Acne treatments may be local (local topical application) or systemic (systemic antibiotics) and generally work by reducing the inflammation in the skin, speeding up skin cell turnover, fighting bacterial infection or a combination of these methods. Sudden discontinuation of acne medication can lead to a recurrence of acne several weeks later.

Acne lotions, gels and washes may dry up sebum, kill the acne bacteria or promote the proper sloughing of dead skin cells. Over-the-counter topical treatments are generally mild. Their active ingredients may include benzoyl peroxide, one of the most commonly used topical treatments. Other ingredients include alcohol and acetone, which are used together to reduce oil concentrations and help kill bacteria.

Prescription lotions used for moderate to severe acne involve retinoids (vitamin A derivatives) that work by increasing cell turnover (Haider and James, 2004) and preventing the clogging of hair follicles. The 3 main topical retinoids are tretinoin, adapalene, and tazarotene. Topical antibiotics work by killing the bacteria that lead to acne and reducing inflammation.

Oral antibiotics may be prescribed for moderate to severe acne. These reduce bacteria and fight inflammation, but may take months to work. They are often used in combination with topical products.

When acne outbreaks coincide with a woman's monthly period, oral contraceptives may help to control the acne as they suppress the excessive androgenic hormone action (Thorneycroft et al, 1999).

Large, inflamed nodules or cysts may be treated by an injection with corticosteroids. It typically takes three to five days after the injection to clear up the treated nodule or cyst.

Other treatment options for acne and the scars left by acne include:

- Extraction of comedones. A whitehead or blackhead is opened and extracted with a sterile, pen-sized device, fine needle or blade
- "Acne surgery," is the surgical drainage and extraction of large cysts. It reduces the pain and decreases the likelihood of scarring
- Chemical peels of glycolic acid and salicylic acid are applied to the skin to loosen blackheads and whiteheads. This removes superficial scars by peeling away damaged skin
- Subcision involves making small cuts under the skin to release scar tissue and help skin to resume normal contours and may cosmetically improve wide, indented scars
- A depressed acne scar is surgically removed and replaced with a patch of skin (punch skin graft) from elsewhere on the patient's body
- Soft tissue fillers. Small quantities of soft tissues (e.g., collagen, polymer implants, fat) are injected under the skin to elevate depressed scars to skin level
- Laser resurfacing. Short pulses of intense light are used to remove the outer, damaged layer of skin and tighten the middle layer, leaving skin smoother.

Physical Therapy Management

This involves application of UVR (Ultraviolet therapy) and advice on diet, hygiene and fitness.

Ultraviolet Radiations

These radiations are generally produced via a high-pressure air-cooled mercury vapor burner which is housed in a reflector which can be angled to obtain maximum absorption of UVR (having wavelength 190-390 nm). Patient is supported in a comfortable position (usually modified sitting) and the lamp is kept at distance usually kept at distance of 45 cm.

Dosage of UVR depends on the aim of the treatment.

To Improve Skin Health

First-degrec erythema (E1) is given 2-3 times a week for 3-4 weeks. It helps in increasing the arterial circulation and provides extra amino acids, oxygen and other nutritive substances to enable the synthesis of healthy skin. Given that epidermal cells pass from basal layer to the surface in 3 weeks. It is safe to give an El to the face, chest and upper back in the line treatment session.

To Promote Peeling

A second- or third-degree erythema (E2, E3) dose is given and repeated only when peeling has stopped. The theory is that affected skin is cleared more quickly and healthy skin will replace it.

The E2 or E3 dose will open up the pilosebaceous openings to promote the discharge of infected material.

It is not very pleasant to have a peeling face so an E2 is generally the maximal dose aimed for. An E3 may be tolerated on the chest or upper back but may be uncomfortable on face. An E2 can be tolerated to the face, upper back and chest but if all areas are red and sore at the same time the patient has difficulty lying down to sleep.

With UVR application the condition clears with this treatment in 6-8 weeks. If there is no improvement in 12 weeks it is probably wise to abandon treatment given because prolonged application of UVR may lead to danger of skin cancer and unlike the PUVA method there is no means of measuring the electromagnetic energy to which the patient has been exposed.

Advice on Diet and Fitness

Follow faithfully any instructions from the doctor or dietitian regarding lifestyle, drugs and diet.

Must participate in outdoor sport and shower scrupulously afterwards to remove sweat and dirt (which could have provided a medium for bacterial growth). Sufferer must wash the affected areas at least twice a day with oil-free soap and be sure to rinse well with cool water.

Prevention

- Washing problem areas with gentle cleansers. It is important to wash the face twice daily with a gentle cleanser. It is also important to remove all makeup from the skin. However, excessive washing and scrubbing can irritate the skin. People with acne are typically advised to avoid facial scrubs, astringents, masks and skin abrasion, as these may irritate the skin and cause or worsen acne.

- Shampooing hair frequently helps to remove the seepage of oil from hair which otherwise could have lead to acne formation around the hairline.
- Avoiding irritants. Oily or greasy substances (e.g., cosmetics, sunscreens, hair styling products, acne concealers) may contribute to the development or worsening of acne. Using water based, noncomedogenic (do not block pores), and oil free lotions may help to avoid this.
- Exercising caution around problem areas. This includes: Keeping hair off the face; avoiding the headphones and telephones to touch on the face; avoiding tight clothing and hats; shaving carefully as razors can irritate skin, and thus shaving should be done gently and done only when necessary.

PSORIASIS

Psoriasis is a common skin condition that causes skin redness and irritation. Most persons with psoriasis have thick, red skin with flaky, silver-white patches called scales.

Psoriasis is a common, chronic skin disorder that can affect any part of the body. It is characterized by raised, inflamed lesions that join together to form plaques (Fig. 4.2A) and patches (Fig. 4.2B) with distinct borders that are covered with flaky scales. It is not contagious, but is related to hereditary factors (Frank et al, 2009).

Incidence of Psoriasis

- Age—common age: 15-30 years
- Sex—both sexes equally affected (onset is typically earlier in women)
- Climate— damp and cold climate
- It also occurs earlier in patients with a family history of psoriasis.

Pathology of Psoriasis

The skin changes that characterize psoriasis are due to the rapid turnover of cells in the epidermis. Normal skin cells mature in about one month. In psoriasis, new cells are produced, grow to maturity and die quickly, severely reducing the cell cycle to about four days.

The skin changes that characterize psoriasis are due to the rapid turnover of cells in the epidermis. New cells are produced, grow to maturity and die too quickly, severely reducing the cell cycle.

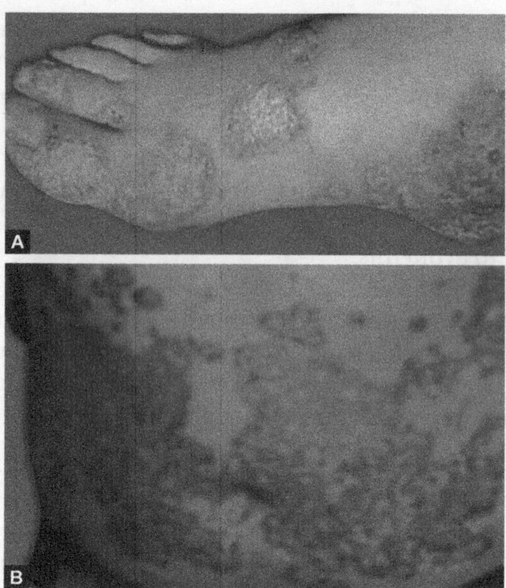

Figs 4.2A and B: (A) Clearly defined plaques on foot; (B) Red color patches on abdominal region (*For color version, see Plate 5*)

Although the cause of this is not known, it is believed to involve a faulty response of the immune system.

There is a genetic factor involved in the development of psoriasis. Because this is believed to be caused by a faulty immune system, psoriasis is considered an autoimmune disease (Fig. 4.3).

Presentation of Psoriasis

Psoriasis is highly variable and its presentation varies from person to person. For some it may not be more than a minor cosmetic problem while for others it may be quite severe, however most cases are mild to moderate. There may be many remissions and flares, but prolonged remissions are rare. In addition, the patient's quality of life may be affected due to cosmetic or associated infection factors.

Complication of Psoriasis

Most cases of psoriasis are not life-threatening, but severe cases may lead to secondary infections, some of which may become more serious as severe psoriasis may also lead to fluid loss and poor circulation

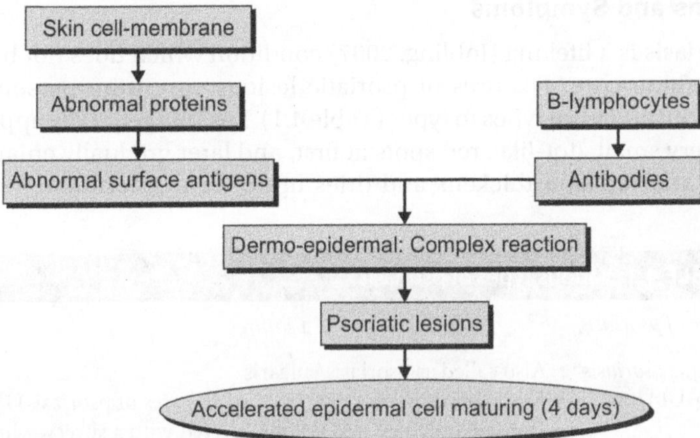

Fig. 4.3: Pathogenesis of psoriasis

(blood flow). In addition, patients undergoing treatments for severe psoriasis may experience adverse side effects from the drugs used.

Classification

The various types of psoriasis are briefed in (Table 4.1).

Risk Factors and Causes

The onset of psoriasis is believed to require a trigger. Triggers may also lead to flares and exacerbations. Common triggers include:

- Skin injury, including cuts, bites, bruises, burns, chafing or sunburns
- Emotional stress
- Viral or bacterial infection (e.g., thrush, HIV, strep throat)
- Certain drugs, including antimalarial drugs, beta blockers (used to treat high blood pressure), lithium, and the prolonged use of steroids (James et al, 2005)
- Climate, including lack of sunlight and dry weather conditions
- Obesity
- Hormonal factors, including hypocalcemia (not enough calcium in the blood) and those involved in pregnancy
- Alcohol and smoking.

Psoriasis triggers factors vary from patient to patient. What triggers psoriasis in one person may not cause symptoms in another.

Signs and Symptoms

Psoriasis is a lifelong (Jobling, 2007) condition which does not have a definite cure. Features of psoriatic lesions vary from person to person, and from types to types (Table 4.1). Lesions generally appear as very small, dot-like, red spots at first, and later gradually enlarge. The affected skin thickens and dries up to form cracks and crust.

TABLE 4.1 Various types of psoriasis

Type of psoriasis	*Features*
Plaque psoriasis (Fig 4.4A)	• Also called as psoriasis vulgaris • Most common psoriasis (80% of all cases of psoriasis) • Rraised, inflamed, red lesions covered with a silvery-white build-up of dead skin cells • Nails may also be affected and may become brittle and dry
Psoriatic arthritis	• Also called as psoriasis arthropica or psoriatic arthropathy • Resembles rheumatoid arthritis (RA) however is milder than RA • Frequently involves fingers and toes • Makes 30% of all incidences of psoriasis
Guttate psoriasis	• Small, distinct, generally widespread red lesions • Onset is most common in children, particularly after respiratory infections (e.g., strep throat)
Inverse psoriasis (Fig 4.4B)	• Also known as skin fold psoriasis, flexural psoriasis or genital psoriasis • Smooth, dry, red lesions form in the folds of skin, commonly in the arm pits, genital area and under the breasts
Pustular psoriasis	• Makes less than 5% of all incidences of psoriasis • Small, sterile pustules appear, dry up and form a scab blisters associated with this form of psoriasis are white and surrounded by red skin
Erythrodermic psoriasis	• Also known as psoriasis universalis • This particularly severe form of psoriasis, and is least common • Characterized by intense redness that covers all or most of the body surface • It often causes dangerously high temperatures and a greatly increased susceptibility to infection, generally requiring hospitalization
When injury to the skin leads to the development of psoriasis, it is referred to as Koebner phenomenon. This may result in any type of psoriasis.	

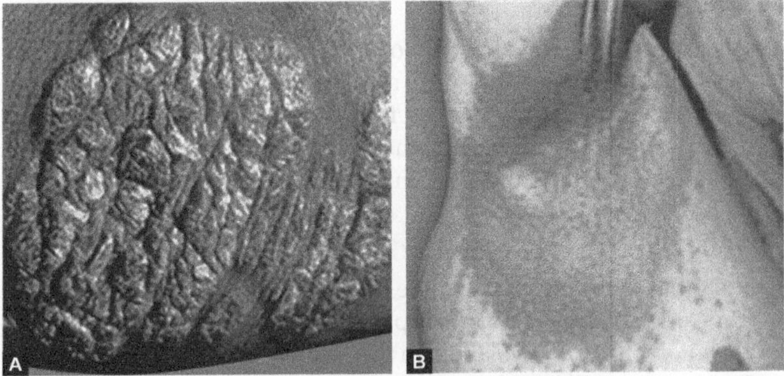

Figs 4.4A and B: (A) Plaque psoriasis; (B) Inverse psoriasis in axilla region (*For color version, see Plate 6*)

These raised patches are typically swollen (edema), red (erythema) and are often itchy. Lesions are typically covered with flaky, silvery, yellow-white scales.

The scales on the surface come off easily and are constantly shed. Those below the surface are more difficult to remove and, when removed, often leave tiny bleeding points (Auspitz's sign). The skin beneath is generally very red and may be tender and painful. Lesions vary in size and shape, but the borders are distinct. There is usually only one or a few patches, but they may cover large areas of skin and merge into each other. The lesions may impair the body movement and flexibility and can be disabling when they appear in certain areas (e.g., palms, soles). The itching associated with severe cases can also disrupt a person's ability to sleep at night (Smitha et al, 2010).

Complications associated with psoriasis:

- Nails often become pitted and discolored. The base of nail gets lifted up at nail bed (onycholysis) and thickening of the nail (nail dystrophy) may also occur.
- Unaffected skin may become thin and easily torn.
- Eyes may have burning sensations, itching or have discharge. Inflammation of the eyelids (blepharitis) or inner eye lining (conjunctivitis) may occur.
- When arthritis is associated with psoriasis, joint involvement occurs after skin lesions are already apparent.

Diagnosis

Psoriasis is diagnosed through observation of the lesions during a physical examination. There are no associated blood tests, although X-rays (images of a body part on film paper or fluorescent screens) may be used to look for early signs of arthritis (joint inflammation). If a diagnosis is not definite, it can be confirmed with a skin biopsy.

Treatment

Factors that determine the course of treatment to be used include:
- Type and severity of psoriasis present
- Location and size of lesions on the body
- Patient's overall health, age and medical history
- Patient's tolerance of specific medication, procedures or therapies
- Patient and physician's opinion or preference.

Treatment of psoriasis may be general, topical, systemic and by physical therapy management.

General Treatment

Since psoriasis has no definite treatment, the reassurance, relaxation and the lifestyle modification is important. The management of psoriasis aims to improve the skin condition and its appearance; reduce inflammation; slow down cellular growth rate. Treatment choice depends on the type, severity, location and the duration of psoriasis. The treatment also varies from person to person and time to time. Few patients may require lifelong therapy.

Topical Treatment

Soften and remove scales
- Relieve pruritus (itch)
- Reduce pain and discomfort
- Slow down rapid cell proliferation.

Topical medications may be used to treat mild to moderate psoriasis. They may be used alone, in combination, or with exposure to ultraviolet light.

Medication choice for topical management of psoriasis:
- Emollients (moisturizers) to restore moisture and flexibility to affected skin and may reduce itching, scaling and inflammation. Increased use may be necessary in dry climates or during winter.

- Coal tar preparations—these may be applied directly to the lesion, added in bath water as a soak, or used in combination with ultraviolet B (UVB) light.
- Corticosteroids—these are the most commonly prescribed medications for psoriasis and recommended during mild to moderate form. Are not recommended in severe psoriasis. Because prolonged use can cause rebound psoriasis, which could be more worse than the original condition.
- Anthralin—reduces increase in skin cells and inflammation.
- Topical steroids, vitamin D_3 derivatives, retinoids (Lorette and Fontès, 2004).

Physiotherapy Management

Phototherapy is often used in the treatment of moderate to severe psoriasis. Natural sunlight or ultraviolet light exposure may help reduce lesions, although care must be taken not to burn. Sunburn can make psoriasis worse.

Methods of delivering ultraviolet light include:
- *Psoralen ultraviolet A radiation (PUVA)*: Psoralen is a medication usually applied topically before exposure to ultraviolet A light. This treatment is give by using Theraktin tunnel having 4 fluroscent tubes. Suberythemal dose are given twice/thrice a week.
- *Narrowband UVB (NB-UVB)*: Intense ultraviolet B light may also reduce lesions. Advantages over PUVA include shorter treatment times and no need for medications. However, it is not widely available (Walters, 1999).

Prevention

Patients with psoriasis can help prevent flares by identifying and avoiding triggers that cause or worsen psoriasis. Following points may be considered to avoid the flaring of psoriasis:-
- Live a healthy lifestyle
- Balanced diet
- Drink plenty of water (at least 8-ounce glasses a day) and get an adequate amount of sleep
- Quit smoking
- Drink in moderation. Patients should limit their consumption of alcohol. Those taking methotrexate should not consume alcohol at all, due to the risk for side effects

- Reduce stress
- Stress management techniques such as yoga, meditation and exercise
- Moisturizers help to relieve dry skin and prevent cracking
- Avoid scratching or picking at lesions to avoid the secondary infections
- Avoid hot water
- Avoid harsh, drying soaps. Non-deodorant and fragrance-free soaps are best
- Avoid rubbing the skin with a towel following a shower or bath. Gently patting the skin dry with a towel will help avoid irritation
- Avoid fabric clothing as they do not allow sweat to escape and aggravate condition. Cotton is the best choice for clothing
- Use of humidifier during a dry day is helpful to maintain moisture in the air.

ALOPECIA AREATA

Alopecia is very common non-contagious autoimmune disease that causes hair loss. It may cause patchy baldness and occur most commonly on scalp (Fig. 4.5). It may occur both in men and women, though it is more common in men (Fabiane and Bergfeld, 2003). Alopecia usually is not painful or life-threatening and patients are often generally healthy otherwise.

Alopecia areata involves patchy loss of hair. The cause of alopecia areata is unknown. It typically occurs first in childhood, and appears as one or more round bald patches on the scalp approximately the size of a quarter. The patches typically occur suddenly. Most of the alopecia are noncicatricial, means that they are reversible (Fabiane and Bergfeld, 2003).

Types of Alopecia

- Alopecia areata—loss of scalp hair in patches. This is most common form. It is in its mild form (<50% hair loss) or extensive form (>50% hair loss). Treatment is more effective in milder form.
- Alopecia totalis—loss of all scalp hair and eyebrows.
- Alopecia universalis—total loss of body hair (including head, face and body). It is rare form.

In few cases pits/dents may develop in fingernails as a result of the disease.

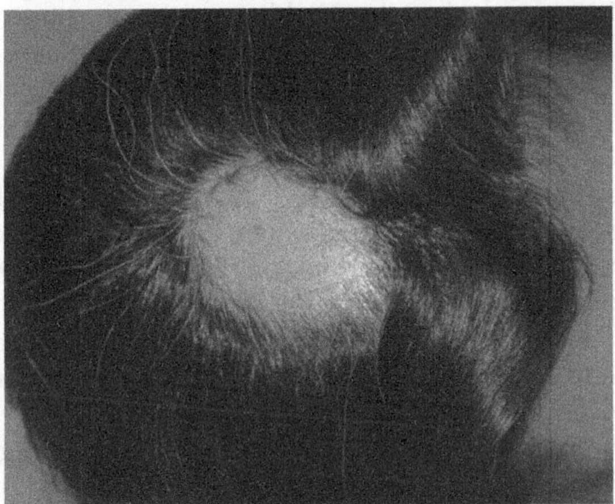

Fig. 4.5: Alopecia areata (*For color version, see Plate 6*)

Hair loss results when more hairs are being shed than regrowth. During the normal cycle of hair growth, approximately 90 percent of the hair on a person's scalp is growing at any one time. This growth (anagen) phase may last several years, with each hair growing about one centimeter per month during this time. When hair stops growing, it enters a resting (telogen) phase of three to four months. Hair is released from the hair shaft and shed from the scalp, initiating the next cycle of growth. Each day about 75 hairs are lost from a healthy person's head and these are replaced by new hair formation.

Risk Factors and Causes

Exactly why alopecia areata occurs is unknown.

- Some sort of biological (e.g., virus) or emotional trigger (e.g., stress) initiates alopecia areata in people genetically predisposed to the disease
- Family history of alopecia
- General anxiety
- Fatigue
- Poor health
- Heredity (universalis is often congenital)
- People with asthma, thyroid disease or certain allergic conditions (e.g., atopic eczema, hay fever)
- Family history of these conditions or other autoimmune diseases (e.g., diabetes, rheumatoid arthritis, vitiligo)

Alopecia areata (patchy baldness) is a noncontagious, autoimmune disease in which white blood cells release chemical messengers known as cytokines to attack healthy cells located in hair follicles. This shrinks the follicle to a point where hair production is considerably reduced. However, new follicle cells being produced naturally by the body are not affected, making hair regrowth possible in all cases. The deep sited inflammation process around the hair follicle is responsible for this condition (Shapiro and Price, 1998).

Children with the disease do not usually have a parent with the condition. It is generally believed that several genes cause alopecia areata. This makes it unlikely that a child born to one or both parents with alopecia areata would inherit all of the necessary genes to develop the disease. In addition, twins with identical genes that cause alopecia areata often do not develop the disease in unison, suggesting other factors besides genetics may play a role in how the disease is triggered.

Signs and Symptoms

Signs and symptoms of alopecia areata may vary depending on the individual, and include:

- Clumps of hair come away in the comb
- Onset is usually insidious
- Hair loss confined solely to the scalp
- Hair loss on the face and body
- Hairs tapered near the scalp (exclamation point hairs)
- The patient can be very distressed, especially when new patches appear as others are recovering
- Bald patches appear in which the skin is very white.

Diagnosis

Diagnosis of alopecia areata is done by a physician on the basis of medical history and physical examination of patch, inspecting the scalp and hair loss pattern. This is sufficient to diagnose and differentiate alopecia areata or a similar disorder (e.g., male pattern baldness, androgenetic alopecia).

Biopsy of hair and scalp samples are studied by biopsy and laboratory analysis if physical assessment fails to detect the diagnosis. Blood tests investigations are used to detect other medical conditions that could hair loss (e.g., hyperthyroidism).

Treatment and Prevention

Treatment of disease focuses on reducing its emotional impact. There is no sureshot cure of this condition. Hair regrowth is always possible for patients, regardless of the severity of hair loss, because follicle production is not affected. Thus, medication is not used to prevent formation of new bald patches but may be useful in regrowing hair. Following are medications prescribed for this purpose:-

- Corticosteroids—it suppresses the immune system and may be given to treat alopecia areata
- Topical immunotherapy—it is effective in faster regrowth of hair, but has chances of frequent hair loss relapse, and episodes of rashes, lymph node swellings
- Minoxidil is also effective in regrowing the lost hair in patients with alopecia areata
- Finasteride—it slows hair loss by inhibiting the conversion of testosterone into dihydrotestosterone (DHT), a hormone that is responsible for causing shrinkage of hair follicles
- Photochemotherapy—drugs, which increase the skin's sensitivity to ultraviolet radiation are given and this is followed by exposure to light.

Physiotherapy Management

The aim of Physiotherapy is to improve general health as well as to improve nutrition to hair follicles.

UVR (Theraktin) may be given as a general body treatment. E1 or Suberythema dosage is given daily for 6-7 treatments.

To improve nutrition UVR (Kromayer) may be given to individual patches with E2 or E3 dosages. Two or three patches may be treated in one session and the patient may attend one or two times a week.

If there is no sign of recovery after 2-3 months then treatment should be stopped and the condition reviewed after 2-3 months. As soon as hair starts to grow in a patch UVR must be stopped to that area.

LEUCODERMA (VITILIGO)

Leucoderma is commonly known as "Vitiligo".

Vitiligo is an acquired skin disorder characterized by depigmented skin patches (called macules) on skin, mucous membrane and hair. It is not a serious medical problem and does not spread from the

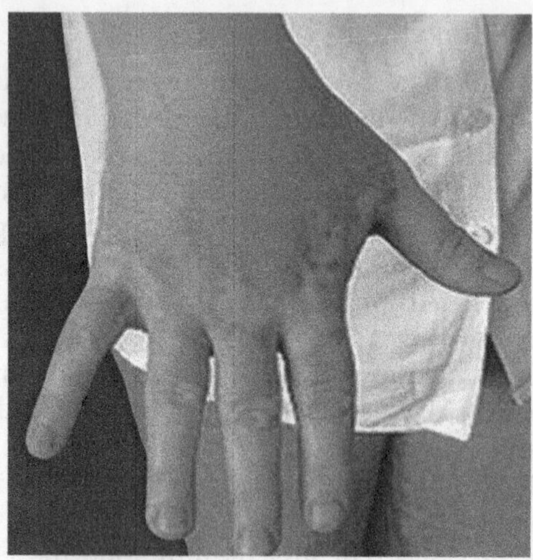

Fig. 4.6: White/light colored skin patch on hand
(*For color version, see Plate 7*)

patients to others. The depigmentation of skin due to malfunctioning or absence of melanocytes (Fig. 4.6).

The onset is in form of appearance of few small white spots, which may progress gradually or rapidly in size and the area. The faster growth of these patches occurs during stress and illness. Depigmentation may progress to involve entire body or in rare cases the skin color may return spontaneously to normal.

Vitiligo is a relatively common disorder which may affect men and women of all races equally. Onset may occur at any age, however onset after the age of 40 is very rare.

The patches of vitiligo may occur on both sides of body (vitilage vulgaris) or on one side of body (segmental vitiligo).

Classification

Vitiligo Vulgaris: This is a common form where depigmented patches occur, scattered, widely distributed, equally on both sides of the body. The vitiligo universlis involve depigmentation of the skin all over the body.

Patches of vitiligo may occur localized on one single area (focal), segmental (one or more patch on one side of body), or mucosal (involve mucosal membrane).

Universal is the complete or nearly complete depigmentation of the skin over the entire body. This type of vitiligo is the rarest.

Risk Factors and Causes

The cause of vitiligo is malfunctioning of melanocytes which could be due to stresses, emotional injury or many other factors, but the exact cause is yet to be identified.

The reason melanocytes disappear or cease functioning is not known, but there are many theories, including:

- Genetics and family history may or may not be present.
- Autoimmune disease may lead to formation of autoantibodies that damage melanocytes, causing the skin to depigment.
- Chemical exposure to phenol also causes skin to lose pigmentation.

Signs and Symptoms

Vitiligo is characterized by hypopigmented or depigmented flat patches of varying size and discrete margins and round, oval or linear shape. The margins are distinct but irregular. Size of macules may vary from very tiny to large portions of the body. Some patches may have hyperpigmentation at the edges (Huggins et al, 2005). The areas most commonly affected include face, hand, groin, mouth, bony prominences. In scalp the macule also involves the patch of hair loss.

Vitiligo patients are otherwise good healthy persons. The other autoimmune conditions which occur with vitiligo are alopecia areata, pernicious anemia, uveitis, diabetes mellitus.

Vitiligo is commonly regarded as a harmless cosmetic skin problem in Western societies, and the importance of treating patients with vitiligo is often underestimated. Generalized vitiligo is a serious skin disorder with an adverse impact on the emotional state, comparable with that of other major skin diseases (May et al, 2009).

Diagnosis

The diagnosis of vitiligo involves a physician taking a medical history, family history, recent stress or illness, depigmentation of hair before macule appearance, any other autoimmune disease, and photosensitivity.

Physical examination includes examination under visible and ultraviolet light. Normal visible light shows white patches, while the examination under Wood's lamp which uses ultraviolet a light reveals characteristic yellow-green or blue fluorescence of true vitiligo patches.

Skin biopsy of a depigmented macule shows absence of pigment present within the melanocytes (pigment producing cells).

Treatment and Prevention

Because the process and cause of vitiligo is unknown, there is no known way to prevent the condition. The treatment is not possible in definite way but this may be controlled to certain extent. The treatment primarily focuses to repigment the skin and control the depigmentation process.

There are many ways to hide the depigmented patches (vitiligo macules), including:

- Cosmetics such as sun protection factors (SPF)
- Tattooing (micropigmentation) of the depigmented patch, however the color frequently may fade over the years
- Self tanning lotions which tan the patch may hide vitiligo macules.

Corticosteroids on topical application are often used early in the treatment of vitiligo. Topical corticosteroids (e.g., hydrocortisone cream) are used most commonly. These seem to help stabilize the progression of depigmentation and may encourage repigmentation in small, localized areas. These are the simplest and safest actual treatment, though not the most effective (Kwinter et al, 2007).

Topical corticosteroids may be used with other treatments, but may thin the skin or cause dilation of blood vessels. They are not recommended for use on the face. In rare cases, oral corticosteroids may be used to stabilize depigmentation and induce repigmentation. However, these have significant potentials for serious side effects (e.g., loss of bone density), especially long-term use, and use in vitiligo treatment remains controversial.

Immunomodulators (drugs that suppress the immune system) have also been successfully used in very localized areas of vitiligo.

Phototherapy Treatment

- Psoralen and long-wave ultraviolet radiation (PUVA). The most common form used for vitiligo. It involves the medication psoralen followed by timed exposure to controlled ultraviolet A light. Psoralen makes the skin very sensitive to light and helps to stimulate melanocytes to divide and fill in areas where pigment was lost. It is usually taken in an oral form, but may be applied topically. However, special care must be taken to avoid severe sun damage with topical applications. Skin cancer is also a potential side effect of PUVA (Gawkrodger DJ, 2008).

- According to the American Osteopathic College of Dermatology (AOCD), PUVA is partially successful in over 50 percent of cases, but total repigmentation occurs in only 15 to 20 percent. The treatment is least likely to work on the hands and feet. Older people and individuals with pigment loss for more than five years are also poor candidates.
- Narrowband UVB (NB-UVB). Controlled treatment with intense ultraviolet B light is used to induce repigmentation. Advantages over PUVA include shorter treatment times and no need for medications. NB-UVB (Gawkrodger DJ, 2008) can be used in children, pregnant or breastfeeding women and people with kidney or liver dysfunction. However, it is not widely available.
- Focused microphototherapy. Ultraviolet B light is shone through a dark pad with tiny holes that is applied to the skin. This can be used to irradiate only the affected skin and results are typically good, but it requires expensive equipment and trained personnel, and is not widely available.

Certain areas have a poorer prognosis in terms of repigmentation. These areas include the lips, fingertips, toes and genitals.

When depigmented macules cover more than half of the body, patients and physicians may chose to depigment the remaining skin. A bleaching agent (e.g., monobenzone) is applied to the normal skin to match it with the depigmented skin. However, the patient's appearance is significantly altered and the skin is made much more sensitive to sun damage. Many patients are allergic to the bleaching agents, so tests must be performed before widespread application. Side effects include contact dermatitis.

Vitiligo macules may occasionally be treated by transplanting (grafting) the patient's own tissue when other treatments fail. This is typically only done on patients with small patches of stable vitiligo. Patients must have a positive minigrafting test, no tendency to scar and be over the age of 12 years.

Vitiligo macules are highly susceptible to sun damage and must be protected. Patients are recommended to wear sunscreens with a sun protection factor (SPF) of at least 30 over all exposed macules, wear protective clothing and avoid the sun during peak hours (10 a.m. to 4 p.m.).

Patients with widespread vitiligo may suffer from depression (Mechri et al, 2006), embarrassment or other emotional distress. These individuals may benefit from including psychological counseling and/or support groups as part of their treatment.

Precautions

- Do not take psoralen empty stomach
- Use protective glasses
- Avoid direct sunlight
- Do not use ointments
- Do not become pregnant or Father of a child.

LEPROSY

Leprosy is a chronic, infectious disease characterized by dermal changes and nerve damage. It is deforming, disabling and stigmatizing condition but not to be fatal. The disease primarily affects the peripheral nerves, eyes and mucous membranes of the nose (So called the cooler regions of the body because its causative organism needs cooler environment, approximately 35°C for its growth). Its incubation period is very long.

In earlier period it was thought to be highly infectious disease and the people infected with the disease were quarantined to isolated leper colonies.

Leprosy occurs very rarely. It is most often seen in tropical and subtropical regions today. This is more prevalent in the areas of poor hygiene. The disease is most common in Brazil, India, Indonesia, Madagascar, Mozambique, Myanmar, Nepal and Nigeria.

Complications of leprosy include sensory loss, ulcer and skin damage, bacterial skin infections, and amputation of fingers and toes due to damage caused by the lack of sensation.

Classification

The form of leprosy a person develops depends on his or her immune response to the infection. In most cases, people are already immune to Mycobacterium leprae and never develop signs or symptoms of leprosy. The disease develops in people whose immune response is less effective. Its progression and the resolution also depend on the individual's immunity.

There are three common forms of leprosy. These are:

1. *Lepromatous leprosy (multibacillary leprosy).* Occurs in immune-deficient patients. This is characterized by multiple skin lesions and the symmetrical (occurs on both sides of the body equally) involvement of the peripheral nerves. Due to the nerve involvement the motor and sensory symptoms appear which involve loss of sensation, muscle weakness and paralysis. This is the most infective form of leprosy.
2. *Tuberculoid leprosy (paucibacillary leprosy).* Occurs in patients with normal immune function. This form is characterized by lesser number of lesions which are asymmetrically affecting the body. Sensory and motor involvement may occur. Skin lesions are few or absent.
3. *Borderline leprosy (dimorphous leprosy)* is the intermediated form. The presenting features may resemble either of the commoner form. It may transform to either of the two depending on the immunity of the body.

Risk Factors and Causes

Leprosy is caused by the bacteria Mycobacterium leprae. The mode of spread is droplet infection via nasal mucosa or via open skin. Most people are not prone to the infection by this bacteria, and short-term exposure will not cause infection. The lesion may develop after years and lead to patch formation. People susceptible to leprosy often have close, long-term contact with an infected person (e.g., a family member). An impaired immune system (or one that is not resistant to the Mycobacterium leprae bacteria) may also be a risk factor.

Signs and Symptoms

It has long incubation period and disease goes unnoticed for many years before the symptoms start appearing.

It primarily affects the cooler areas of the body (peripheral nerves, mucous membranes in the nose).

Skin lesions may be reddened or hypopigmented. Lesions lack the sensations and may lead to trauma due to hot or sharp objects. These lack the healing tendency and may develop into sores.

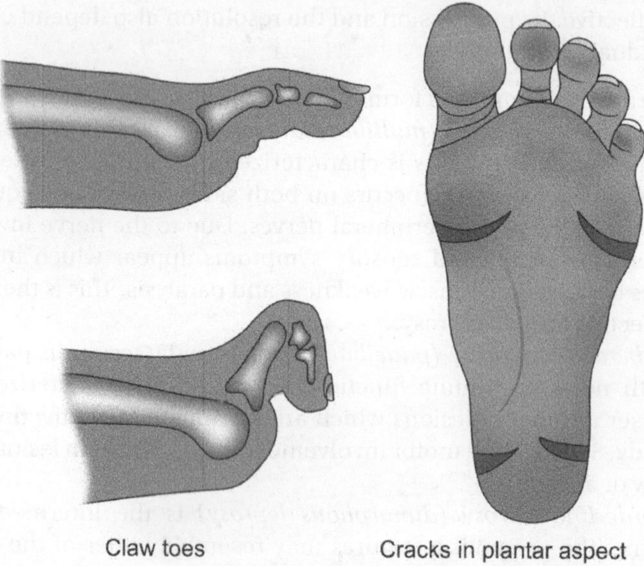

Fig. 4.7: Deformities in leprosy

Numbness may be the first symptom to develop. In fact, numbness may develop years before skin lesions occur. In some cases, the nerves may be enlarged or painful. Due to the motor weakness or paralysis the numerous deformities (Fig. 4.7) may occur such as claw hand, foot drop, claw toes, ptosis (drooping of the upper eyelid) and lagophthalmos (inability to close the eye). In dry foot, cracks of the hard skin are commonly seen. These cracks are very painful and in numb foot, they may get too deep and form ulcer by getting infection.

The thickened nasal mucosa causes recurrent nasal infection or snuff nose. In some cases collapse of the nose may occur. Eye tissues may become inflamed and laryngeal (voice box) involvement may lead to hoarseness.

The lack of sensation in the lower extremity may lead to plantar ulcers in weight bearing area of foot. Most of these ulcers (up to 75%) occur in forefoot and remaining (25%) occur in mid and hind foot. (Fig. 4.8).

The different forms of leprosy have specific signs and symptoms (Table 4.2). These include:

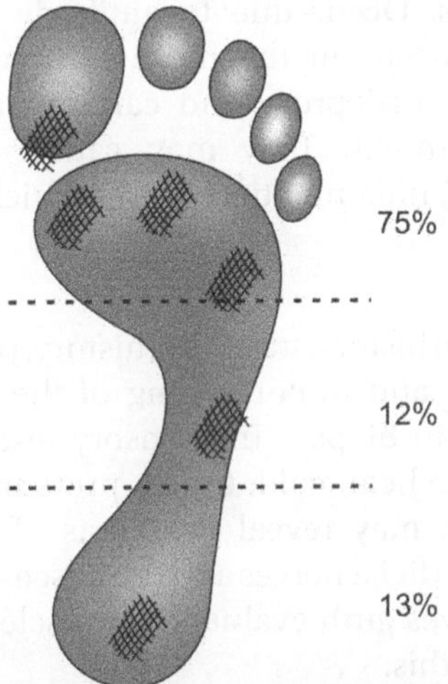

Fig. 4.8: The distribution of plantar ulcers in leprosy

TABLE 4.2 Types of leprosy

Type of lepsory	*Symptoms*
Lepromatous	• Poorly-defined macules, papules, nodules and plaques (raised patches) common on the face, buttocks and lower extremities • No sensory impairment • Eyebrows may be lost
Tuberculoid	• Few (less than five) or no skin lesions form • Slightly raised plaques that are localized, asymmetrical and well-defined, with sharp borders • Lesions may also become dry and hairless • Sensation is completely absent
Borderline	• Features are between lepromatous and tuberuloid forms
Indeterminate	• Few hypopigmented patches with partial sensory loss

Leprosy is slowly progressive and may have period of remission (called reactions) which may cause tissues to become inflamed (red, swollen and hot). There are two general types of reaction, including:

- Type 1 (reversal) reactions. These may cause neuritis (inflammation of a nerve), increased inflammation in established lesions, acute nerve pain or tenderness, loss of nerve function and the formation of new lesions.

- Type 2 reactions. Occur due to antibody activity against the bacteria. These occur in the more extreme lepromatous and borderline forms of leprosy and can occur while a patient is undergoing treatment. They may cause: vasculitis, myalgia, malaise, swelling, inflammation of eye/testicles or skin tissue.

Diagnosis

Diagnosis is based on history, travelling history, physical examination of patches, sensory and motor testing of the region supplied by suspected nerve, skin biopsy. The sensory testing involves checks the sensation for the heat, cold, touch, pressure and the pain. The palpation of nerves may reveal the areas of muscle thickening, enlargement of superficial nerves and the abscess accumulation. The motor testing involves girth evaluation, muscle strength, weakness or deformity due to this.

Samples of skin for examination are typically taken from within a lesion. Smears may be taken from lesions on the ears, elbows or knees. A mucous sample from inside the nose may also be taken. Laboratory examination of these samples may detect the presence of the bacteria that cause the disease or other characteristic changes. In most cases, multiple samples from many different lesions will be needed.

Conditions that may be mistaken for leprosy include:

- *Psoriasis*: A skin disease characterized by red patches covered in silvery scales. Some lesions of psoriasis may resemble those of leprosy.
- *Sarcoidosis*: A rare disease characterized by protein deposition in various body tissues. Skin involvement may resemble leprosy.
- *Cutaneous T-cell lymphoma*: Cancer of certain cells in the skin. Lesions may resemble those characteristic of leprosy.

Treatment and Prevention

Leprosy was thought for many years to be incurable, but this is no longer the case. Patients are now considered cured after completing the treatment regimen. Furthermore, after treatment has begun, the patient is no longer infectious to others.

Early diagnosis and treatment is important. Left untreated, the disease can cause significant damage to the skin, nerves, limbs and eyes. Neurological (nerve) damage may be difficult to repair, although physical therapy may help. In some cases, surgery may be required to restore nerve function. In cases of very deep ulcers if the infection reaches up to bones, it may lead to osteomyelitis and may necessitate the amputations (Fig. 4.9) to prevent the spread of infection to other regions of the body.

Though skin lesions typically clear up within a year of therapy, reconstructive surgery may be required for advanced cases where deformity occurs. The management of the disease is complex and may require expert consultation. There are several centers for the care and treatment of the disease located throughout the United States.

Leprosy is treated with multiple medications. The primary drugs used are antibiotics (e.g., dapsone, rifampin, clofazimine). A combination of two or more antibiotics may be recommended. These and most other drugs used in therapy may pose some risks to the fetus in pregnancy but are generally considered safe. Active treatment may last from six months to two years. The patient is closely observed for up to five years after treatment ends. Typically, there are few relapses.

Reactions are treated when they arise. Type 1 (reversal) reactions are treated with oral corticosteroids. Type 2 reactions are treated with corticosteroids and, at times, thalidomide. This drug is not safe for use in women who are or may become pregnant.

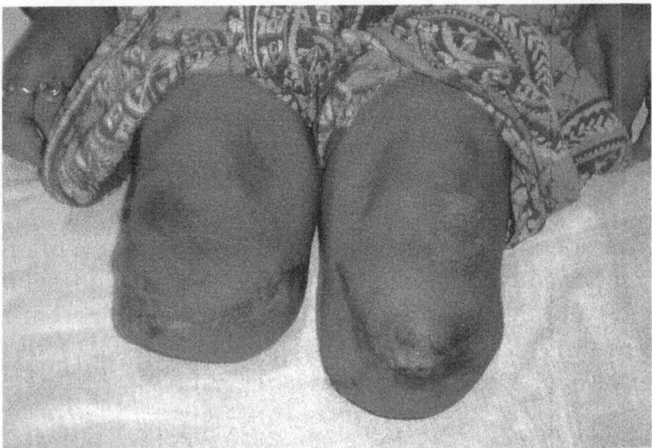

Fig. 4.9: Bolow knee amputation secondary to leprosy
(*For color version, see Plate 7*)

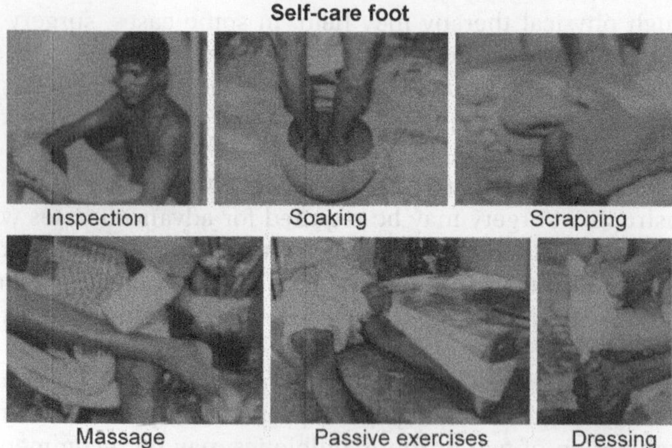

Fig. 4.10: The physiotherapy management of the leprosy

Preventing the spread of leprosy involves early diagnosis and treatment of those who are infected. Family members and others who have had close, long-term contact with a leprosy patient should have annual examinations for five or more years after last contact with the infected person.

The aims of the physiotherapy management of the leprosy (Fig. 4.10) involves:

- Prevention of muscle paralysis: The maintenance of the muscle strength
- Prevention of joint deformity: The proper splinting, positioning of the joint, prevention of the muscle imbalance
- Prevention of ulcer formation: Regular inspection of skin, SSO (scrapping, soaking and oiling); avoid prolonged walking and standing, avoid growth of the skin cracks and erosion
- The pre-operative management of the patient: Prevention of the joint contracture; strengthening of the to be transferred muscle; improve the flexibility of muscle; the passive range of motion exercises.
- The post-operative management of the patient.

Treatment of ulcers:

- Dressing: To keep ulcer clean, protect from dirt and flies and to absorb discharge from ulcer

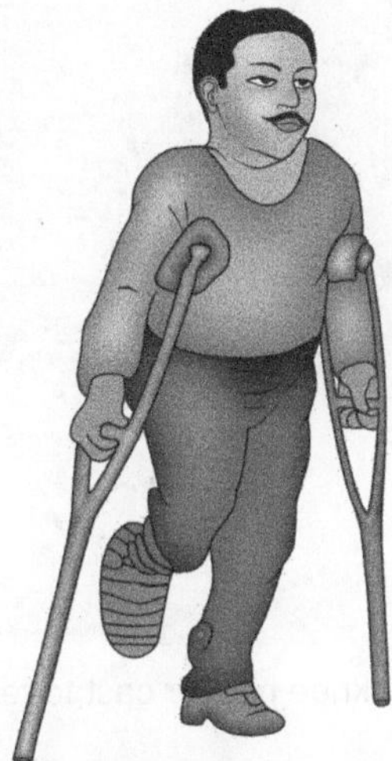

Fig. 4.11: Use of crutch to relieve pressure on ulcer

- Rest: Rest is important to relieve the pressure on ulcer, alternative mean of rest may be the use of crutch (Fig. 4.11)
- Plaster boot
- Blow-knee POP with walking iron (Fig. 4.12)
- Aids/appliances
- Surgery.

Management of Foot Drop

The involvement of the common peroneal nerve leads to foot drop where the patient can not clear the foot from the ground during stance phase of gait. This can lead to the formation of ulcer of forefoot, plantar flexion contracture or the unstable joints of foot. The management of this involves the use of specialized foot supporting orthosis with a special spring (Fig. 4.13) and leg band attached to pull the forefoot from dropping down.

Surgical Management

In cases of deep ulcers, full thickness involvement, and the irreversible muscle paralysis the reconstructive surgical procedures are used. The common used reconstructive procedures involve the skin grafting to cover the ulcers, tendon transfers to improve

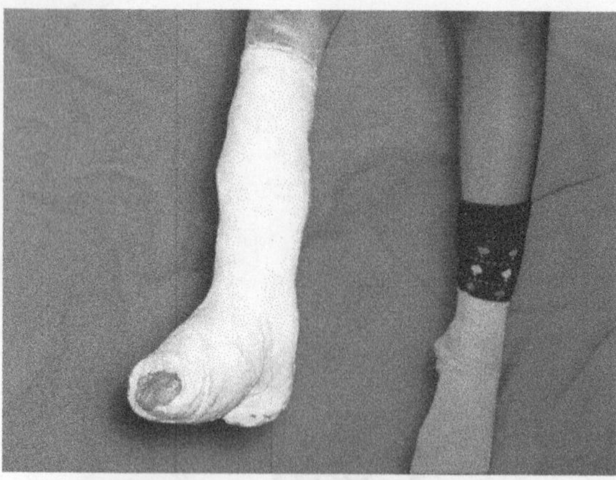

Fig. 4.12: Use of below-knee plaster cast to relieve pressure on ulcer

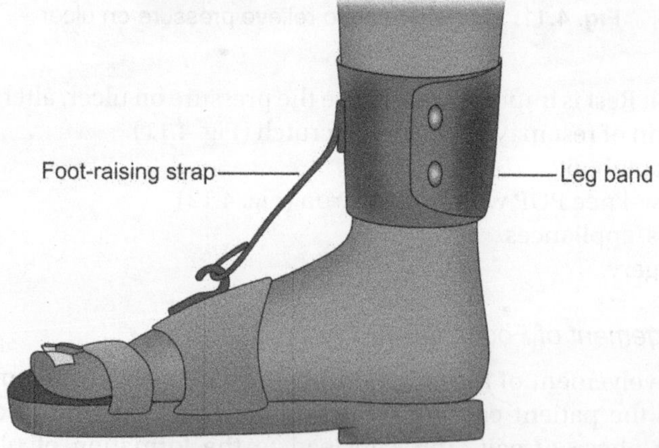

Fig. 4.13: The foot supporting orthosis with attached spring and leg band to prevent the dropping of forefoot

the muscle strength, the ulcer reconstruction to improve cosmetic appearance.

Preventive Education to Patient Regarding Sensory Loss

- Patient to wear shoes instead of slipper, as it provides better protection from some sharp/hot object
- Reduce walking and standing for prolonged time at stretch as it can lead to the damage of skin due to sustained pressure

- Daily foot inspection—to avoid any new formation of any corn, blister or cracks
- Keep the skin clean and soft—to avoid any infective organism from invading in to the wounds/cracks
- Avoid sitting cross legged
- Avoid cracks, corns and blisters—as they can always progress into more deeper lesions, and complete skin thickness involvement.

SEXUALLY TRANSMITTED DISEASES

Sexually transmitted diseases (STDs) are among the most common infectious diseases in the United States. STDs spread through sexual activities which may include vaginal intercourse, anal intercourse, oral sex (mouth-to-genital contact) or any other form of intimate contact involving genitals. The other modes of spread are sharing sexual devices that are not washed or not covered with a barrier like condom. In some cases, certain STDs (e.g., pubic lice, scabies) are also spread through contact with an infected person's clothes, towels or linens. Although it is uncommon, some STDs (e.g., genital herpes) have also been spread through contact with toilet seats and hot tubs.

The common sources of the infection include body fluids, include semen, vaginal fluids and blood of the infected person. These can enter the body through tiny cuts or tears in the mouth, anus or genitals. STDs that are spread through blood, such as human immunodeficiency virus (HIV) and hepatitis or by sharing the needles used for taking intravenous drugs.

STD is one of the fastest growing diseases, yet they mostly stay unnoticed in early stages.

Anyone involved in sexual activity is at risk of contracting an STD. The indulgence in multiple sex partner and unprotected sex further increases its risk. This includes sexual activity between a man and woman or between people of the same gender. This can occur at any age and in age gender yet young people (of age between 15-24 years) are particularly affected. The transmission is more common from men to women due to the larger surface area of vagina and its ability to act as reservoir of the infectious fluid.

Complications of STD may involve the foul smelling infectious discharge, sore and ulcers, the massive sepsis in body, liver failure or death. Also the risk of other infections is also increased. Complications are more in women and further it can transmit to the infant during or before birth as the STD can cross placenta.

Classification

Sexually transmitted diseases (STDs) are caused by three types of organisms. These organisms include:

- *Parasites*: These are very small organisms that get nourishment from the infecting host. Examples of sexually transmitted parasites include: Pubic lice, trichomoniasis, scabies.
- *Viruses*: These complex molecules invade the cells of their host, where they are capable of growing and multiplying. Viral STDs are commonly transmitted during sexual activity, including vaginal intercourse, anal intercourse and oral sex (mouth-to-genital contact). Include HIV (Human immune deficiency virus), genital herpes virus, hepatitis virus, human papillomavirus.
- *Bacteria*: These single-celled organisms cling together in colonies to feed from the body of their host. They are commonly transmitted through sexual activity, including vaginal intercourse, anal intercourse and oral sex. Many sexually transmitted bacterial infections also increase the risk of HIV transmission. Examples of sexually transmitted bacterial infections include: Chlamydia, gonorrhea, chancroid and syphilis.

Risk Factors and Causes

Any person participating in sexual activity is at risk of becoming infected with a sexually transmitted disease (STD). However, there are certain factors that increase this risk including:

- Participating in unprotected vaginal intercourse, anal intercourse or oral sex (mouth-to-genital contact)
- Having multiple sexual partners. The more sexual partners a person has, the greater their risk of being exposed to an STD. Having multiple partners also makes it less likely that a person knows about each partner's sexual history and drug habits
- Having a sexual partner with a history of many sexual partners
- Not knowing the sexual history of all sexual partners
- Illegal intravenous drug use. HIV/AIDS and some other STDS can be transmitted by sharing needles.

Signs and Symptoms

Common signs and symptoms of sexually transmitted diseases (STDs) include: pain in the pelvic region, pain during urination or defecation, whitish abnormal discharge from vagina or penis, pain in pelvic area during intercourse, burning sensation during urination or intercourse. In more advance cases the sore and blister can appear in genital or anal area.

Other possible signs and symptoms of STDs include:

- Pain in the anus (in people who engage in anal intercourse)
- Sore throat [in people who engage in oral sex (mouth-to-genital contact)]
- Scaly rash on the palms of the hands and soles of the feet (e.g., syphilis)
- Dark-colored urine or loose, light-colored stool
- Yellow eyes and skin (jaundice)
- Swollen lymph nodes
- Fever with body aches or night sweats
- Unusual infections
- Unexplained fatigue (extreme tiredness) or weight loss.

Early detection of the symptoms and signs can help in the prevention of its progression. Some of the common signs and symptoms of STDs mimic those caused by urinary tract infections (UTI) and genital infections.

Although the recognition of symptoms allows a disease to be diagnosed earlier, many STDs have no symptoms or have symptoms that are not easily recognizable. The lack of symptoms is especially common in women.

All sexually active people are encouraged to have regular medical checkups and STD screening tests. The earlier an STD is diagnosed, the earlier treatment for the disease can begin. Early treatment is important because STDs may cause serious complications if left untreated.

Diagnosis

Sexually transmitted diseases (STDs) may be diagnosed before symptoms develop during routine medical checkups or when the patient requests testing. To diagnose an STD, the history and the detailed history of the intercourse is important. The physical examination of the genitals is also important. If sores or discharge are present, the physician may use a swab to collect samples for examination. The samples will then be tested for the presence of various microorganisms. The swabs may be collected from vagina, cervix.

After an STD is diagnosed, the patient should inform present and past sexual partner(s) about the diagnosis. This is necessary because all sexual partners will require testing and treatment.

Treatment

The method used to treat a sexually transmitted disease (STD) depends on the cause of the disease. STDs caused by bacteria, such as chlamydia, syphilis and gonorrhea, are usually treated with antibiotics. STDs caused by parasites are also treated with medications or over-the-counter drugs. Current medications allow for most STDs caused by bacteria and parasites to be cured when treated early.

STDs caused by viruses, such as HIV/AIDS, genital herpes and human papillomavirus (HPV), are treated differently then those caused by bacteria or parasites because usually they cannot be cured. Instead, medical treatment is used to control the disease. Drugs may be used to reduce the severity of symptoms and the frequency of outbreaks but they are often unsuccessful. For a virus such as HPV, which may cause the development of warts on the skin, treatment may focus on removing the warts with chemicals or surgery.

Having a curable STD may not prevent a person from developing the disease again. Individuals being treated for an STD are encouraged to abstain from all sexual activity until treatment is complete. Abstinence is necessary during this period to prevent reinfection.

Prevention

The only 100-percent effective way of preventing STDs is abstinence (not engaging in any form of sexual activity). For people who choose to participate in sexual activity, the risk can be lowered by using condoms and limiting their number of sexual partners. The risk is significantly lowered by having one sexual partner who does not have any other sexual partners and who does not have a STD.

Prevention methods for sexually transmitted diseases (STDs) include:

- Correctly using a male latex or polyurethane condom with every act of vaginal intercourse, anal intercourse and oral sex (mouth-to-genital contact). Although male latex condoms are not 100 percent effective, they significantly reduce the risk of transmission. Female condoms offer some protection from

STDs, but are not as effective as male latex condoms. Condoms do not provide protection against sores on areas not covered by the condom. Using a water-based lubricant with condoms will reduce breakage.

- Refusing to have sex with someone who will not use a condom.
- Washing the genitals with soap and water after sexual activity. This may help to eliminate parasites and bacteria that may have contacted the genitals.
- Urinating after sexual activity. This may help to eliminate bacteria that may have entered the urethra.
- Performing regular genital self-examinations to become familiar with the normal appearance of the genitals. This knowledge will help to identify any symptoms that may develop if a person is exposed to an STD.
- Abstaining from sex during a woman's menstrual period. During menstruation, women who have HIV/AIDS are more infectious and women who do not have the disease are more likely to become infected. Using a condom during menstruation can reduce this risk.
- Vaccinations for human papilloma virus (HPV) and the hepatitis B virus.
- Avoiding anal intercourse. The rectum and anus contain a large amount of bacteria. Contact with these bacteria can cause STDs in both women and men. In addition, the mouth, vagina and penis should not be exposed to any object that has been in contact with an anus or rectum. If anal intercourse is preferred, a male latex condom should always be used.
- Using caution when sharing sex toys. Because STDs can be transmitted through shared bodily fluids, individuals should use condoms with sex toys when appropriate.

People are encouraged to discuss their sexual history with their sexual partners and to ask their partners about their history. These discussions are important regardless of gender because people who engage in sexual activity of any kind are all at risk for STDs. Partners should also discuss drug habits, and whether testing for STDs is necessary. These screening tests can be conducted during routine medical checkups. Testing is particularly important at the beginning of a new sexual relationship.

Because a partner may be dishonest about their drug use, sexual history or the fact they have (or have not) been tested, people are encouraged to look for signs and symptoms of STDs on their partner.

Although many STDs do not always have noticeable symptoms, people should never engage in sexual activity with a partner who is visibly showing symptoms of an STD. In addition, people are encouraged to abstain from engaging in sexual activity with a partner who is being treated for a curable STD. The disease may be transmitted at any time until the course of treatment is complete.

BIBLIOGRAPHY

1. Bataille V, Snieder H, MacGregor AJ, Sasieni P, Spector TD. The influence of genetics and environmental factors in the pathogenesis of acne: A twin study of acne in women. J Invest Dermatol. 2002;119:1317-22.
2. Capitanio B, Sinagra JL, Ottaviani M, Bordignon V, Amantea A, Picardo M. Acne and smoking. Dermato-endocrinol 2009;1(3):129-35.
3. Fabiane Mulinari-Brenner, Wilma Bergfeld. Hair loss: Diagnosis and management. Cleveland Clinic Journal of Medicine. 2003;70(8).
4. Gawkrodger DJ, Ormerod AD, Shaw L, Mauri-Sole I, Whitton ME, Watts MJ, Anstey AV, Ingham J, Young K. Guideline for the diagnosis and management of vitiligo. British journal of 2008;159(5):1051-76.
5. Haider A, Shaw JC. Treatment of Acne Vulgaris. JAMA, 2004;292:726-35.
6. Huggins RH, Schwartz RA, Janniger CK. "Vitiligo". Acta Dermatovenerologica Alpina, Panonica, et Adriatica 2005;14(4):137-42,144-5.
7. Jobling R. "A patient's journey: Psoriasis". Br Med J 2007;334(7600):953-4.
8. Ju Q, Zouboulis CC, Xia L. Environmental pollution and acne: Chloracne. Dermato-endocrinol. 2009;1(3):125-8.
9. Kwinter J, Pelletier J, Khambalia A, Pope E. "High-potency steroid use in children with vitiligo: A retrospective study". Journal of the American Academy of Dermatology 2007;56(2):236-41.
10. Lorette G, Fontès V. Prescribe topical treatments for psoriasis. Rev Prat. 2004;15:54(1):40-2.
11. May W, Linthorst Homan, Phyllis I Spuls, John de Korte, Jan D Bos, Mirjam A Sprangers, JP Wietze van der Veen. The burden of Vitiligo: Patient characteristics associated with quality of life. 2009;61(3)411-20.
12. Mechri A, Amri M, Douarika AA, Ali Hichem BH, Zouari B, Zili J. "Psychiatric morbidity and quality of life in Vitiligo: a case controlled study (Psychiatric morbidity and quality of life in Vitiligo: a case controlled study)" (in French). La Tunisie Médicale 2006;84(10):632-5.
13. Nestle FO, Kaplan DH, Barker J. Review article: Mechanisms of Disease. Psoriasis. N Engl J Med. 2009;361:496-509.
14. Shapiro J, Price VH. Hair regrowth: therapeutic agents. Dermatol Clin, 1998;16:341-56.

15. Smitha Gowda, Orin M Goldblum, W Vaughn McCall, Steven R Feldman. Factors affecting sleep quality in patients with psoriasis. Journal of American Academy of Dermatologist. 2010; 63(1):114-23.
16. Thiboutot D, Chen W. Update and future of hormonal therapy in acne. Dermatology. 2003;206:57-67.
17. Thorneycroft IH, Stanczyk FZ, Bradshaw KD, Ballagh SA, Nichols M, Weber ME. Effect of low-dose oral contraceptives on androgenic markers and acne. Contraception 1999;60(5):255-62.
18. Van YH, Lee WH, Ortiz S, Lee MH, Qin HJ, Liu CP. All-trans Retinoic Acid Inhibits Type 1 Diabetes by T Regulatory (Treg)-Dependent Suppression of Interferon-{gamma}-Producing T-cells without Affecting Th17 Cells. Diabetes 2009;58:146-55.
19. Walters, et al. Suberythemogenic narrowband UVB is markedly more effective than conventional UVB in treatment of psoriasis vulgaris. Journal of the American Academy of Dermatology. 1999;40(6)893-900.
20. William J, Timothy B, Dirk E. Andrews' Diseases of the Skin: Clinical Dermatology (10th ed.). Saunders. 2005.
21. Zaenglein AL, Thiboutot DM. Expert Committee Recommendations for Acne Management. Pediatrics 2006;118:1188-99.

CHAPTER

5

Deficiency Disorders

■ RICKETS

Rickets is a disorder in children due to the deficiency of adequate mineralization of bones during development age, before the skeletal maturity. This leads to the weakening of bones and making them prone to undergo deformity and fracture.

Causes

This disorder occurs in children and following could be the reasons behind it:

- Vitamin D deficiency
- Calcium deficiency in diet (Malnutrition, starvation, lactose intolerance, pure vegetarian diet, the child who is fed purely on mother milk may develop calcium deficiency)
- Severe diarrhea, fluid loss, diarrhea (Inadequate calcium absorption in body)
- Hormonal imbalance—in case of low serum calcium, the hormonal reactions force bones to loose minerals and calcium, phosphates, thus making them dematerialized and prone to fracture
- Inadequate sunlight exposure also makes one prone to develop rickets because in absence of sunlight the calcium absorption in body does not occur
- Liver malfunctioning—in case of liver malfunctioning, the vitamin D cannot be converted into its active form
- Rapid growth—if between 6 to 24 month of age the rapid growth occurs, body need high stock of calcium for bone mineralization, thus if calcium is deficit, the rickets will develop
- Genetic links is found and generations may be affected (Signe Sparre et al, 2009). It occurs when the kidneys are unable to

hold onto the mineral phosphate. Rickets may also be caused by kidney disorders that involve renal tubular acidosis.

Symptoms

- Bone pain or tenderness in the bones of (Aggarwal and Gulathi, 2009) arms, legs, pelvis and spine
- Delayed formation of teeth, defects in the structure of teeth; holes in the enamel, dental caries
- Decreased muscle tone (loss of muscle strength) due to rickets hypotonia
- Progressive weakness due to weak attachment of muscles at bones
- Impaired growth because the weak bones lead to impaired bone development and stunted growth
- Increased bone fractures due to poor minerals in bones
- Muscle cramps and muscle weakness due to lower levels of calcium. The excessive weakness of muscles makes the child to appear floppy
- Short stature (adults less than 5 feet tall) due to the poor development of the bones
- Skeletal deformities (Fig. 5.1): Asymmetrical or odd-shaped skull; bowed legs or knock knees due to the pressure on the weak bones by the body weight; expansion of the anterior rib ends at costochondral junction ribcage (rachitic rosary); breastbone pushed forward (pigeon chest); pelvic deformities; spine deformities (spine curves abnormally, including scoliosis or kyphosis)
- The abnormal thinning and softening of skull bones lead to "Craniotabes" (Signe Sparre et al, 2009)
- The weak bones of ribs are pulled by muscles to produce flaring over the diaphragm, which is known as Harrison groove
- Lack of muscle strength and weakness will reduce the physical activity of child, which will reduce the necessary stress on the bones for development. As a result of this bone weakness progresses further
- Child tends to stay in supine lying position for prolonged period due to weakness, this will cause weakness of abdominal muscles and the "Protruding abdominal belly" while assuming standing position.

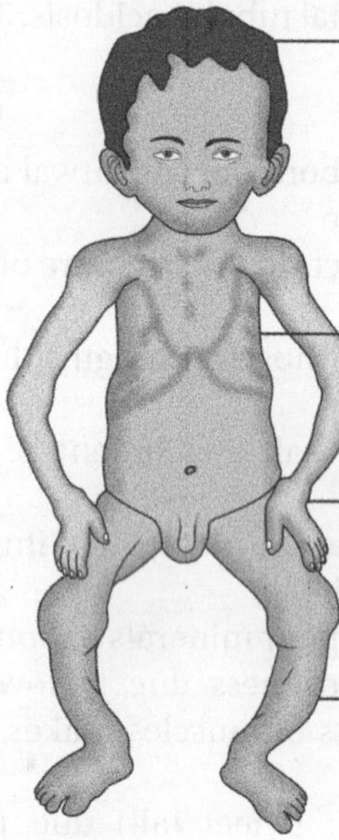

Signs of rickets

Soft spot on baby's head is slow to close

Bony necklace

Curved bones

Big, lumpy joints

Bowed legs (knees bent out)

Fig. 5.1: Features of child with rickets

Signs and Tests

Vitamin D insufficiency is defined as serum 25(OH)D <50 nmol/l, vitamin D deficiency as serum 25(OH)D 12.5–25 nmol/l and severe vitamin D deficiency as serum 25(OH)D<12.5 nmol/l (Lips 2004).

Nutritional rickets involves severe vitamin D deficiency or vitamin D deficiency and at least one of the following: raised plasma alkaline phosphatase (ALP), raised serum parathyroid hormone (PTH), or low serum calcium (Ca) (Shaw, 2003).

Vitamin D-dependent rickets type 1 (VDDR type 1) is defined as: raised plasma ALP, raised serum PTH, low to normal serum Ca, low plasma PO_4, serum 1,25-dihydroxyvitamin D ($1,25(OH)_2D$) <15 pmol/l, and serum 25(OH)D within the reference range of 50–178 nmol/l (Kim et al, 2007).

X-ray examination reveals the—widening of the anterior ends of ribs, flattening of growing ends of bones (Epiphysis); cupping of metaphysis due to absent or delayed calcification; deformities of bones.

A physical exam reveals tenderness or pain in the bones (due to poor mineralization), rather than in the joints or muscles.

Laboratory investigations include serum calcium; bone X-rays, serum alkaline phosphatase, serum phosphorous.

Widening of the epiphysis may be confused with the metastasis or the bone cancer thus needs to be ruled out.

Other tests and procedures include the following: Calcium (ionized). Parathyroid hormone testing, urinary calcium evaluation.

Treatment

The goals of treatment are to relieve symptoms and correct the cause of the condition. The cause must be treated to prevent the disease from returning. Treatment involves increasing dietary intake of calcium, phosphates and vitamin D.

Patients with nutritional rickets, the rickets heal upon treatment with vitamin D (Signe Sparre et al, 2009). Vitamin D_3 is the easily absorbable and commonly used supplement form.

Replacing calcium, phosphorus, or vitamin D that is lacking will eliminate most symptoms of rickets. Dietary sources of vitamin D include fish, liver, and processed milk. Exposure to moderate amounts of sunlight is encouraged. If rickets is caused by a metabolic problem, a prescription for vitamin D supplements may be needed.

The kids, who are fed purely on breast milk and not exposed to sunlight, must be given vitamin D supplement from two months age till the time when they start taking milk supplements.

Physiotherapy

The goal of the physiotherapy intervention focus, to relieve pain/ muscle spasm to prevent the deformity, prevent muscle tightness or contractures. Positioning or bracing may be used to reduce or prevent deformities. The physiotherapy interventions are also important in post surgical cases who have been managed for correction of deformities and also in regaining optimal functions/ preventing muscle wasting.

Relieve pain/muscle spasm
- Hotpacks
- Cryotherapy
- Soft tissue manipulations
- Ultrasonic therapy
- IFT/TENS

Prevention of deformities/fractures

- Taping
- Orthosis
- Brace
- Cast

Prevention/correction of contracture

- Stretching – manual/self/PNF

Posture correction/re-education

- Posture corrective exercises

Regaining optimal functions/preventing muscle wasting

- ROM exercises
- Joint mobilization
- Hydrotherapy
- Conditioning exercises
- Balance and coordination exercises
- Flexibility exercises

Prognosis

The disorder may be corrected by replacing vitamin D and minerals. Laboratory values and X-rays usually improve after about 1 week, although some cases may require large doses of minerals and vitamin D.

If uncorrected cases the deformities and stunted height may be irreversible.

Complications

- Chronic skeletal pain due to the weak attachments of muscles with bones and the poor strength of the bones.
- Skeletal deformities as the soft bones undergo irregular shape and the deformity when they are subjected to weight bearing.
- Skeletal fractures, may occur without cause.

OSTEOPOROSIS

Osteoporosis is a disorder which is characterized by global osteopenia in body and increased porosity of bones, along with increased weakness and brittleness. It is very common older adults and occurs when low levels of calcium, phosphorus and other minerals cause bones to lose mass. The early stage of decreased bone density is called osteopenia.

Osteoporosis is a severe public health problem that affects all strata of the global community. It can lead to increased risk of fractures - most often in the spine, hip or wrist - that cause sudden, searing pain. Falls or minor events such as coughing, bending over or sneezing can break osteoporotic bones.

Anatomy

In human body the bones are of two types: the cortical bone and the trabecular bones. The former one is the stiffer, compact bone and makes the shaft of long bones. This is primarily responsible for making the weight bearing component and the strong attachment points to muscles and ligaments. The trabecular bone is spongy bone where the trabeculae are arranged in the direction of tension. It is filled with blood and bone marrow.

In normal healthy bones the remodeling process occurs regularly, where small component of the bone is damaged due to wear and tear and is removed by osteoclasts, and the new bone matrix is laid by the action of osteoblasts. This is the life-long process of creating new bone (formation) and breaking down old bone (resorption). The resorption and formation of bone are essential in repairing small fractures and replacing bone. The relative working between osteoblastic and osteoclastic activity determines the bone density and quality. When osteoclastic activity supermines the activity of osteoblasts, then the bone density is reduced and the osteoporosis occurs.

There are two main types of osteoporosis (Harrop et al, 2004):

1. *Primary*: Caused by aging (senile osteoporosis) or by unknown factors (idiopathic osteoporosis).
2. *Secondary*: Caused by another disease, a medical treatment or lifestyle factors.

Postmenopausal women are at higher risk of developing osteoporosis because lower levels of the hormone estrogen weaken bones. However, the disease also affects men and - in rare cases - children.

Risk Factors and Potential Causes

Osteoporosis is result of the loss of non organic minerals including calcium, phosphorus and other minerals. This loss leads to the loss of stiffness of bones and the reduced ability of these bones to absorb shock. When the excessive external load is applied, then the bone fails to dissipate the stress and undergoes disruption of its architecture and sustains fracture because of its porous and weak nature.

Estrogen hormone is believed to decrease the bone absorption rate. Thus, when women reach menopause, bone resorption and bone loss is accelerated further. Bone loss related to menopause usually lasts for about 10 years. In contrast, the testosterone hormone promotes muscle growth and puts excessive stress on the bones to accelerate their growth. However, by age 65, men lose bone at the same rate as women. The risk of developing osteoporosis depends on the amount of bone mass developed between 25 and 35 and how rapidly it is lost during aging.

Many risk factors have been identified for the osteoporosis:

- Women are at higher risk of osteoporosis than men. Hormonal and the bone mass factors play role
- Genetic association is found
- Renal osteodystrophy or renal diseases impair the calcium uptake
- Sedentary lifestyle and lack of exercise
- Smoking habits
- In female athlete the amenorrhea, anorexia and the reduced bone mass density is common and is known as 'female athlete triad'
- Race—people with fair skin, such as Caucasians and Asians, are most likely to experience osteoporosis. African-Americans and Hispanics have lower incidences, but risk remains fairly high
- Hormones—lifetime exposure to estrogen is a factor for women
- The medical problems which may impair the mobility and make one sedentary such as rheumatoid arthritis, heart disorders, renal problems (excessive loss of calcium from body), diabetes, fracture, neurological problems, amenorrhea
- Medications—long-term use of some corticosteroids or other immunosuppressants damages bones
- Radiotherapy for cancer causes osteoporosis.

Signs and Symptoms

The osteoporosis is not a disease per se therefore it is not easily detected in its initial phases. Client may have complaint of back pain and the weakness of some muscles. The later stage manifestation may include apparent radiological features, loss of height due to the damage to individual vertebral bodies, stooping forward of the posture due to the loss of height of anterior portion of the vertebral body. With the more and more of the mineral contents of the bones, the higher risk of fracture occurs and even a trivial trauma such as simple fall from chair may cause multiple fractures. The fractures of pelvic bone, femur or spine may be life fatal due to the massive loss of blood (thus leading to shock) and the damage to spinal cord respectively.

The most common site of fracture is femur neck, vertebral bodies and distal end of radius (Colle's fracture). The femur neck fracture is most notorious and fails to heal in absence of surgical interventions. If left untreated, this fracture makes person bed confined and secondarily leads to multiple morbid conditions life deep vein thrombosis (DVT), cardiac problems, cardiovascular deconditioning, emboli dislodgement and the chances of stroke.

Diagnosis

Early detection of osteoporosis is important because early treatment can slow the progress of the disease. However the early diagnosis is not always possible because lack of clinical manifestations and the failure to report the problem to physician. Most of the time the problem of osteoporosis is detected at the time of X-ray taking due to some other ailments or the fracture.

When suspected the osteoporosis in the prone age groups the careful history documentation regarding the medicines, calcium intake, dietary style, lifestyle habits, hormonal imbalance, etc. may play role. The risk of idiopathic fractures and the alteration in the client's eight is also relevant.

The other possible medical causes such as myelomas, hormonal imbalance, kidney problems also have to be ruled out.

Bone density is the parameter that can be determined best *in vivo*, has a high precision, and correlates well with the biomechanically determined bone strength (it explains approximately 70% of bone strength (NIH, 2001) the World Health Organization (WHO) has defined osteoporosis on basis of BMD (WHO, 1994) using a classification system suggested in 1994 by an expert panel of the WHO (Kanis, 1994; WHO, 2003).

- The bone mass density is the DEXA scan (dual energy X-ray absorptiometry). The most popular method of gauging bone density in patients suspected of osteoporosis. It measures the density of bones. The different X-ray beams are made to pass through body and received using X-ray detector. The amount of beam passed through bones is measured, coded and imaged to reveal patient bone density.

WHO definition of osteoporosis, based on bone mineral density and T-scores using DEXA of the proximal femur and spine (WHO, 1994; Thomas & Majumdar, 2003).

T-score > – 1	Normal
T-score < – 1, > – 2.5	Osteopenia
T-score < – 2.5	Osteoporosis
T-score < – 2.5	Severe (Established) Osteoporosis

- *The BMD evaluation reveals two scores*: The T-score and a Z-score. The T-score compares bone density to peak density of young healthy. A T-score of greater than minus-1 is considered normal. A T-score of minus-1 to minus-2.5 is considered osteopenia, and a risk for developing osteoporosis. A T-score of less than minus-2.5 is diagnostic of osteoporosis. The Z-score is used to compare bone density score to other people of same age, weight, ethnicity, and gender. This is useful to determine secondary osteoporosis.
- *Single-photon absorptiometry*: Used to measure bone density of the forearms and heels.
- *Dual-photon absorptiometry*: Used to measure bone density of the hips and spine.
- *CAT scan (computed axial tomography)*: A noninvasive test which takes multiple cross-sectional images of bones and measures the bone shape, structure and density. However this exposes the client to high dose of radiation.

People of the prone age (both males and females) over 70 year age must undergo the screening for osteoporosis.

Treatment

If secondary osteoporosis is suspected then the causative problem and pathology has to be resolved first using medical treatment or by removing cause. Client must take proper diet, must indulge in regular exercise, should take calcium and vitamin D supplements, should avoid the fracture risk activities, must avoid falls.

The recommended medications for osteoporosis:

- Bisphosphonates—reduce bone resorption and increase bone density. It is the prophylactic therapy in prone patients and those who are at higher risk of secondary osteoporosis due to cancer, radiotherapy, bed confinement, steroidal therapy.

- Hormonal drugs. These include:
  - Calcitonin (Fortical, Miacalcin): This is a hormone naturally from the thyroid gland. It reduces the bone resorption rate specially in post menopausal women. It is given by nasal spray. Useful to prevent spinal fracture but not the peripheral bone and hip bone fracture.
  - Teriparatide (Forteo): This injectable synthetic version of parathyroid hormone helps to regulate calcium and phosphate metabolism in bones. It may be prescribed to women or men at high risk for fractures. Side effects may include nausea, dizziness and leg cramps.
  - Testosterone therapy: This may benefit men who have or are at high risk for osteoporosis because of low levels of testosterone.

Hormone replacement therapy (HRT) had long been the primary treatment for osteoporosis in women. By taking estrogen or combined estrogen and progesterone replacements, women have been able to slow down or halt the loss of bone mass associated with menopause. However, recent studies link long-term HRT to serious risks including breast cancer (Chlebowski, 2009) and blood clots. As a result, many experts no longer recommend HRT as a primary means of controlling osteoporosis.

Physiotherapy management for osteoporosis rests upon:

- Improving the balance so as to tackle with the fall.
- Improving muscle strength to improve the mobility.
- Enhance mobility and the functional status.
- The education regarding healthy lifestyle, diet and the exercises.
- The symptomatic management of associated pain.
- The deep diathermy and the deep heat must be avoided as they can reach upto bones and may further cause the loss of minerals from bones.
- In case of spinal fracture the proper bracing, proper education and the protected mobility maintenance is important.
- In severe kyphosis and the forward stoop posture maintenance of lung vital capacity and breathing status is important.
- The stretching of the tightened muscles helps to prevent the further deformity.

- The improvement of muscle endurance especially in the postural muscles is important to maintain the body posture against gravity.
- In cases where the surgical interventions have been done to correct deformity, to change the joints, correction of spinal fractures, the pre and postoperative physiotherapy is also important.
- The indulgence in regular exercise helps to preserve the bone mass and its density. Also this is important to improve the bone density status.
- The type of exercises that is supposed to be most important include the low-to-moderate intensity aerobic activity with special emphasis on improving the endurance.
- The high impact activities must be avoided due to higher risks of developing the stress and gross fractures in bones.

Prevention

- Regular exercise. Regular physical activity low-to-moderate intensity for a long duration (about 30 minutes a day) helps to preserve bone strength and density. It also slows down the bone loss rate. The type of activity could involve brisk walking, mild jogging, weight bearing activity, stair climbing, sports like football and dancing, aerobic activity.
- The proper diet is also important. The dietry supplements in population with additional demands such as growing children pregnant females, breastfeeding mother, old age is highly important. The diet that must be encouraged in all population groups include milk, cheese, fruit juices, soya supplements, almonds, spinach and other green vegetables, eggs, cereals, fatty fish.
- Healthy lifestyle habits also include to avoidance of alcohol, smoking. The consumption of omega-3 fatty acids.
- The daily exposure to sunlight also helps to synthesize the vitamin D in the body.
- The prevention of morbidity focuses on the reduction of the fall incidence so as to avoid many fracture.
- Considering wearing hip pads. Fat or muscle that pads the hips helps to reduce hip fractures. Researchers are investigating whether external hip pads may provide a cushion that lessens the risk of fracture when a person falls. Initial results in studies involving nursing home residents have been encouraging.

In addition, research shows that men who take the cholesterol-controlling drugs known as statins may be less likely to suffer osteoporotic fractures. Studies have produced mixed results on whether statins affect women's risk of such fractures.

DIABETES

Diabetes mellitus is a disorder that affects the body's ability to make or use insulin. Insulin is a hormone produced in the pancreas that helps transport glucose (blood sugar) from the bloodstream into the cells so they can break it down and use it for fuel. People cannot live without insulin.

Diabetes results in abnormal levels of glucose in the bloodstream. This can cause severe short-term and long-term consequences ranging from brain damage to amputations and heart disease.

The root causes of diabetes are complex. Most cases begin with one of two processes:

- *Metabolic*: Unhealthy lifestyle factors such as overeating, physical inactivity and obesity can impair the body's ability to use insulin. This is called insulin resistance. Uncontrollable risk factors including genetics, family history and age can also be involved. Metabolic forms of diabetes include:
  - *Type 2 diabetes*: This accounts for 90 to 95 percent of diabetic cases, according to the US National Institutes of Health (NIH). Some of these patients have had prediabetes that went uncontrolled. Once considered a disease of middle and old age, type 2 is also becoming more common in youths as the incidence of childhood obesity grows.
  - *Gestational diabetes*: Hormonal changes contribute to this condition, which can develop in any previously nondiabetic woman during pregnancy, especially those who are overweight.
- *Autoimmune*: The body's immune system can mistakenly destroy the insulin-producing beta cells of the pancreas. The causes of autoimmune diabetes are poorly understood, but genetics and family history play a role, and viruses or other environmental factors are believed to figure in. Autoimmune forms of diabetes include:
  - Type 1 diabetes. Formerly known as juvenile diabetes, this form generally develops in children and young adults.
  - Latent autoimmune diabetes of adulthood. This variation of type 1 can occur later in life.

- Individuals with autoimmune diabetes who overeat, are sedentary, gain weight or have certain genes can, like people with metabolic forms of diabetes, develop insulin resistance. This state is known as double diabetes.

Diabetes can also result from another disease, such as pancreatitis, or even from a medical treatment, including pancreatectomy (surgical removal of the pancreas) or certain medications. This is known as secondary diabetes. In addition, there are uncommon inherited disorders that cause diabetes, such as maturity-onset diabetes of the young and Wolfram syndrome. Most cases of diabetes last the rest of a person's life. However, gestational diabetes generally ends when the pregnancy does, and some cases of secondary diabetes are also temporary.

Diabetes involves chronic levels of abnormally high glucose (hyperglycemia). Many patients, especially those with type 2 diabetes, also have elevated blood pressure (hypertension), chronic high levels of insulin (hyperinsulinemia) and unhealthy levels of cholesterol and other blood fats (hyperlipidemia). All of these factors contribute to the long-term complications of diabetes, which include:

- *Vascular disease (diabetic angiopathy), atherosclerosis, heart conditions and stroke.* These cardiovascular disorders are the leading cause of death in people with diabetes.
- *Kidney disease (diabetic nephropathy)*: Diabetes is the chief cause of end-stage renal disease, which requires treatment with dialysis or a kidney transplant.
- *Eye diseases*: These include diabetic retinopathy, glaucoma and cataracts. Diabetes is a leading cause of visual impairment and blindness.
- *Nerve damage (diabetic neuropathy)*: This includes peripheral neuropathy, which often causes pain or numbness in the limbs, and autonomic neuropathy, which can impede digestion (gastroparesis) and contribute to sexual dysfunction and incontinence. Neuropathy may also impair hearing and other senses.
- *Impaired thinking*: Many studies have linked diabetes to increased risk of memory loss, dementia, Alzheimer's disease and other cognitive deficits. Recently some researchers have suggested that Alzheimer's disease might be "type 3 diabetes," involving insulin resistance in the brain.

- *Infections and wounds*: Foot conditions and skin disorders, such as ulcers, make diabetes the leading cause of nontraumatic foot and leg amputations. People with diabetes are also prone to infections including periodontal disease, thrush, urinary tract infections and yeast infections.
- *Cancer*: Diabetes increases the risk of malignant tumors in the colon, pancreas, liver and several other organs.
- *Musculoskeletal disorders*: Conditions ranging from gout to osteoporosis to restless legs syndrome to myofascial pain syndrome are more common in diabetic patients than nondiabetics.
- *Pregnancy complications*: Diabetes increases the risk of preeclampsia, miscarriage, stillbirth and birth defects.
- *Emotional difficulties*: Many but not all of the studies exploring connections between diabetes and mental illness have found increased rates of depression, anxiety and other psychological disorders in diabetic patients. In addition to chronic hyperglycemia, diabetic patients can experience acute episodes of hyperglycemia as well as hypoglycemia (low glucose). Severe cases can cause seizures, brain damage and a potentially fatal diabetic coma. Acute glucose emergencies include:
  - *Insulin shock*: This advanced stage of hypoglycemia is typically due to excessive amounts of insulin medication or certain anti-diabetic agents.
  - *Diabetic ketoacidosis*: A lack of insulin can force the body to burn fats instead of glucose for energy. The result is a toxic byproduct called ketones, along with severe hyperglycemia.
  - *Hyperosmolar hyperglycemic nonketotic state*: This involves severe hyperglycemia and dehydration.

These dangerous glucose complications are most common in patients with unstable diabetes, but they can develop even in individuals who do not realize they have diabetes. About one-third of the estimated 20.8 million Americans with diabetes have not yet been diagnosed, according to the US Centers for Disease Control and Prevention (CDCP).

The incidence of diabetes has soared worldwide in recent years and is expected to keep growing, with the greatest increase seen in metabolic forms of diabetes, notably type 2. This is blamed largely on the rise of obesity and the global spread of Western-style habits: physical inactivity along with a diet that is high in calories, processed carbohydrates and saturated fats and insufficient in fiber-rich whole foods. The aging of the population is also a factor. However, other factors, such as environment may also be contributing, because cases of autoimmune diabetes (type 1) are also becoming more common.

The word "diabetes" stems from a Greek term for passing through, a reference to increased urination (polyuria), a common symptom of the disease. "Mellitus" is the Latin word for honeyed, a reference to glucose noted in the urine of diabetic patients.

Diabetes mellitus is sometimes referred to as sugar diabetes but usually is simply called diabetes. There is also a rare disease called diabetes insipidus (water diabetes) in which the kidneys release too much water. Like diabetes mellitus, it has excessive urination as a symptom, but these two endocrine disorders are otherwise unrelated.

Classification

There are several forms of diabetes. Scientists are still defining and categorizing some of these variations and establishing their prevalence in the population. Types of diabetes include:

- *Type 1 diabetes*: An autoimmune disease in which the immune system mistakenly destroys the insulin-making beta cells of the pancreas. It typically develops more quickly than other forms of diabetes. It is usually diagnosed in children and adolescents, and sometimes in young adults. To survive, patients must administer insulin medication regularly. Type 1 diabetes used to be called juvenile diabetes and insulin-dependent diabetes mellitus (IDDM). However, those terms are not accurate because children can develop other forms of diabetes, adults sometimes develop type 1, and other forms of diabetes can require insulin therapy. A variation of type 1 that develops later in life, usually after age 30, is called latent autoimmune diabetes of adulthood (LADA).

  Sometimes patients with autoimmune diabetes develop insulin resistance because of weight gain or genetic factors. This condition is known as double diabetes.
- *Type 2 diabetes*: A disorder of metabolism, usually involving excess weight and insulin resistance. In these patients, the pancreas makes insulin initially, but the body has trouble using this glucose-controlling hormone. Eventually the pancreas cannot produce enough insulin to respond to the body's need for it.

Type 2 diabetes is by far the most common form of diabetes, accounting for 85 to 95 percent of cases in developed nations and an even higher percentage in developing nations, according to the International Diabetes Federation. This disease may take years or decades to develop. It is usually preceded by prediabetes, in which levels of glucose (blood sugar) are above normal but not high enough yet for a diagnosis of diabetes. People with prediabetes can often delay or prevent the escalation to type 2 diabetes by losing weight through improvements in exercise and diet, as the Diabetes Prevention Program and other research projects have demonstrated. Type 2 diabetes used to be called adult-onset diabetes and non-insulin-dependent diabetes mellitus (NIDDM). Those terms are not accurate because children can also develop this disease, and some patients require insulin therapy.

- *Gestational diabetes*: A temporary metabolic disorder that any previously nondiabetic woman can develop during pregnancy, usually the third trimester. Hormonal changes contribute to this disease, along with excess weight and family history of diabetes. About 4 percent of pregnant women develop gestational diabetes, according to the American Diabetes Association. Gestational diabetes can cause problems for the mother and baby, including preeclampsia, premature delivery, macrosomia (oversized infant), and jaundice and breathing difficulties in the infant. This disease typically ends when the pregnancy does, but it increases the risk of type 2 diabetes later in life for the mother and the child.
- *Secondary diabetes*: Diabetes caused by another condition. The many potential sources of secondary diabetes range from diseases such as pancreatitis, cystic fibrosis, Down syndrome and hemochromatosis to medical treatments including corticosteroids, other immunosuppressives, diuretics and pancreatectomy.
- *Maturity-onset diabetes of the young (MODY)*: An uncommon disease caused by a genetic defect inherited from a parent. It is usually diagnosed before age 25 in people of normal weight. MODY is sometimes classified as a form of type 2 or secondary diabetes but is often considered a separate condition.

Unstable diabetes, also known as brittle or labile diabetes, is a term that may be used to describe any case of poorly controlled diabetes regardless of the type.

All of these conditions involve diabetes mellitus ("sugar diabetes"). Diabetes insipidus ("water diabetes") is an unrelated endocrine system disorder in which the kidneys release too much water.

Risk Factors and Causes

The causes of diabetes are complex and only partly understood. This disease is generally considered multifactorial, involving several predisposing conditions and risk factors. In many cases genetics, habits and environment may all contribute to a person's diabetes.

To complicate matters, there can be contrary risk factors for the various forms of the disease. For example, autoimmune diabetes (type 1 and latent autoimmune diabetes of adulthood, LADA) is more common in white people, but metabolic diabetes (type 2 and gestational diabetes) is more common in people of other races and ethnicities. Type 1 is usually diagnosed in children, but advancing age is a risk factor for type 2 and gestational diabetes.

Insulin resistance, prediabetes and metabolic syndrome are strong risk factors for type 2 diabetes. Other diabetic risk factors and causes include:

- *Genetics and family history*: Certain genes are known to cause maturity-onset diabetes of the young (MODY) and Wolfram syndrome. Genes also contribute to other forms of diabetes, including types 1 and 2.
- *Weight and body type*: Overweight and obesity are leading factors in type 2 diabetes and gestational diabetes. Excess fat, especially around the abdomen (central obesity), promotes insulin resistance and metabolic syndrome.

  Most people with autoimmune diabetes (type 1 and LADA) are of normal weight, and excess weight has not traditionally been considered to be related to these conditions. However, recent research indicates that obesity may hasten the development of type 1 diabetes and that the increasing rate of type 1 diabetes may be at least partly due to the rise of childhood obesity. Furthermore, patients with autoimmune diabetes who gain weight are susceptible to insulin resistance and double diabetes.
- *Sex*: Little or no research has been conducted to explain this trend.
- *Level of physical activity*: Lack of regular exercise is blamed for much of the twin global epidemics of obesity and diabetes.

- *Diet*: The effect of diet in the development of diabetes is controversial. Some studies have linked heavy consumption of soft drinks and other simple carbohydrates to risk of metabolic diabetes, and foods low in the glycemic index, such as whole grains, to reduced risk. Yet the ADA states that eating foods containing sugar does not cause the disease. The culprit, rather, is the weight gain due to sedentary habits and excess intake of calories, according to the ADA.
- *Other diseases*: Medical conditions including high blood pressure, hyperlipidemia (unhealthy levels of cholesterol), polycystic ovarian syndrome, asthma and sleep apnea have been linked to type 2 diabetes. Celiac disease (gluten intolerance) and other autoimmune diseases have been linked to type 1. The many conditions that may cause secondary diabetes include pancreatitis, hemochromatosis, endocrine disorders including hyperthyroidism, Cushing's disease and acromegaly, and genetic conditions including cystic fibrosis, Down syndrome and some forms of muscular dystrophy.
- *Hormones*: These chemical messengers can contribute to diabetes in various ways. For example, stress hormones such as cortisol have been linked to fluctuating glucose levels in type 2 diabetes, and stress hormones in women during pregnancy have been linked to risk of type 1 diabetes in the child. The release of growth and sex hormones during adolescence may make some teens more susceptible to diabetes. A wide range of hormonal treatments including anabolic steroids, growth hormone, estrogens, injected contraceptives, androgen deprivation therapy for prostate cancer and corticosteroids have been linked to secondary diabetes.
- *Medical treatments*: In addition to hormonal therapies, medications including diuretics, beta blockers (another class of antihypertensives), immunosuppressives, antiretrovirals (AIDS/HIV drugs) antipsychotics, lithium, and some antidepressants, anticonvulsants and chemotherapy drugs have been linked to an increased risk of secondary diabetes. Pancreatectomy and radiation therapy may also result in secondary diabetes. Drugs including pentamidine (used to treat pneumonia) and L-asparaginase (used to treat leukemia) have been linked to type 1 diabetes.
- *Other chemicals*: In addition to these pharmaceuticals, some studies have linked PCBs, other pollutants and certain pesticides

including the defoliant Agent Orange and dioxin (its active ingredient) to insulin resistance and type 2 diabetes. Common consumer plastics and plastics ingredients including phthalates and bisphenol A have also been linked to insulin resistance in some cases. Exposure to agricultural pesticides during pregnancy has been tentatively linked to gestational diabetes. A rat poison called pyriminal has been linked to type 1 diabetes.
- *Other environmental factors*: Some researchers theorize that free radicals may contribute to the development of type 1 and possibly other forms of diabetes. Free radicals are formed as a result of chemical reactions in the body. Smoke, air pollution and even genetics contribute to the formation of free radicals. When these radicals build up, they can destroy cells, including those involved in the production of insulin. Cold weather is another possible environmental factor in type 1 diabetes. This disease occurs more commonly in cold climates and develops more frequently in the winter than the summer.
- *Viruses*: Some people are diagnosed with type 1 diabetes after a viral infection. Viruses thought to be related to type 1 diabetes include mumps, rubella and coxsackie virus (related to the virus family that causes polio and hepatitis).
- *Smoking*: Cigarette smoking is a risk factor for type 2 diabetes and possibly other forms of diabetes.
- *Alcohol*: Excessive use of alcohol is a risk factor for diabetes. For example, it can cause pancreatitis. However, some research has found that light drinking may decrease the risk of becoming diabetic.

Most of these risk factors can be described as either uncontrollable, such as genetics and age, or controllable, such as exercise and diet. Some, such as obesity, may involve genetics and lifestyle choices. People cannot alter their uncontrollable risk factors, but they can lower their risk of developing diabetes by reducing controllable risk factors through improved health habits.

Signs and Symptoms

Diabetes often goes undetected because symptoms can be attributed to many other causes and some patients experience no symptoms or fail to heed warning signs. Possible indicators of diabetes include:
- Excessive thirst (polydipsia)
- Excessive urination (polyuria) and dehydration

- Excessive hunger or appetite (polyphagia)
- Unexplained weight loss
- Blurred vision, nearsightedness or other vision problems
- Frequent infections, including skin infections, thrush, gingivitis, urinary tract infections and yeast infections
- Slow healing of sores
- Skin problems, such as itchiness or acanthosis nigricans
- Fatigue, lethargy or drowsiness
- Shakiness or trembling
- Mood swings or irritability
- Dizziness or fainting
- Numbness, tingling or pain in the feet, legs or hands.

Type 1 diabetes can develop rapidly and often occurs after an illness, but symptoms may be mistaken for the flu or other common conditions. Type 2 diabetes can take many years to develop and sometimes becomes apparent only after long-term complications occur, such as sexual dysfunction or leg pain that is due to diabetic neuropathy or claudication (caused by peripheral artery disease).

Some people, especially young people with type 1 diabetes, go undiagnosed until they are brought to a hospital with an emergency condition called diabetic ketoacidosis. Indicators of diabetic ketoacidosis include sweet fruity-smelling or wine-smelling breath, confusion and heavy labored breathing (Kussmaul breathing). Sometimes patients are diagnosed with diabetes only after suffering other serious complications including insulin shock, hyperosmolar hyperglycemic nonketotic syndrome or diabetic coma.

To help prevent such complications, people are advised to undergo periodic screening for diabetes with glucose tests, especially if they have risk factors.

Diagnosis

Blood sugar level testing is used for diagnosing the diabetes.

Often when people have a physical examination they are screened for diabetes with a fasting plasma glucose test (FPG). An FPG is usually performed in the morning because this makes it easier for the patient to fast for the required eight hours.

Glucose is measured in milligrams per deciliter (mg/dL) of blood. FPG results below 100 mg/dL are normal. Glucose between 100 and 125 mg/dL is considered prediabetes. Glucose above 125 mg/dL indicates diabetes. To confirm diagnosis, another glucose test should be performed on another day, according to the National Institute of Diabetes and Digestive and Kidney Disorders.

If glucose testing determines that a patient has diabetes, additional tests may be offered to establish the type. For example:

- A C-peptide test can distinguish autoimmune from metabolic diabetes. People with type 2 diabetes have C-peptide, which is a byproduct of insulin production, but people with type 1 diabetes and latent autoimmune diabetes of adulthood do not or have a very low level.
- Autoantibody testing can reveal misguided antibodies present in autoimmune but not metabolic diabetes.
- Genetic tests can help diagnose conditions such as maturity-onset diabetes of the young and Wolfram syndrome.
- Other tests, such as thyroid blood tests, may be ordered to find the cause of secondary diabetes.

During pregnancy, usually during the 24th to the 28th week, women may be screened for gestational diabetes with a glucose challenge test, which evaluates the body's ability to metabolize sugar. Blood is drawn an hour after the patient drinks a solution containing 50 grams of glucose. If results are abnormal, an additional, more complicated blood test called an oral glucose tolerance test (OGTT) is used to confirm diabetes.

Treatment

The regular check-up by multidisciplinary experts is needed in a diabetic patient.

Diabetes care teams essentially include a dietician, ophthalmic surgeon, endocrinologist, dentist, physiotherapist, cardiologist, vascular expert, neurologist.

The autoimmune variety of diabetes (Type I) needs regular insulin therapy for lifelong. The secondary diabetes needs the cure of the associated causative medical problem. Forms of insulin administration include syringe injections, insulin pumps, insulin pens, jet injectors and inhaled insulin.

Many patients are prescribed hypoglycemic agents for type 2 diabetes. Oral diabetes medications include:

- Alpha-glucosidase inhibitors
- Biguanides
- Meglitinides
- Sulfonylureas

- Thiazolidinediones
- A new group called DPP-4 inhibitors.

There are also injected medications known as incretin mimetics and synthetic amylin. Synthetic amylin is the only drug other than insulin approved to treat type 1 diabetes.

In addition, patients may be prescribed a glucagon kit. Glucagon is a hormone that acts against insulin and can be injected in cases of severe hypoglycemia or insulin shock.

Patients with diabetes are often prescribed other medications, including antihypertensives and cholesterol drugs, to treat related conditions. Antihypertensives such as ACE inhibitors and angiotensin-II receptor blockers can help prevent kidney disease (diabetic nephropathy) and are sometimes recommended even for patients who do not have elevated blood pressure. Patients who have or are at high risk for heart conditions may be advised to take low-dose aspirin daily.

People with diabetes need to perform glucose monitoring according to the schedule devised by their care team. Some patients use a glucose meter occasionally, but others, especially those using insulin or antidiabetic agents, must test several times a day. Patients at risk for diabetic ketoacidosis are advised to perform ketone tests.

In addition to these self-tests, patients will have glycohemoglobin tests or fructosamine tests periodically performed by their physician to assess long-term control of glucose. It is also essential to have regular dilated eye exams and dental care, and periodic tests of kidney function such as microalbuminuria testing and glomerular filtration rate.

Physiotherapy

Diet and exercise (Chipkin et al, 2001) are crucial in managing diabetes, especially type 2 diabetes. Some patients with metabolic forms of diabetes are able to control their disease using only these lifestyle interventions, which help the body use glucose (blood sugar) and prevent or reduce hyperglycemia. The aerobic exercise and the resistance training (Castaneda et al, 2002) are used as important adjuncts to manage diabetes.

Other important aspects of treating and monitoring diabetes include for physiotherapist:

- Nutrition counseling
- Daily foot care and skin care

- Regular physical examinations and foot examinations
- Regular blood pressure readings and cholesterol tests
- A pneumonia vaccination and annual flu shots
- Additional medical care before, during and after pregnancy
- Cardiac and neurological testing as needed.

OBESITY

Obesity is a condition in which people have an excess of body fat and body weight in proportion to their height. In last two decades the incidence of obesity has increased very rapidly due to the increasing machine usage, reduced physical labor, and dietary habits changes. Obesity is a complex, multifactorial, chronic disease involving environmental (social and cultural), genetic, physiologic, metabolic, behavioral, and psychological components.

Obesity is problem of global concern. Worldwide, more than 300 million adults are obese, according to the World Health Organization (WHO, 2000). The terms "obesity" and "overweight" are often used interchangeably. However, there is a distinct difference between the two. Overweight refers to an excess body weight that includes fat, bone, muscle, and/or body water. Thus, a weight lifter with good amount of muscle mass may be labeled as overweight even if he lacks body fat. The term obesity is defined in respect to the body weight and the person's height and the body mass index (see Table 5.1).

Obesity can act as a significant risk factor for causing the number of health problems such as:

- *Coronary heart disease (Boger et al, 2006)*: Obesity is associated with fibrinolytic activity and plasma fibrinogen concentrations, which have been implicated in the onset and course of ischemic heart disease (Meade et al, 1979). Moreover, obesity appears to increase cardiac work load and intravascular volume (Hubert, 1983) and to alter glucose and lipid metabolism (Robert et al, 1998). Increased cardiac work load in a heavier person may precipitate an acute event or elicit symptoms if the coronary circulation is already compromised. The burden of excess weight on the heart also has been shown in autopsy studies in which relative weight was independently related to heart size. Obesity has also been associated with the extent of coronary atherosclerosis.

- *Cancer (Goodman et al, 1997)*: Obesity raises the risk of breast, uterine, cervical, ovarian and gallbladder cancer in women; and colon, rectum and prostate cancer in men.
- *Diabetes*: Excess fat makes the body resistant to insulin, the hormone that helps it maintain proper blood sugar levels. Studies have shown that both obesity and type 2 diabetes impair insulin-induced suppression of glycogenolysis and gluconeogenesis and that the degree of impairment correlates with plasma free fatty acid (FFA) concentrations (Basu et al, 2005).
- *Fatty liver disease*: Obesity causes fats to accumulate in the liver, leading to inflammation and scarring of the liver that can result in cirrhosis.
- *Gallbladder disease*: Obesity increases levels of cholesterol, which can be deposited in the gallbladder, raising the risk of gallstones (Stampfer et al, 2005) due to the formation of the lithogenic bile (Park et al, 2003).
- *High blood pressure (Carl Lavie et al, 2009)*: Fatty tissue relies on oxygen and nutrients in the blood to survive. Blood flow through the body must increase to meet this demand, which raises blood pressure.
- Joint overuse and the abnormal stresses due to excessive body weight.
- Sleep apnea and other breathing problems.

The risk of death and associated illness increases as the degree of obesity and overweight increases. One study estimated that between 280,000 and 325,000 deaths annually in the United States could be attributed to overweight and obesity (Allison et al, 1999). Over 80% of these deaths occur among people with a BMI > 30 kg/m^2.

Other health conditions linked to obesity include: Pregnancy complications (e.g., high birth weight), increased surgical risk, weak pelvic floor muscles, and difficulty in breathing while lying supine or during sleep.

People also tend to gain more weight if they are older and/or have a low metabolic rate. Women often have a more difficult time losing fat than men, and may have particular trouble losing weight from the hips and thighs. Other factors (e.g., genetic, socioeconomic, psychological, medical factors) are also involved in obesity, but the relationship among these factors and the extent to which each contributes to obesity is less understood.

Causes

High calories diet causes the increased energy intake as compared to the energy consumption (Vainio and Bianchini, 2002), this further forces the excessive energy to be stored in adipose tissues in form of fat cell. The number of fat cells increases fastest during late childhood and early puberty, when the child is growing. Thus, if the more weight and the obesity during childhood can lead to the rigid form of obesity which is difficult to be managed with, as this is associated with the higher number of fat storing cells. Additional fat cells may continue to develop throughout a person's lifetime whenever the person consumes more energy than is expended.

A combination of high-fat, high-calorie diet (Vainio and Bianchini, 2002) including large quantities of refined sugar and sedentary lifestyle (FAO guidelines, 2002) (including lack of regular exercise) is one of the main causes of excessive energy intake compared to energy output, an imbalance that tends to lead to obesity.

The genetic factors and the somatotype of the individual is also closely responsible for obesity. Although dietary fat receives a lot of attention from consumers and health professionals, a certain amount of fat is required for a balanced diet. Obese children under three years of age without obese parents are at low risk for obesity in adulthood, but among older children, obesity is an increasingly important predictor of adult obesity, regardless of whether the parents are obese. Parental obesity more than doubles the risk of adult obesity among both obese and non obese children. Further if one parent is obese then child will be obese in 40% cases and this incidence doubles if both parents are obese (Robert Whitaker et al, 1997).

The common theories to explain obesity are:

- *Set point theory*: In some people due to non specific risk factors the setting point (Harris, 1990) at which the one feels satisfaction of hunger, is set at higher values. This setting point is determined by leptin hormone. In such person even after taking meal the feeling of satisfaction of hunger is not perceived, thus they tend to eat more. This increase the energy intake while compared to the energy consumed. Thus, it leads to obesity. This theory is not being challenged by conflicting results of other studies (Roland Weinsier, 2000).

- *Fuel efficiency theory*: It believes that in past generations during evolution, the some species and races faced the starvation due to limit food supply. In such people the genes adapted to store energy and use it efficiently. The future generations of them yet contain these efficient genes, thus they tend to have higher energy reserves. They even if consume little food, the energy stock is high and it aids to the obesity risk.

The obesity is complex and multifactorial in origin. The multiple personal, genetic, social, environmental and health factors play complex interaction to cause obesity. Some of these factors are as follows:

- *Age*: In aged people the metabolism slows down and even small amount of meal acts the reserve for food storage in body.
- *Sedentary lifestyle*: In less active individuals the reduced muscle activity demands less energy, thus there is higher reserves available of energy as compared to the utilized reserves. Thus it creates calorie excess and leads to increased storage of fat and the obesity.
- *Bullemia nervosa*: The psychological disorder linked to overeating leads to calorie excess in body and causes obesity. Similarly higher intake of calorie too causes obesity. Other psychological problems like anxiety, tension, depression also leads to obesity.

Hormonal problems like hypothyroidism, hypo cortisone in body reduces metabolic rate and cause obesity.

Other pathology like diabetes, fracture, cardiac problems, pulmonary condition may force one to confine to bed and thus further increase the obesity risk.

Individual differences like less muscle mass, less metabolic rate due to genetic component also lead to obesity among individuals of same phenotype and demographic characteristics.

Diagnosis

Because the direct measurement of body fat is difficult, the body mass index (BMI), a simple weight-to-height ratio (kg/m^2), is typically used to classify overweight and obese adults. Consistent with this, the WHO has recently published international standards for classifying overweight and obesity in adults. Obesity is defined as a BMI $\geq 30\ kg/m^2$, but it can be further subdivided on the basis of the severity of the obesity (Table 5.1).

TABLE 5.1 WHO classification of obesity

BMI range	*Classification*
<=18.5	Underweight
18.5 to 24.9	Normal
25.0 to 29.9	Overweight
30.0 to 39.9	Obese
40+	Extreme/morbid obesity

However, BMI is only an estimate of body fat and does not take a number of factors into account, including the amount of muscle mass. Extremely muscular individuals (e.g., body builders, weightlifters, athletes) may have a high BMI but are not obese and do not have increased risks for disease. Conversely, BMI may not provide an accurate measurement of people who have high concentrations of abdominal fat or those with low muscle mass (e.g., the elderly).

Waist measurement may be used in combination with BMI to calculate a person's risk for diabetes.

The following chart provides healthy versus obese ranges for men and women:

	Healthy	Obese
Men	< 37 inches (94 cm)	> 40 inches (102 cm)
Women	< 32 inches (81 cm)	>35 inches (89 cm)

A third tool for estimating body fat is the waist-to-hip ratio. This ratio is determined by measuring the circumference of the waist and dividing it by the circumference of the hips. If the stomach measurement is 1.5 times larger than the hip measurement, indicating abdominal or visceral fat (android obesity), the risk of various diseases (e.g., diabetes, cardiovascular disease) is increased.

These are general tools that can be objectively used to measure obesity include skin-fold caliper evaluation, bioelectric impedance analysis, DEXA scan, hydrostatic weighing, MRI scan of abdominal cross-section.

Treatment

For most people, weight gain can be prevented or controlled by adequate diet and exercise. Ideally, good habits begin in childhood, because studies have shown that overweight children are likely to carry this condition into adulthood.

People who are obese usually can gain significant health benefits by losing weight. The key is to change the person's energy balance so that energy output exceeds the energy intake. When this occurs the size of the person's fat cells shrinks, leading to modest but significant weight loss.

Even losing as little as 5 percent to 7 percent of total body weight can result in a dramatic decrease in risk for health conditions such as diabetes, cardiovascular disease and stroke. A relatively small weight loss can also lower blood pressure, total and low-density lipoprotein (LDL, so-called "bad") cholesterol levels, triglyceride levels and blood sugar. In addition, modest weight loss may cause high-density lipoprotein (HDLs, so-called "good") cholesterol to increase.

It is important to note that people who are obese often have trouble losing significant amounts of weight and keeping the weight off. When an obese person loses weight, the size of fat cells shrinks, but the number of fat cells does not diminish. Over time, many of the shrunken fat cells may fill again, leading to weight gain. It is for this reason that people with an average number of fat cells tend to have a better chance of maintaining weight loss than those who have higher numbers of fat cells.

In addition, research indicates that each person has an inner mechanism that establishes an individual's weight or body composition at a "set point." When a person gains or loses weight, the body's metabolism adjusts to restore the person's weight to its original level.

Still, people who are obese can often maintain modest weight loss by adhering to a healthier diet and engaging in regular physical activity. Modest weight loss of one-half to 2 pounds a week (0.23 to 0.91 kilograms) is often easier to maintain over time than sudden and massive weight loss. And even people who have trouble losing weight can often prevent further weight gain by adopting healthier lifestyle habits. These habits can reduce the disease risks associated with obesity.

The management and treatment of obesity requires permanent changes to the diet. In order to lose weight, numerous options are available, including:

- *Diet pills*: Some diet pills are available over the counter, and others require a physician's prescription. Over-the-counter medications may contain ingredients that increase the heart rate and/or blood pressure or cause other side effects. In addition, their ability to help reduce body weight has not been proven. Anyone considering use of these drugs should discuss the potential risks with a physician. Herbal supplements that claim to promote weight loss also appear to be largely ineffective. Prescription diet pills may be recommended for some patients. However, most people who use them regain the weight when they stop taking the medication. Also, the long-term effects of taking these drugs are not known.

- *Other medications*: If a healthy diet, exercise, stress management and counseling are ineffective in managing weight, medications may be prescribed. One drug (sibutramine) used to treat obesity affects levels of certain hormones (e.g., serotonin and noradrenaline) in areas of the brain associated with food intake and satisfaction. This temporarily decreases the urge to eat and, with appropriate diet and exercise, supports weight loss efforts. The prescription medication orlistat is used in combination with a low-fat diet to help lose weight and maintain the loss by blocking the absorption of dietary fat. There are some drawbacks to obesity medications. These drugs can produce serious side effects, such as high blood pressure in the blood vessels of the lungs and valvular heart disease. The medications should be used by patients whose treatments are closely monitored by a qualified physician.
- *Surgical intervention*: In certain cases, surgery may be used to treat people with clinically severe obesity who have not lost weight by other medical therapies. One surgical technique is gastric bypass surgery, in which part of the small intestine is bypassed as food passes out of the stomach. The gastric bypass involves significant changes in how much food and drink can be consumed, and people are encouraged to learn all about the surgery before having it done. For all surgical candidates, an integrated medical program must be in place to provide guidance on diet, physical activity and support before and after the surgery. Not all people are good candidates for surgery.
- *Avoiding smoking and alcohol use*: These unhealthy strategies are often used to relieve stress. They do not solve whatever problem is at hand, and often make situations worse (e.g., by causing new health problems). By using healthy stress management

techniques instead of using alcohol excessively or smoking, individuals can reach weight loss goals more quickly.

People who are trying to shed the excess weight associated with obesity are encouraged to avoid crash diets and fasting. Crash diets that suddenly and dramatically reduce calorie intake deprive the body of important nutrients that can cause health problems. Meanwhile, fasting tends to cause weight loss that is mostly water-based and also deprives the body of important nutrients.

Physiotherapy

- *Regular exercise*: Exercise without an associated change in diet will likely reduce weight by only a few pounds. However, people who exercise regularly are more likely to adhere to a change in diet, both of which help to prevent further weight gain. Physical exercise of at least 150 minutes a week along with a balanced diet is crucial for long-term weight loss. Aerobic exercise, such as walking, swimming or stair climbing, can help to keep weight off while at the same time providing many other benefits to an individual's overall health and well-being. Even if people exercise regularly and do not lose weight, they can reduce abdominal obesity and the chances of developing cardiovascular disease, insulin resistance and high blood pressure.
- *A well-balanced diet*: For weight loss to occur, people must take in less energy (the calories taken in from the diet) than they use or burn (the calories used in daily activities and exercise). To get rid of one pound of body fat requires using or burning an additional 3,500 calories. For example, a deficit of 500 calories a day can result in losing a pound a week. For most people, a balanced diet containing no more than 2,000 calories a day for women and 2,500 for men is recommended. Crash diets are not recommended as they can end up leading to additional health problems including nutrition deficiencies.
- *Counseling*: Several studies have confirmed that obese patients who receive nutritional counseling from a dietitian achieve better weight-loss outcomes, including better metabolic control and reduced waist circumferences. In addition, some people have trouble controlling food intake not because of hunger, but because of emotional needs. People who use food to fill a feeling of emptiness, to comfort themselves or to gain a sense of control may benefit from speaking to a qualified counselor about the

situation. Inpatient programs are available, in which people stay overnight as they relearn to eat only when hungry and to satisfy emotional needs through other means.

BIBLIOGRAPHY

1. Aggarwal A, Gulati D. Early adolescent nutritional rickets. J Orthop Surg (Hong Kong). 2009;17(3):340-5.
2. Allison, DB. Annual deaths attributable to obesity in the United States, JAMA. 1999;282:1530-8.
3. Basu R. Obesity and type 2 diabetes impair insulin-induced suppression of glycogenolysis as well as gluconeogenesis, Diabetes. 2005;54(7):1942-8.
4. Beck-Nielsen SS, Brock-Jacobsen B, Gram J, Brixen K Jensen TK. Incidence and prevalence of nutritional and hereditary rickets in Southern Denmark. European Journal of Endocrinology. 2009;160(3):491-7.
5. Bogers RP, Hoogenveen RT, Boshuizen H, Woodward M, Knekt P, Van Dam RM, Hu FB, Visscher TLS, Menotti A, Thorpe RJ, Jamrozik K, Bemelmans WJE. Overweight and obesity increase the risk of coronary heart disease: A pooled analysis of 30 prospective studies. In the IEA-EEF European Congress of Epidemiology 2006 Epidemiology and Healthcare Practice, 28th June - 1st July. 2006;107.
6. Castaneda C, Munoz-Orians L, Patricia L Gordon RN, Joseph Walsmith, Mona Foldvari, Roubenoff R, Katherine L Tucker, Miriam E Nelson. A Randomized Controlled Trial of Resistance Exercise Training to Improve Glycemic Control in Older Adults With Type 2 Diabetes. Diabetes Care 2002;25(12):2335-41.
7. Chipkin S, Klugh S, Chasan-Taber L. Exercise and diabetes. Cardiology Clinics. 2001;19(3)489-505.
8. Chlebowski Rowan T, Kuller Lewis H, Prentice Ross L, Stefanick Marcia L, Manson JoAnn E, Gass Margery, Aragaki Aaron K, Ockene Judith K, Lane Dorothy S, Sartov Gloria E, Rajkovic Aleksandar, Schenken Robert, Hendrix Susan L, Ravdin Peter M, Rohan Thomas E, Yasmeen Shagufta, Anderson Garnet, the WHI Investigators. "Breast Cancer after Use of Estrogen plus Progestin in Postmenopausal Women." N Engl J Med. 2009;360(6):573-87.
9. Eckel Robert H, Krauss Ronald M. American Heart Association Call to Action: Obesity as a Major Risk Factor for Coronary Heart Disease. Circulation. 1998;97:2099-100.
10. FAO. The Developing World's New Burden: Obesity, Food and Agriculture Organization, United Nations, Geneva, Switzerland, 2002, http://www.fao.org/FOCUS/E/obesity/obes2.htm. 2002.

11. Goodman MT, Hankin JH, Wilkens LR. Diet, body size, physical activity, and the risk of endometrial cancer. Cancer Research 1997;57(22): 5077-85.
12. HARRIs RBS. Role of set-point theory in regulation of body weight. FASEB 1990;4:3310-8.
13. HB Hubert, M Feinleib, PM McNamara, WP Castelli.. Obesity as an independent risk factor for cardiovascular disease: A 26-year follow-up of participants in the Framingham Heart Study. Circulation. 1983;67:968-77.
14. Kanis JA. Osteoporosis and its consequences. In R Marcus (Ed.), Osteoporosis (pp. 1–20). Cambridge, MA: Blackwell Science. 1994.
15. Kim CJ, Kaplan LE, Perwad F, Huong N, Sharma A, Choi Y, Miller W, Portale A. Vitamin D 1α-hydroxylase gene mutations in patients with 1α-hydroxylase deficiency. Journal of Clinical Endocrinology and Metabolism. 2007;92:3177-82.
16. Lavie Carl J, Milani Richard V, Ventura Hector O. Obesity and Cardiovascular Disease: Risk Factor, Paradox, and Impact of Weight Loss. J Am Coll Cardiol. 2009;53:1925-32.
17. Link TM, Majumdar S. Osteoporosis imaging. Radiol Clin N Am. 2003;41:813-39.
18. Lips P. Which circulating level of 25-hydroxyvitamin D is appropriate? Journal of Steroid Biochemistry and Molecular Biology 2004;89-90: 611-4.
19. Meade TW, Chakrabarti R, Haines AP, North WRS, Stirling Y: Characteristics affecting fibrinolytic activity and plasma fibrinogen concentrations. Br Med J 1979;1:152.
20. NIH Consensus Development Panel on Osteoporosis Prevention and Therapy. Osteoporosis prevention, diagnosis, and therapy. JAMA. 2001;285:785-95.
21. Park YW, Zhu S, Palaniappan L, Heshka S, Carnethon MR, Heymsfield SB. The metabolic syndrome: Prevalence and associated risk factor findings in the US population from the Third National Health and Nutrition Examination Survey,1988-1994. Arch Intern Med. 2003;163:427-36.
22. Shaw NJ. Vitamin D deficiency rickets. Endocrine Development. 2003;6:93-104.
23. Stampfer MJ, Maclure KM, Colditz GA, Manson JE, Willett WC. Risk of symptomatic gallstones in women with severe obesity. American Journal of Clinical Nutrition. 1992;55:652-8.
24. Vainio H, Bianchini F. IARC handbooks of cancer prevention. Weight control and physical activity. Lyon, France: IARC Press. 2002;6.
25. Weinsier Roland L, Nagy Tim R, Hunter Gary R, Darnell Betty E, Hensrud DD, Weiss Heidi L. Do adaptive changes in metabolic rate favor weight regain in weight-reduced individuals? An examination of the set-point theory. American Journal of Clinical Nutrition. 2000;72(5):1088-94.

26. Whitaker Robert C, Wright Jeffrey A, Pepe Margaret S, Seidel Kristy D, Dietz William H. Predicting Obesity in Young Adulthood from Childhood and Parental Obesity. The New England Journal of Medicine, 1997;337(25):869-73.
27. WHO, Obesity: Preventing and Managing the Global Epidemic, Report of WHO Consultation on Obesity, Technical Report Series No. 894, World Health Organization, Geneva, Switzerland. 2000. p. 256.
28. WHO. Technical report: Assessment of fracture risk and its application to screening for postmenopausal osteoporosis. A report of a WHO study group. Geneva: World Health Organization. 1994.
29. World Health Organization. Prevention and management of osteoporosis. Technical Support Series, no. 921. Geneva, Switzerland: Author. 2003.

CHAPTER

6

Psychiatric Conditions

PSYCHOSIS

Psychosis (abnormal condition of the mind) is defined as grossly impaired reality testing which does not apply to minor distortions of reality that involve matters of relative judgments.

According to DSM-IV-TR classification (Diagnostic and Statistical Manual of Mental Disorders, year 2000 revision) of mental disorders, schizophrenia and mood disorders have been grouped separately.

SCHIZOPHRENIA

This is most common form of psychosis. This is characterized by disturbances in thought and verbal behavior, perception, affect, motor behavior and relationship to external world.

The diagnosis of schizophrenia is based entirely on the psychiatric history and mental status examination. There is no laboratory test for schizophrenia diagnosis.

Clinical Features

- Withdrawal from social relationship
- Disturbance of thought and speech—unusually long period of silence or unusual interruption in other's talks
- Failure of goal directed behavior.
- Loss of memory—most affected feature (Saykin, et al. 1994)

Disorders of Perception

- *Hallucinations*: The patient experiences sensation from any of the five senses, however actual source of the stimulation is lacking (Horowitz, 1975). He may hear sounds, or see objects which in fact are not present or exist. The visual hallucinations are most common, but tactile, gustatory, auditory (also called as paracusia) and olfactory hallucinations are uncommon.

- *Illusions*: Illusions are distortion of real images or sensations.
- Hallucinations and delusions result from the patient attributing his own actions to an external agency. This error is due to an inability to distinguish between external events and perceptual changes caused by his own actions (Chris Frith, 1996).
- Disorder of affect
- Negative symptoms
- Disorders of motor behavior example, increased or decreased psychomotor activity/spontaneity/inertia/stupor/excitement/restlessness/agitation
- *Rigidity of thoughts*: Process includes flight of ideas, thought blocking, impaired attention, poverty of thought contents, poor abstraction ability,
- Improper posture.

The symptoms must have been present for at least a week and there must have been signs of a more general disturbance for at least 6 months (Johnstone, 1991).

Clinical Types

1. *Paranoid*: Preoccupied with the one or more delusion. It is characterized by tense, suspicious, guarded, reserved and sometime aggressive behavior.
2. *Hebephrenic*: Also known as disorganized type schizophrenia. It is characterized by marked regression to primitive, uninhibited and unorganized behavior. Common age is before 25 year.
3. *Catatonic*: Marked disturbance in motor function. May include stupor, rigidity, posturing, excitement, negativism.
4. *Residual*: Absent of true symptoms. Eccentric behavior, emotional blunting, illogical thinking are common features.
5. *Undifferentiated*: When patient does not exhibit the clear features of any of the above mentioned variety of schizophrenia.
6. *Simple schizophrenia*: Characterized by gradual insidious loss of drive and ambition, withdrawal from social and work related situations.

Etiology

Genetic factors: Not well-established, however some genes are linked to be responsible for schizophrenia (Owen M, 2007).

- Biochemical theories
- Altered neurophysiology

- Stress psychological theories
- Sleep deprivation has also been associated with the psychosis (Chan-ob, 1999; Sharma, et al. 2003).

Management

The strategy used for the management of psychosis depends on the clinical type, clinical presentation, severity of symptoms and the underlying pathology.

Antipsychotic medications may be the first line of management and sometimes hospitalization is needed.

Cognitive behavior therapy is being used effectively for management of psychotic symptoms (Cooper and Mick, 2008). This includes goal oriented systematic procedure to manage dysfunctional emotions. It includes multiple methods of behavior therapy and cognitive therapy. It is a very slow process and need to recognize the client's thought, reactions, feelings, behavior associated with different events. This is possible by maintaining a diary by patient himself to clearly document these responses. The client has to learn when the responses and thought go out of control. Relaxation, distraction, thought stopping, mental diversion are common methods used for behavioral modification. These treatments may be used as adjunct to the pharmacological treatments, antidepressant drugs and the mood stabilizing medicines.

The severe cases associated with depression may need the ECT (electroconvulsive therapy) to alleviate depression.

Schizophrenic patients need a very long period of supportive environment at family.

During management must—establish eye to eye contact, to make sure they are paying proper attention to your commands. Expose them with the practical situation. Show them that you felt good when they cooperated your commands. May give the feedback, reinforcing, praise for their compliance and cooperation.

A method to improve neurocognitive functioning is an important step in improving rehabilitation outcomes. When neurocognitive deficits are targeted for direct intervention, it is thought that gains in functioning may be made and that such gains will enhance the success of other rehabilitation effort (Silverstein, et al. 2001).

Method to deal with neurocognitive deficits in schizophrenia involves dichotic listening to demonstrate auditory selective attention deficits (Silverstein, et al. 2001) in schizophrenia, and also to enable patients to practice attending to relevant stimuli and ignoring irrelevant stimuli (Spaulding, et al. 1986). In dichotic listening, two different auditory stimuli (usually speech) are presented to the participant simultaneously, one to each ear, normally using a set of headphones. Participants are asked to attend to one or (in a divided-attention experiment) both of the messages. They may later be asked about the content of either message (Wikipedia, 2010).

The most widely reported approach to neurocognitive remediation of schizophrenia has been group-based therapy as developed by Brenner, et al. (1994). This intervention targets skills in a hierarchical fashion, beginning with conceptual differentiation (executive functioning) and moving through social perception, verbal communication, basic social skills, and interpersonal problem-solving segments. Skills are targeted through group practice and problem solving using a series of exercises that increase in complexity over time (Silverstein, et al. 2001). However, this is not an appropriate treatment for patients with severe attention impairment.

Previous studies support the use of behavioral techniques to improve cognition.

These methods may include:

- Monetary reinforcement for correct responding to improve performance of attention (Kern et al. 1995)
- Operant procedures to increase attention span during brief, structured social interactions (Massel et al. 1991)
- The reinforcement schedule and contingencies may be tailored as per the client's level of functioning. Progression is made by systematic and gradual approach, and this really can make performance more meaningful (Silverstein, et al. 1991).
- Shaping procedures as neurocognitive rehabilitation methods allows the clinician/researcher to achieve these goals. Shaping is the application of several fundamental techniques of learning to bring about new behavior or to modify a certain aspect of an existing behavior (Silverstein, 2001). As such, shaping can be viewed as a method to achieve operant conditioning, with attention being the response that is targeted. The primary technique involved is differential reinforcement of successive approximations (Silverstein, et al. 1991).

In acute phase they may be under the strong influence of some auditory and visual delusions. Therefore in acute stage too much of auditory and visual stimuli must be avoided as it creates more confusion and tendency to regress instead of cooperation.

Chronic cases of Schizophrenia may have associated depression with this condition. Such patients have:

- Greater need for counseling, thus detailed history must be documented.
- It is important to settle a rapport with patient, and relax his anxiety thus must devote adequate time to the patient.

MOOD DISORDERS

A mood disorder involves the disturbance of person's mood, and this may lead to underlying features. The word is introduced by the DSM IV TR classification system.

Classification of Mood Disorders

- Manic episode
- Depressive episode
- Bipolar mood disorder
- Persistent mood disorder
- Other mood disorder.

Clinical Features

- Manic episode
  - Elevated, expansive or irritable mood, euphoric
  - Elated mood
  - Increased psychomotor activity, e.g. restless, overactive, manic stupor
  - Increase talkative
  - Decreased sleep
- Depressive episode
  - Loss of interest
  - Depressive ideation/cognition
  - Anxiety
- Psychomotor activity
  - Decreased in younger patient (less than 40 years)
  - Restlessness, agitation, etc. in older patients

- Headache, vague body symptoms, body ache, etc.
- Delusion, hallucination in severe form
- Tendency to commit suicide.

Etiology

- Genetic hypothesis
- Biochemical theories
- Neuroendocrine theory
- Sleep abnormalities
- Brain changes
- Stress
- Psychosocial theories.

Management

- Antidepressants
- ECT
- Lithium
- Antipsychotics
- Psychosocial treatments
- Cognitive behavior therapy
- Behavior therapy
- Group therapy
- Counseling
- Rehabilitation.

NEUROTIC STRESS-RELATED AND SOMATOFORM DISORDER

Sometime, the mental disorder may be manifested by physical symptoms and may mimic some physical disease or injury, whose cause cannot be identified. Since these features are not due to underlying organic pathology therefore the medical laboratory tests are either normal or don't reveal the cause of symptoms.

- Phobic anxiety disorders
- Other anxiety disorders
- OC disorders
- Reaction to stress and adjustment disorders
- Dissociative disorders
- Somatoform disorders
- Other neurotic disorders.

■ DEMENTIA

Dementia is a pathological condition characterized by the significant deterioration of person's cognitive ability in otherwise normal individual. This is significantly more while compared to that what could be expected due to normal aging process.

Meaning of the word "dementia" is "deprived of mind". Dementia is a non-specific problem and includes signs and symptoms according to the affected areas of brain. Accordingly the features may involve impaired memory, language, personality, attention and problem solving (rationale thinking).

Etiology

- Parenchymal brain disease
- Vascular dementia
- Tonic dementia
- Metabolic dementia
- Endocrine causes
- Deficiency dementia
- Dementia due to infection
- Neoplastic dementia
- Hydrocephalic dementia.

Clinical Features

- Impaired intellectual functions
- Impairment of memory
- Neglect of self care
- Delusions
- Disorientation
- Emotionally labile
- Impaired thinking.

Physiotherapy Management

The aim of physiotherapy is to enhance information processing and thus improve motor reaction.

It must be kept in mind that most of dementia patients involve the aged population therefore the physiotherapy interventions don't significantly differ from the other interventions of the elders, however the methods of intervention may vary for each of these two set of people.

The interest of the client must always be born in mind.

Common techniques used while dealing with dementia patients are:

- Body awareness training
- Functional mobility training
- Music and movement therapy
- Sitting and positioning for activity and comfort
- Vocational training.

PHYSIOTHERAPY MANAGEMENT FOR GENERAL PSYCHIATRIC CONDITIONS

Framework used in physiotherapy interventions in mental health which provide a conceptual basis for analyzing patient's condition and choosing preferred line of treatment.

- Transfer of training framework
- Sensory integration framework
- Rehabilitative frame of reference
- Compensatory frame of reference
- Cognitive rehabilitation frame of reference
- Biomechanical frame of reference for associated motor deficits
- Neurological rehabilitative frame of reference.

Physiotherapy Treatment Approaches

- Remedial
- Adaptive/compensatory
- Patient, family, caregiver and significant other's education.

Physiotherapy Assessment in Mental Health

- History
  - Medical history
    - History of present illness
    - Past psychiatric history
    - Treatment history
  - Family history
  - Personal History
    - Perinatal history
    - Childhood history
    - Play history
    - Occupational history
    - Sexual and marital history
    - Premorbid personality

- Mental status examination
  - General appreanece and behavior
  - Speech
    - Rate and quantity
    - Volume and tone
    - Flow and rhythm
  - Mood and affect
  - Thought
    - Stream and form
    - Content
  - Perception
  - Cognition
    - Consciousness
    - Orientation
    - Attention
    - Concentration
    - Memory
    - Intelligence
    - Abstract thinking
  - Insight
  - Judgment
- Standardized cognitive and perceptual assessment
  - Canadian occupational performance measure
  - Short form health survey
  - Reintegration of normal living index (RNL)
  - Functional independence measure (FIM)
  - Allen cognitive level test (ACL)
  - Rivermed behavioral memory test
- Regular neuro-motor/biomechanical assessments
  - Motor strength and tone
  - Gait
  - MMT
  - Coordination
  - Contracture/deformity
  - Endurance
  - BADL and IADL
  - Cardiopulmonary examination
  - Sensory examination
  - Posture (dynamic and static)
  - Biomechanical assessments

Physiotherapeutic Intervention

- For increased psychomotor activity
  - Heavy resistance training with other precautions.
- For restlessness
  - Relaxation techniques (Jacobson progressive relaxation techniques)
  - Exercise therapy
  - Breathing exercises
  - Biofeedback
- Lack of concentration
  - Fine motor skill
  - Medication
  - Relaxation
  - Puzzles
- Low, depressive mood
  - Distraction activity
  - Jogging
  - Therapeutic play/music/art
  - group exercise/therapy
- Inactivity
  - Group therapy
  - Scheduling and charting routine
  - Maintaining activity
  - Conditioning methods
  - Mild aerobic exercise training
- Phobia and anxiety
  - Biofeedback
  - Environmental modifications
  - Relaxation technique
  - breathing technique
  - distractive exercise /activities
  - conditioning methods (operant and classical conditioning)
- Panic attacks
  - Respiratory control techniques
  - Distraction
  - Biofeedback
  - Relaxation
  - Meditative techniques
  - Graded activity and exercises
  - Environmental modification
  - Cognitive behavioral techniques
- Cognitive perceptual intervention.

Finding a method to improve neurocognitive functioning is an important step in improving rehabilitation outcomes (Silverstein, 2001).

- Memory cueing for patients
- Family, caregiver education
- Mnemonics
- Environmental modification
- Rehearsal
- Visual imagery
- Semantic elaboration
- Body imaging
- Flow charts for daily tasks
- Environmental modifications.

Visual Perception and Praxis Interventions

- Environmental/contextual modifications
  - Lighting
  - Contrast
  - Color
  - Pattern
  - Print size
  - Working distance
  - Magnification
- Ocular motor exercises
- Visual scanning training
- Sensori-motor experience reinforcement along with visual experience
- Spatio-motor cueing
- Constraint induced therapy (visual patching)
- Body awareness training
- Tactile cues

Behavioral Disorders

- Behavior modification techniques
- Group therapy
- Conditioning techniques (operant and classical conditioning)
- Cognitive adaptation training (Velligan and Bow-Thomas 2000)

Obsession/Compulsion/Delusion

- Environmental modification
- Conditioning techniques
- Cognitive behavioral therapy

- Cognitive enhancement therapy (Hogarty and Flesher 1999)
- Graded group therapy
- Relaxation techniques
- Biofeedback.

Affective Symptoms

- Rapport building
- Conditioning
- Rationale-emotive technique
- Distraction
- Group work
- Cognitive behavioral techniques
- Interpersonal therapy
- Family and marital therapy.

Physical/Biomechanical Interventions

- Exercise therapy
- Deformity correction
- Strengthening
- Tone normalization
- Gait training
- Postural correction
- Sensory re-education
- Coordination training.

BIBLIOGRAPHY

1. Chan-Ob, Boonyanaruthee. "Meditation in association with psychosis". Journal of the Medical Association of Thailand. 1999;82(9):925-30.
2. Chris Frith. Neuropsychology of schizophrenia: What are the implications of intellectual and experiential abnormalities for the neurobiology of schizophrenia? British Medical Bulletin. 1996;52(2): 618-26.
3. Cooper and Mick. Essential Research Findings in Counselling and Psychotherapy: The Facts are Friendly. 2008.
4. Dichotic listening. From Wikipedia, the free encyclopedia. http://en.wikipedia.org/wiki/Dichotic_listening. Accessed on. 2010;15:8.
5. Hogarty GE, Flesher S. Practice principles of cognitive enhancement therapy for schizophrenia. Schizophrenia Bulletin. 1999;25(4):693-708.
6. Horowitz MJ. "Hallucinations: An Information Processing Approach". in West LJ, Siegel RK. Hallucinations; behavior, experience, and theory. New York: Wiley. 1975.

7. Jeffrey Poland (2002). DSM-IV Sourcebook. Review of book by Thomas A Widiger, Allen J Francis, Harold Alan Pincus, Ruth Ross, Michael B First, Wendy Wakefield Davis. American Psychiatric Association, 1996.
8. Johnstone EC. Disabilities and circumstances of schizophrenic patients-a follow-up study. Br Journal of Psychiatry 1991;159(Suppl 13).
9. Kern RS, Green MF, Goldstein MJ. Modification of performance on the span of apprehension, a putative vulnerability marker to schizophrenia. Journal of Abnormal Psychology. 1995;104:385-9.
10. Massel HK, Corrigan PW, Liberman RP, Milan MA. Conversation skills training of thought-disordered schizophrenic patients through attention focusing. Psychiatry Research. 1991;38:51-61.
11. Owen MJ, Craddock N, Jablensky A. The genetic deconstruction of psychosis. Schizophr Bull 2007;33:905-11.
12. Saykin AJ, Shtasel DL, Gur RE. Neuropsychological deficits in neuroleptic naive patients with first-episode schizophrenia. Arch Gen Psychiatry. 1994;51:124-31.
13. Sharma Verinder, Dwight Mazmanian. 2003. Retrieved 2006-09-27.
14. Silverstein SM, Anthony AH, Paul Stuve. Shaping attention span: an operant conditioning procedure to improve neurocognition and functioning in schizophrenia. Schizophrenia Bulletin. 2001;27:2.
15. Spaulding WD, Storms L, Goodrich V, Sullivan M. Applications of experimental psychopathology in psychiatric rehabilitation. Schizophrenia Bulletin. 1986;12(4):560-77.
16. Velligan DI, Bow-Thomas CC. Two case studies of cognitive adaptation training for outpatients with schizophrenia. Psychiatric Services. 2000;51:25-9.

CHAPTER

7

Respiratory Conditions

INTRODUCTION

Respiration term means the exchange of gases between body and environment, between different cells, and the metabolic process to release energy from the food particles. Depending on the level of consideration of gas exchange it can be classified as follows:

At cellular level respiration means the metabolic processes whereby certain organisms obtain energy from organic molecules; processes that take place in the cells and tissues during which energy is released and carbon dioxide is produced and absorbed by the blood to be transported to the lungs.

The breathing means respiration is a general term used to describe gas exchange within the body and can be categorized as either external respiration or internal respiration.

External respiration involves gas exchange between environment and respiratory organs. A single complete act of breathing in and out is considered to be single cycle of respiration. The bodily process of inhalation and exhalation; the process of taking in oxygen from inhaled air and releasing carbon dioxide by exhalation. This is also called as ventilation. It involves the coordinated activity between different muscles, ribs cage movements, costo-vertebral movements, upper and lower respiratory tract.

Internal respiration involves gaseous exchange between pulmonary capillaries and the tissues lying in immediate surroundings. During this the fresh oxygen from arterial blood diffuses into the tissues for oxygen utilization, and the carbon dioxide from the tissues is diffused into the capillaries.

STRUCTURE OF HUMAN RESPIRATORY SYSTEM

Upper Respiratory Tract

The upper respiratory tract is made of nasal cavity, pharynx and larynx.

Nasal Cavity and Pharynx

- The function of the nasal cavity and pharynx is:
  - To filter off to remove the dust particles from the inspired air by entrapping them in hair of the passage
  - To humidify the inspired air so as to avoid the drying of the nasal mucosa
  - To warm the inspired air to the body temperature level. This is possible by the vascular supply of the nasal mucosa
  - The cilia and mucus lining of the nasal cavity passage trap and remove the foreign particles from inspired air
  - During illness or by breathing through mouth, the mucosa of nasal cavity dry out, the cilliary movement gets inhibited due to increased viscosity
  - The posterior wall of pharynx when irritated, elicits the protective cough reflex to avoid any foreign material to enter into the respiratory tract.

Larynx

During inspiration it contracts to close the epiglottis and preventing the entering of food, foreign particles into trachea.

Lower Respiratory Tract

It consists of the respiratory tract beyond nasopharynx, and is made of tracheobronchial tree and the terminal respiratory units (Fig. 7.1). The tracheobronchial tree consists of the conducting branches which are made of approximately intial 16 branch generations and the respiratory branches which are made of millions alveoli and make terminal 6 branch generations of tree.
The lower respiratory tract consists of followings:

Trachea

- Rounded, flexible tube having semicircular rings in anterior wall. The posterior wall is smooth and has ciliated epithelial cells and goblet cells to secret mucus
- Trachea bifurcates into bronchi.

Mainstem Bronchi

- The right one is vertical and large diameter, while the left one is oblique and relatively lesser in diameter

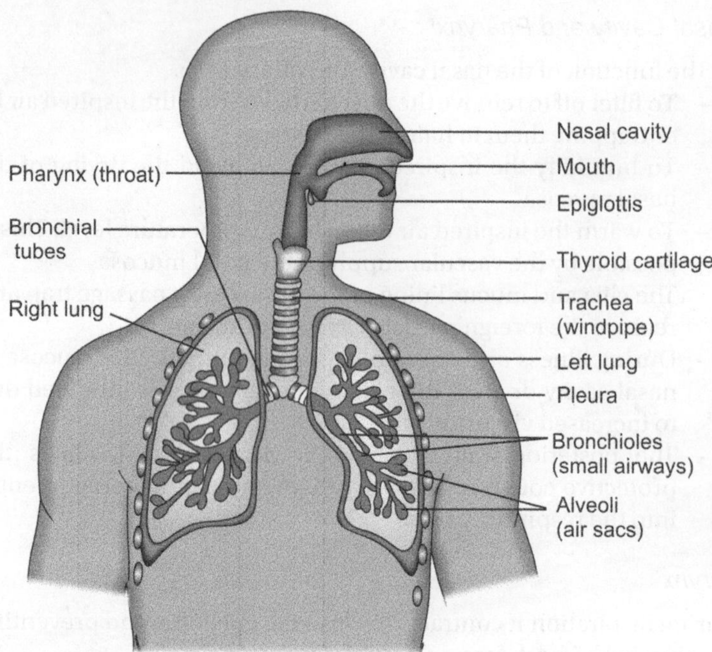

Fig. 7.1: Components of respiratory system in human

- The right bronchi further branches into three lobar bronchi for the three lobes of right lung
- The left bronchi further branches into two lobar bronchi for the two lobes of left lung.

Lobar Bronchi

Lobar bronchi are three on right side and two on left side. Have greater amount of cartilage thus they keep the airway to each lobe of lung patent.

Segmental Bronchi

- There are 10 segmental bronchi on the right and 8 on the left
- They have scattered hyaline cartilage for maintaining patency, smooth muscle for allowing the constriction and dilation, elastic fibers, and a capillary network (Gartner 2001).

Bronchioles (Fig. 7.2)

- Segmental bronchi divide into bronchioles
- These have less cartilage and ciliated epithelial cells.

Terminal Bronchioles

- Bronchioles divide into the terminal bronchioles which don't have ciliated cells
- They branch repeatedly and form respiratory bronchioles which form alveolar ducts having smooth muscles and narrow lumen.
- These duct lead into alveoli

Alveoli (Fig. 7.2)

- These are balloon like structures which are millions in number and are supplied by alveolar ducts and sacs. These provide the interface for the gaseous exchange to occur at alveolar-arterial membrane, between the lungs and the surrounding environment.

Function of the Lower Respiratory Tract

- The lower respiratory tract conducts air to and from the alveolar system for gas exchange.

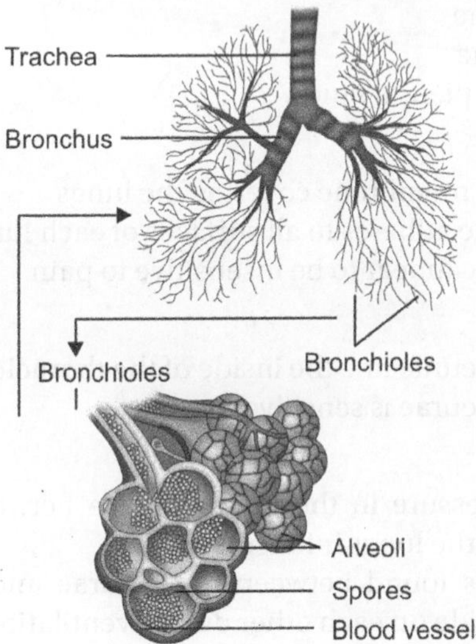

Fig. 7.2: Structure of trachea-bronchial tree and alveoli

- Responds to the stimulus for the cough reflex to clear the larger airways.

The Lungs and Pleurae

The gross anatomy of respiratory system includes lungs and pleurae.

Lungs

Lungs are the basic organs of human respiration. Lungs are made up of the following components:
The right lung consists of:
- Three lobes—the upper, middle and lower
- Ten bronchopulmonary segments.

The left lung consists of:
- Two true lobes—the upper and lower—and a slip of lung called the lingual
- Eight bronchopulmonary segments
- Lingual is not considered a "true" lobe of the lungs.

Pleurae

Pleurae is the covering of each lung. Pleurae are made up of the following components:
- Visceral pleurae
- Parietal pleurae
- Pleural space (pleural fluid).

Visceral pleurae
- It is the serous membrane covering the lungs
- This membrane adheres to all surfaces of each lung
- Visceral pleura appear to be insensitive to pain.

Parietal pleurae
- The parietal pleurae line the inside of the thoracic wall
- The parietal pleurae is sensitive to pain.

Pleural space
- A negative pressure in the minute space between the pleurae serves to keep the lungs inflated.

Pleural fluid is found between the pleurae and lubricates the pleurae as they slide on each other during ventilation.

Thorax and Chest Wall: Structure and Function

The structure of thoracic cage (chest wall):

- Along the posterior aspect of the thorax, the dorsal portions of the ribs articulate with the 12 thoracic vertebrae at the costotransverse and costovertebral joints.
- Along the anterior aspect of the thoracic cage, the first to seventh ribs articulate directly with the sternum via the costal cartilage.
- The eighth to tenth ribs have cartilaginous attachments to the rib above, whereas the eleventh and twelfth are floating ribs.

The main functions of the thoracic cage (chest wall) are:

- The thoracic cage protects the internal organs of respiration, circulation and digestion.
- The thoracic cage provides the site of attachment for the muscles of ventilation to mechanically enlarge the thorax for inspiration or to compress the thorax for expiration and thus participates in ventilation of the lungs.
- The thoracic cage provides site of attachment for upper extremity muscles, which function during lifting, pulling, or pushing activities.

Muscles of Ventilation (Respiratory Muscles)

The muscles responsible for the respiration have their attachements on thorax and ribs, and by their action they regulate the movement of air into and out from the lungs during inspiration and expiration respectively. These muscles can be classified as primary or accessory muscles. The primary inspiratory muscles are those which are recruited during tidal breathing and include the diaphragm muscle, scalene and the external intercostals muscles.

The diaphragm is main inspiratory muscle and is supplied by phrenic nerve having root value C3, C4, C5. This muscle alone can carry out the 70–80% of the whole work of breathing in tidal breathing state. This causes the vertical increase in the thoracic cavity size during inspiration, as due to its contraction the central tendon is pulled downward to become flatten from its dome-shaped position. During inspiration air flows through specific path (Flow chart 7.1).

The scalene muscles start contracting during onset of inspiration and may contract even stronger when diaphragm is weak. The scalene lifts the first two ribs and pulls the sternum upward and forward to increase the AP and lateral diameter of thoracic cavity by "pump-handle movment" (Fig. 7.3).

Flow chart 7.1: Path air takes in respiratory tract

The oxygen rich fresh air is inspired in via nasal cavity

↓

After filteratiion, warming and the humidification via upper respiratory tract This air enters nasopharynx, larynx, and then directed into trachea

↓

The air is further filtered by cilia in trachea, also the mucus in trachea removes dust particles or any foreign particle

↓

Air enters into bronchi, then segmental brochioles, respiratory brochioles and then into alveoli

↓

At alveoli-capillary, the capillary lining has more carbon dioxide and less oxygen. At this interface the oxygen from the inspired oxygen rich fresh air gets diffused into the capillaries of the opposing membrane, the corbon dioxide diffuses back in reverse direction

↓

The air having higher quantity of carbon dioxide now leaves lungs, moves upward and finally expired out of lungs via upper respiratory tract

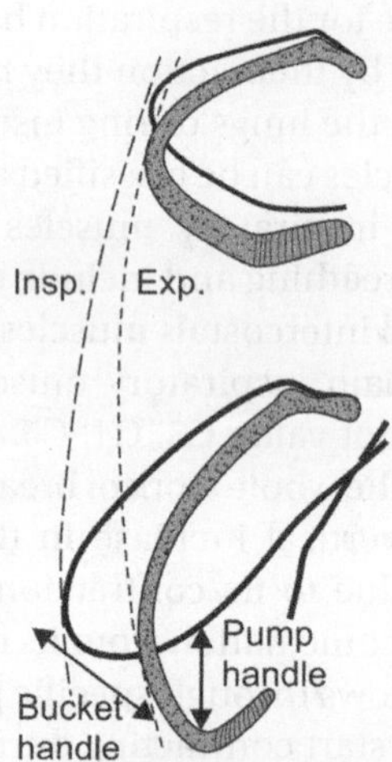

Fig. 7.3: Pump-handle movement of ribs during inspiration

Accessory muscles of inspiration are those which are recruited only during deep, forced, or labored breathing. These include those which can further increase the diameter of thoracic cavity to create negative pressure inside lungs to pull the air inward. These muscles include sternocleidomastoid, trapezius, pectorals (minor and major), subclavius.

There are no primary expiratory muscles as expiration is a passive process which occurs due to recoiling back of the diaphragm tendon in resting state. However, during forceful expiration the accessory muscles may play role which include rectus abdominis, transverse abdominis, obliques (internal and external), pectoralis major, quadrates lumborum and internal intercostals. Thus forceful expiration is an active type of expiration.

The movements of pump handle and bucket handle components of rotation progressively decrease as the number of measured level of ribs increases. The value of pump handle movement is around 11degree and that of bucket handle movement is about13 degrees at third rib level. Their value decreases up to level of 7th rib to 7 and 10 degrees respectively (Wilson, et al. 1997).

The composition of air that we breathe in is:

- Nitrogen — 78%
- Oxygen — 21%
- Carbon dioxide — 0.03 - 0.04%
- Hydrogen — traces
- Noble gases — traces.

Lung Volumes and Capacities

The pulmonary function testing essentially deals with the documentation of various volumes and capacities related to lungs. The lung volumes and capacities may be varied by age, gender, body weight, disease, training or deconditioning. Values of these volumes and capacities are important to reflect any pathological process and the mechanical functioning of lung tissues.

The various terms associated with the pulmonary function testing and the spirometry (Fig. 7.4) are as follows:

- Tidal volume (TV)
  - It is the volume of air inspired and expired during relaxed breathing at rest.

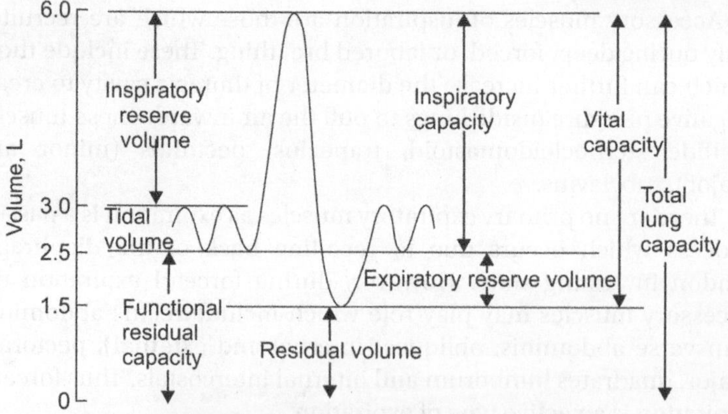

Fig. 7.4: Various volumes and capacities related to pulmonary functioning

- Tidal inspiration is the air, which is inspired in during respiration at rest.
- Tidal expiration is the air, which is expired out during respiration at rest.
- Its value is approximately 500 mL
- Approximately 350 mL of this tidal volume reaches the alveoli and participates in gas exchange.

• Inspiratory reserve volume (IRV)
  - It is the amount of air that can be further forcefully inspired in after the end of a tidal inspiration (approximately 3000 mL).

• Expiratory reserve volume (ERV)
  - ERV is the amount of air that can be further exhaled forcefully after the end of tidal expiration (approximately 1000 mL).

• Residual volume (RV)
  - It is the amount of air left in the lungs after a maximum expiration (approximately 1500 mL).
  - RV increases with age, restrictive and obstructive pulmonary diseases.

• Inspiratory capacity (IC)
  - It is the maximum amount of air that can be breathed in after a resting expiration. This is the combined result of TV and IRV (approximately 3000+500=3500 mL).

• Functional residual capacity (FRC)

- It is total amount of air remaining in the lungs after a resting (tidal) expiration (approximately 2500 mL).
- It is the sum of the ERV and RV.

• Vital capacity (VC)
  - The maximum amount of air which can be inspired in and then expired out forcefully after the end of tidal expiration. Vital capacity (VC) is the sum of the TV, IRV, and ERV (approximately 4500 mL).

• Total lung capacity (TLC)
  - TLC is the total amount of air contained in the lungs after a maximum inspiration. It is approximately 6000 mL in a healthy young adult. TLC is the combined result of four volumes, which are TV, IRV, ERV and RC.

Mechanics of Ventilation

During inspiration the thorax enlarges in all three planes due to the:

• *Increased anteroposterior (AP) diameter* of chess wall. This occurs by the pumb-handle movement (Fig. 7.3) of the ribs at costovertebral joints. This projects the sterna forward along with the reduction in the thoracic kyphosis.

• *Increased lateral/transverse dimensions of the thorax cavity*: It occurs due to the elevation and the outward turning of the midshaft portions of the ribs. This occurs by the bucket-handle motion when the ribs flare/open outward by the increase in the costo-chondral junction. This occurs due to the movement of the lower ribs (8–10 ribs).

• *Increase in vertical dimension of thoracic cavity*: The vertical dimension of the thoracic cavity increases when the diaphragm contracts to pull the central dome downward, by piston action. This dimension further is increased by the elevation of ribs.

These three increases in dimensions are initiated by the muscular efforts therefore inspiration is considered to be an active process. Due to the increase in all three dimensions the negative pressure is generated inside the thoracic cavity because the pressure inside thoracic cavity is lower than the atmosphere, and this tends to suck the air in from the outer environment.

At the end of inspiration, the expiration process starts where the contracted muscles relax. The diaphragm relaxes and the flattened tendon returns back to its dome shape, this recoiling reduces the vertical diameter of the thoracic cavity. The elevation of ribs and the forward projection of sternum return to their neutral state and thus the transverse and AP dimensions too reduce. The overall result is the reduction of the size of thoracic cavity, and the increased pressure inside the thorax. This increased pressure in the thorax causes the air to move out of lungs. Thus the expiration is resulted from the relaxation of those muscles which contracted at the time of inspiration. Thus expiration is considered to be a passive process.

RESPIRATORY NEURAL CONTROL

The neuronal control of breathing is separate during inspiratory and expiratory phases. This control involves the respiratory control nuclei located in the medulla and pons. The ventral medullary nuclei control the voluntary forced exhalation and acts to increase the force of inspiration (Fig. 7.5). Dorsal medullary nuclei control the timing and movement of inspiration.

Medullary center is responsible for controlling the automatic breathing, consists of I neuron for inspiratory signaling and E neurons for expiratory signaling.

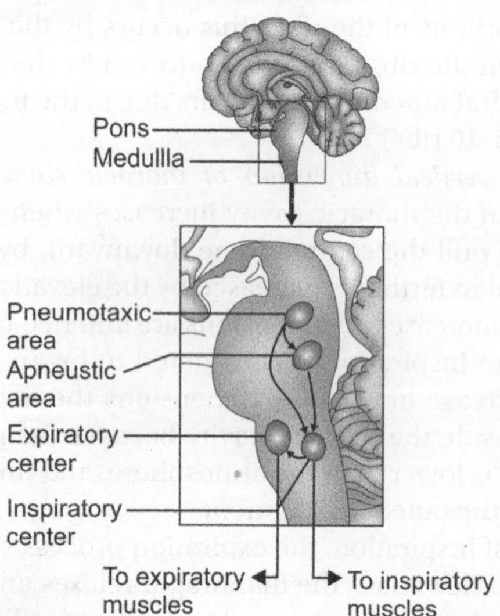

Fig. 7.5: The neural control of respiration

- I neurons — stimulate neurons that innervate respiratory muscles (to bring about inspiration)
- E neurons — inhibit I neurons (to 'shut down' the I neurons and bring about expiration).

Pontine apneustic center stimulates I neuron to facilitate inspiratory process and prolongs inspiratory phase during long deep breath. The pontine pneumotaxic center inhibits apneustic center, and thus inhibits inspiratory process. Pneumotaxic center is also responsible for fine tuning of respiratory rate.

RESPIRATORY CHEMICAL CONTROL

The chemical control of the respiration is also very important. This is based on the relative amount of oxygen and carbon dioxide in

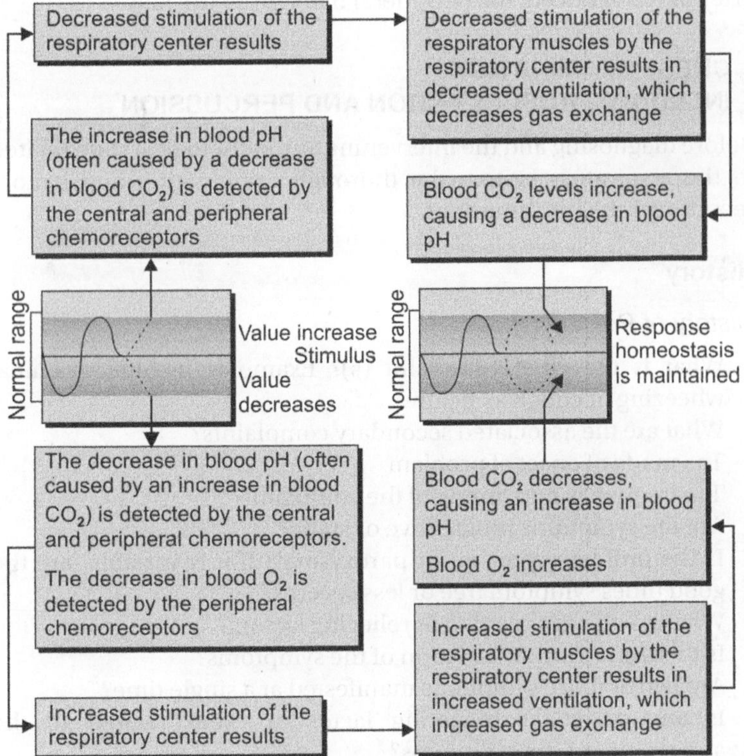

Fig. 7.6: Chemical control of respiration

the blood. The chemical control of respiration is exerted by blood pH, oxygen concentration in arteries, level of carbon dioxide in blood (Fig. 7.6). Chemoreceptors for respiration are located in carotid artery and arch of aorta. Receptors located near arch of aorta respond to level of oxygen in blood, while those located in the medulla respond to level of carbon dioxide in blood. The control of respiration by nervous system and chemical control works by negative feedback mechanism. As the oxygen consumption in body exceeds the rate of removal of carbon dioxide, the accumulation of CO_2 starts in body.

As the concentration of oxygen in blood falls or the concentration of carbon dioxide in blood rises, the respiratory drive is increased which in turn increases the depth and rate of respiration to wash out excessively accumulated carbon dioxide. When the carbon dioxide level in blood falls, the vasoconstricting influence of this CO_2 on arterioles is reduced, the peripheral blood pressure falls.

CHEST EXAMINATION, INCLUDING AUSCULTATION AND PERCUSSION

Before diagnosing and the intervening any pathological state related to the respiratory system the thorough examination and history recording is highly important.

History

History of Present Illness

- What is the chief complaint (s)? Examples include dyspnea, wheezing or cough as below.
- What are the associated secondary complaints?
- The mode of onset of problem
- The frequency and timing of the complaint?
- Are the symptoms progressive or static?
- Is the problem constant or paroxysmal? If it is variable, are the good times symptom free or less severe?
- What are the aggravating or relieving factors?
- Is there any diurnal variation of the symptoms?
- Are two or more symptoms manifested at a single time?
- Is any particular triggering factor or event related to the appearance of the symptoms?

- How severely does it affect the patient's life (quality of life questionnaire, satisfaction levels need to be documented)?
- History of sudden, unexplained weight loss or fever for prolonged time?

History of Past Illness

- Is there particular history related to any pathology?
- Has the client been diagnosed with some other medical pathology in past?
- How the previous pathology managed?
- To what extent the symptoms of previous pathology have been recovered?
- In the past, had there been any history of asthma, wheezing, recurrent fever, malignancy, tuberculosis, sudden onset chest pain, recurrent chest pain or recurrent breathlessness
- Does the client had any history of any particular allergen? Do the symptoms vary with some particular factors like pollens, dust, food, drugs, seasonal transition?

Drug History

- What all medications has the client received in past?
- Any history of use of inhalers, steroids, other drugs.

Family History of Disease

Some respiratory diseases such as asthma, emphysema, allergic conditions and cystic fibrosis can have genetic cause. This needs to be documented carefully.

Some other diseases may be contagious and might be spread from the other members of family. Example tuberculosis, viral fever may spread from the infected member of the family

Examination

On the basis of the history, the probable set of causative conditions have been usually shortlisted before examination. These possible conditions may be further narrowed down on the basis of examination. The examination also helps down to determine the required investigations.

The examination consists of observation, auscultation, percussion and the palpation.

Observation

- Is the patient conscious and oriented?
- Is the breathing spontaneous or it is assisted?
- Look any sign of labored breathing. If excessive usage of accessory muscles is done then these muscle will be prominent.
- Look at the skin, chin to find any indication of unexplained significant weight loss.
- Look out for any sign of peripheral or central cyanosis. In case of central cyanosis the lips and the oral mucosa appear bluish. The central cyanosis results when at least 5 mg of deoxygenated hemoglobin is present per 100 mL of blood. In case of peripheral cyanosis the lips and oral mucosa are normally colored but the nail bed may appear bluish
- Look out for sign of central and peripheral edema. In case of central cause of edema, the massive and multiple regions of edema will be apparent. Also the pitting may be evident due to the excessive protein accumulation. In case of peripheral edema usually one particular extremity may reveal fluid accumulation.
- If edema is apparent then look out for the surrounding veins enlargement or the enlargement of the associated lymph node.
- Type of breathing need to be carefully observed. Is the breathing spontaneous? Is the client struggling for breathing? Does the client appear exhausted and tired due to excessive labored breathing?
- Is the patient relaxed or seems excessively anxious? Is the respiratory rate normal, or excessive or significantly low?
- Is the breathing normal or it is associated with the wheezing or rhonchi?
- Is the chest wall movement normal or less or excessively during breathing?
- Does the chest appears hyperinflated or barrel shaped? Is there any evidence of pigeon chest, or drawing in of chest?
- Is there any evidence of paradoxical breathing?
- Is there any evidence of the change of nail shape? Is there any clubbing or parrot beaking of the finger? Are nail shape normal or altered?
- Look out for any prominent lymph nodes in neck region.
- Is there any abnormal deviation of spine in sagittal or coronal plane? If deviation is present, is it structural or the correctable deviation?

Tactile Examination

- Carefully check the radial pulse. Check for the pulse volume, rhythm, fibrillation. Is the pulse rhythmic and regular, or it is thread and shaky?
- Is body temperature normal? Or is it hyperpyrexia?
- Is there any asymmetry between the chest wall movement of both side?
- Is the chest expansion adequate or it is less than normal? May use the inch tape method to document the chest wall expansion at different levels? (Figs 7.7A and B)
- Is there any evidence of the deviation of the trachea from its normal central position?

Percussion

Percussion is performed by keeping the non-dominant hand over the testing region of chest wall, and then taping the middle finger of this hand by the middle/index finger of dominant hand (Fig. 7.8). The area thus examined includes the regions overlying different lobes of lungs. During percussion, the type, intensity and quality of sound is recorded. This may have clinical implications.

The dull sound may indicate collapse or the consolidation of the underlying lobe. The high resonating sound may reveal the hyperinflation due to entrapment of air in the lungs.

Auscultation

Auscultation is performed with the help of stethoscope to hear the various abnormal or abnormal breathing sounds. This is important

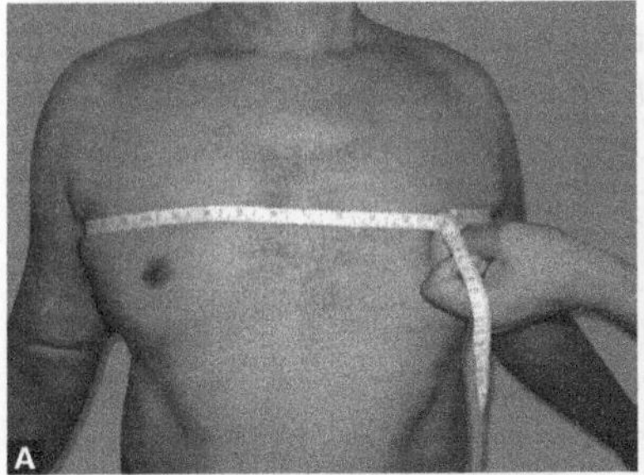

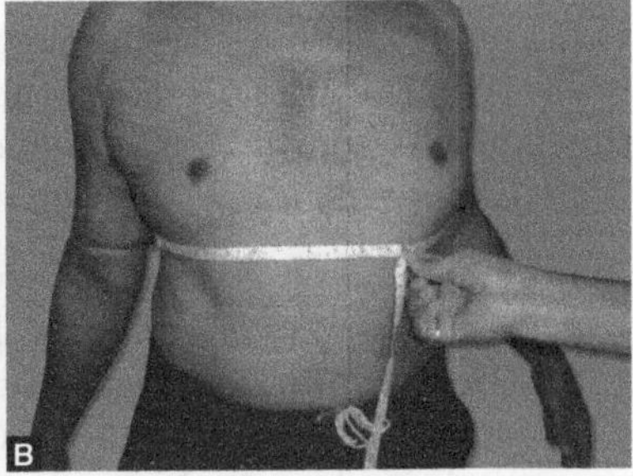

Figs 7.7A and B: Measurement of chest expansion at different levels: (A) For upper lateral coastal expansion; (B) For lower lateral coastal measurement

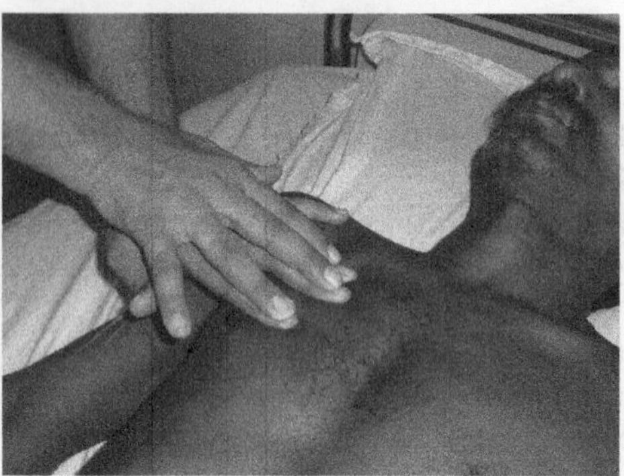

Fig. 7.8: The method to perform percussion of respiratory system

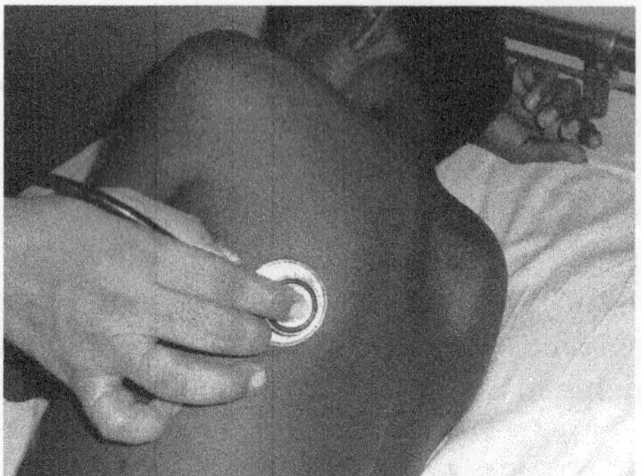

Fig. 7.9: The method to perform auscultation of respiratory system

to examine regional ventilation, the sound attenuation at different levels (Fig. 7.9). The normal breath sounds can be auscultated over the large airways due to the high degree of turbulence produced by large amount of air flow through these airways.

In normal conditions during auscultation:

- The expiratory phase appears shorter than inspiratory phase
- The breath sounds cant be heared beyond segmental bronchi
- Breath sounds are quiter at base of lung while compared to the upper/apical areas, because more lung volume at base causes absorption of the sounds.

Normal sounds are vesicular, and appear like sound of breeze passing through leaves of tree. These are heard in both inspiration and expiration.

The rhonchi are abnormal musical sounds due to the narrowing of airways and high turbulent flow. These occur when the air passes through narrow airways in similar way as musical sound appear in fluke. This occurs mostly in expiratory phase however in severe cases it may appear in inspiratory phase as well. Pure inspiratory rhonchi with normal expiration suggests obstruction outside airways and may be in larynx.

Rales are the abnormal crackling sound which mimic the rubbing of wet polythene films against each other. These result from the opening of small airways and alveoli in case of the pathological state of lung parenchyma.

- Basal rales, which clear on few deep breaths normal
- Basal rales which don't disappear on deep breath pulmonary congestion
- Rales over the large area of lungs pulmonary edema or pulmonary fibrosis.

Bronchial breathing is abnormal suggests consolidation or fibrosis. The sounds of bronchial breathing are generated by turbulent air flow in large airways and similar sounds can be heard in healthy patients by listening over the trachea. The sounds are not normally conducted to the chest wall because they are absorbed by air filled alveoli and lung parenchyma. However in case of consolidation or fibrosis, these sounds are not absorbed and get conducted more effectively to the chest wall, thus can be heared over chest wall.

Wheezing are produced due to the vibration of walls of narrowed airway while air gushes through it. These are produced when the client makes a effort to inspire or expire air across narrowed airways, thus it is associated with increased work of breathing.

VARIOUS INVESTIGATIVE PROCEDURES (INVASIVE AND NONINVASIVE) USED IN THE DIAGNOSIS OF VARIOUS RESPIRATORY DISORDERS

- Radiological examination of the chest: It is most common primary diagnostic measure. It may help to:
  - Locate lesion which can't be identified by the physical examination

- Abnormal signs, e.g. early tuberculosis or tumor
- Determining size and position of pulmonary, pleural and mediastinal lesions than can be obtained from physical examination
- To determine whether some part of lung is collapsed or consolidated
- To find any evidence of pulmonary congestion and the calcification in lung parenchyma
- Size shape position of heart
- Evidence of pulmonary congestion
- To locate any regions having accumulation of secretions and fluid
- Any evidence of fracture of ribs or thorax cage injury
- The position of diaphragm.

- CT scan and tomographical examination
  - These are helpful to determine the location of lesion within lung parenchyma across any plane
  - These are also important to locate if any tumor, fluid accumulation.
- Bacteriological and cytological examination
  - *Sputum culture*: Culture examination can help to identify the infecting organism, and also by further antibody testing the suitable curative antibiotics medicine can be prescribed. Cytological examination can also identify any cancer cells, blood cells or any pus cell presence
  - *Pleural fluid*: This can be tested in similar way for the infective organism or cancer pathology.
- Serological examination
  - Helpful to diagnose variety of infections and allergic conditions.
- Hematological examination
  - Hemogram can be helpful to identify if any hidden infection is present in body or not.
- Skin tests
  - The tuberculin test and Kveim test may be of value in the diagnosis of tuberculosis and sarcoidosis respectively. Prick tests are useful in the investigation of allergic diseases.
- Laryngoscopy
  - The larynx is inspected by laryngoscope to judge its opening and closing.
- Bronchoscopy
  - The trachea and larger bronchi are directly visualized and inspected up to the origin of segmental bronchi.

- Bronchography
  - The bronchi are outlined by injecting contrast dye agents and taking radiographs.
- Lymph node biopsy
  - Histological examination of an enlarged lymph node to rule out tuberculosis, cancer, other infective and non-infective pathology.
- Pleural biopsy
  - In patients with pleural effusion, it is possible to obtain a specimen of parietal pleura and studied in laboratory conditions to find the cause of a pleural effusion.
- Lung biopsy
  - When a diagnosis cannot be made in any other way it may be necessary to obtain a specimen of lung tissue for histological examination either by formal thoracotomy or by drill biopsy through the chest wall.
- Tests of pulmonary function
  - These can be helpful to determine the functioning or the anatomical mechanical pathology influencing the lung parenchymatous tissues. The spirometry (Fig. 7.4) testing can determine the various volumes and capacities of the lung
  - The peak flow rate, the forced expiratory volumes can be helpful to differentiate various restrictive and obstructive pulmonary diseasaes.
- Analysis of arterial blood
  - The concentration of oxygen, carbon dioxide, various ions, and the pH value of blood sample can be determined with the help of ABG (arterial blood gas) analyzer. This permits the simple measurements to reveal various possible causes of carbon dioxide retention and the cyanosis or altered metabolic/ consciousness state of the patient. This also allows to measure the oxygen saturation level of the blood.
- Chest expansion measurement: Chest wall expansion measurements are taken in standing position, during relaxed and deep breathing. Thoracic excursion equals thoracic circumference at the end of forced inspiration minus thoracic circumference at the end of forced expiration. Chest expansion can be measured at three levels (Fig. 7.7):
  - Upper lateral costal level: Placement of inch tape at 4th costal cartilage and normal value should be 2 to 3 cm

– Lower lateral costal level: The inch tape is placed at 7th costal cartilage, and normal value is around 4–5 cm.
– Diaphragmatic level: Inch tape is placed at 9th costal cartilage, normal value is 7–8 cm.

This method of chest expansion measurement is found to be highly reliable in men (Bockenhauer, et al. 2007).

VARIOUS RESPIRATORY CONDITIONS AND THEIR PHYSIOTHERAPY MANAGEMENT

The goals of pulmonary physical therapy management in respiratory dysfunction are to:

- Maximize the pulmonary function within possible limits
- Prevent or at least minimize the airway obstruction and accumulation of secretions that could interfere with normal respiration/oxygen transport
- Maximize the oxygenation of tissues
- Promote airway clearance, improve cough effectiveness
- Improve ventilation through mobilization and drainage of secretions
- Improve endurance, general exercise tolerance, and overall well-being
- Improve quality of life
- Minimize the risk of secondary conditions
- Maintain respiratory efficiency and reduce energy costs during respiration through breathing retraining
- Maintenance of proper posture and to prevent or correct postural deformities associated with pulmonary or extrapulmonary disorders
- Maintain or improve chest mobility
- Encourage relaxation in the anxiety patients to minimize the labored breathing
- To mobilize the thorax and the shoulder girdle so as to encourage correct posture and to improve the length tension relationship of respiratory muscles.

Obstructive Airways Disease vs Restrictive Pulmonary Disease

Chronic obstructive pulmonary diseases (COPD) include diseases manifested due to varying degree obstruction in the airflow into and out of lungs. Thus there occurs increased airway resistance the amount of air flow gets reduced. The peak meter and spirometry show reduced peak expiratory flow rate (PEFR), forced expiratory volume in one second (FEV1). The FVC (forced vital capacity) also gets reduced which is the maximum amount of air a person can expel from the lungs after a maximum inspiration.

In normal airway condition about 70% of FVC can be exhaled out in first second forcefully after the forceful deep inspiration (FEV1) thus FEV1/FVC ratio should be more than 0.7, but in case of COPD due to obstruction, this ratio reduces down (Rabe, et al. 2007) to less than 0.7. This ratio does not improve even if the diameter of bronchi is increased by taking bronchodilator medicines.

Because the airflow across lungs now receives obstruction thus the residual volume, the volume of air left in the lungs following full expiration, is greatly increased in COPD, while the vital capacity remains relatively normal. This leads to clinical sign of chest over-inflation, and appearance of "barrel shape chest". In severe disease the flattening of diaphragm is apparent in chest X-ray.

The common obstructive lung diseases are acute bronchitis, asthma, bronchiolitis (in infants) and bronchiectasis.

COPD commonly refers specifically to emphysema and chronic bronchitis. Most patients with COPD have characteristics of both conditions to varying degrees. Both of these conditions are not reversible. Asthma the third type of obstructive disease is a reversible form of obstruction.

Risk Factors

- The most common and well established risk factor for COPD is cigarette smoking.
- Alpha 1-antitrypsin deficiency results in the proteolytic protease enzymes mediated inflammatory damage to alveolar walls, and leading to abnormal permanent dilatation of alveoli resulting in emphysema.

Four physical signs, including increased activity of strap muscle (sternothyroid, sternohyoid, thyrohyoid, omohyoid muscle), indrawing of supraclavicular fossae in inspiration, loss of pump-handle movement and loss of bucket-handle movement are associated with lower pulmonary functioning of the COPD patients. In such cases, the long term prognosis is poor, risk of exacerbation of symptoms is higher, and the need of oxygen therapy at home is possible (Miyagi, et al. 1990).

Diagnosis

- Diagnosis is established through pulmonary function testing
- Spirometry is useful to determine FEV1/FVC ratio
- FEV1/FVC ratio if less than 70%
- Chest X-ray rules out other pulmonary conditions
- For emphysema CT scan is helpful
- Hyperinflation is seen.

Management

- Long-term management is by bronchodilators and corticosteroids in inhaled form
- Depending on severity, the patient may require oxygen supplementation at home
- Smoking has to be strictly avoided
- Severe emphysema can be treated with lung volume reduction surgery (LVRS).

Restrictive Lung Disease

In case of restrictive lung diseases (RLD) the ability of lungs and chest wall to expand (the pulmonary and thoracic wall compliance) reduces resulting in incomplete lung expansion (due to increased lung stiffness) are characterized by a loss of lung compliance, causing incomplete lung expansion (i.e. via increased lung 'stiffness'). Due to this stiffness the pulmonary volumes and capacity reduce down leading to drop in total lung capacity, inspiratory capacity and vital capacity. The inspiratory volumes and capacities are affected while the expiratory volumes and capacity remain almost unchanged. Thus in contrast to OPD, in RLD the values for tidal volume (TV), expiratory reserve volume (ERV), functional residual capacity (FRC) and respiratory volume are unchanged. The FEV1 and FCV for a patient with RLD will be decreased however FEV1/FVC ratio will be normal or increased for a RLD patient.

CHRONIC BRONCHITIS

Bronchitis is an inflammation of the bronchi in the lungs. This is associated with varying degree of airway constriction, cough, expectoration and high risk of respiratory infections (Andrea, et al. 2000).

Classification

- Acute bronchitis may last for several days and weeks and usually is the result of infections due to viruses or bacteria
- Chronic bronchitis is part of true COPD.

Chronic bronchitis is defined clinically as a persistent cough that produces sputum (phlegm) and mucus, for at least three months in two consecutive years.

Signs and Symptoms

- Chronic bronchitis results in expectorating (productive) cough
- Shortness of breath (dyspnea) due to reduced airways oxygenation
- Wheezing due to narrowing of airways secondary to sputum production
- If infection is associated, it results in chest pains, fever, and fatigue
- Mucus is normally green or yellowish green.

Causes

The risk factors include tobacco consumption, smoking, prolonged exposure to fumes, asbestos.

Diagnosis

Auscultation finds decreased intensity of breath sounds, wheeze and prolonged expiration.

Treatment

- *Antibiotics*: During acute exacerbations of chronic bronchitis, antibiotics are used depending on the sensitivity of the sputum culture.
- *Bronchodilators and corticosteroids*: to manage acute exacerbations of chronic bronchitis.
- *Risk factor elimination*: Smoking cessation
- *During acute exacerbation* the considerable infection may lead to inflammatory narrowing of airway lumen to cause obstruction, inadequate gas exchange and carbon dioxide accumulation. Which in turn leads to drowsiness, confusion state and exhaustion. The artificial ventilator support may be needed in form of ventilators or IPPB(intermittent positive pressure breathing)

Also vigorous physiotherapy helps to clear out secretions and maximize oxygenation of tissues.

During acute exacerbation the chest percussion techniques may increase the bronchoconstriction and may aggravate the problem (Campbell, et al. 1975; May and Munt,1979), therefore during this phase the percussion techniques must be avoided.

To speed up the process of sputum clearance the postural drainage technique is most commonly used however its efficacy is found to be less than the efficacy of the *Flutter device* (Andrea, et al. 2000), which provides oscillatory positive expiratory pressure. The main purpose of using this device is to control the expiratory rate and to prevent the compression of airways and paroxysmal cough (Andrea, et al. 2000; Swift, et al. 1994).

COR PULMONALE

Chronic cor pulmonale is defined as right-heart hypertrophy or right-ventricular dilatation and/or chronic right-heart failure, secondary to disorders of the respiratory system (Rundsch, 1993). It includes the 'Hypertrophy of the right ventricle resulting from diseases of lungs affecting the function and/or structure of the lung, except when these pulmonary alterations are the result of diseases that primarily affect the left side of the heart or of congenital heart disease. Pathogenetic mechanisms involve hypoxic pulmonary vasoconstriction, mechanical narrowing of vessels and obstruction of the pulmonary vascular bed(Runcsch, 1993).

Risk Factor

- The most common risk factor for cor pulmonale is long-standing pulmonary disease such as chronic bronchitis or bronchiectasis.
- Pulmonary hypertention secondary to respiratory infection and pulmonary congestion which makes right ventricle to pump harder to push deoxygenated bloods into pulmonary arteries.

Diagnosis

- Chest X-ray shows right ventricle hypertrophy and enlargement along with dilatation of the pulmonary arteries.
- In advance stage right ventricular failure develops, due to the continuous overwork and fatigue along with and continuing hypoxia.

EMPHYSEMA

Emphysema is a chronic obstructive pulmonary disease (COPD), which involves permanent damage to alveoli of the lungs. Due to damage the elastic recoiling of alveoli is lost and they can't deflate completely, thus they don't completely empty leading to entrapping of air in alveoli. Due to this they can't be filled with fresh air (Cassart and Estenne, 2007), thus adequate oxygen supply to the body gets impaired.

Two common types of emphysema (Fig. 7.10) involves:

- Centriacinar (centrilobular) involves the damage mainly around the respiratory bronchioles. This is more common among coal miners and smokers.
- Panacinar (panlobular) where tissue loss and damage occurs throughout the acinus particularly affecting the lower half of the lungs. It mainly occurs with ageing.

Causes

Emphysema is caused by loss of elasticity (increased compliance) of the lung tissue, from destruction of structures supporting the alveoli, and destruction of capillaries feeding the alveoli.

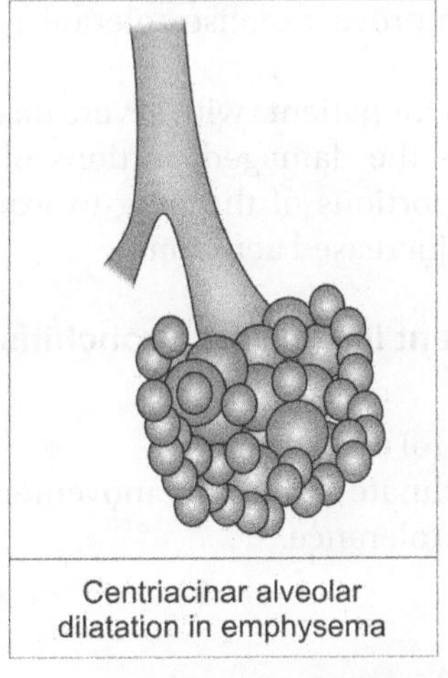

Centriacinar alveolar dilatation in emphysema

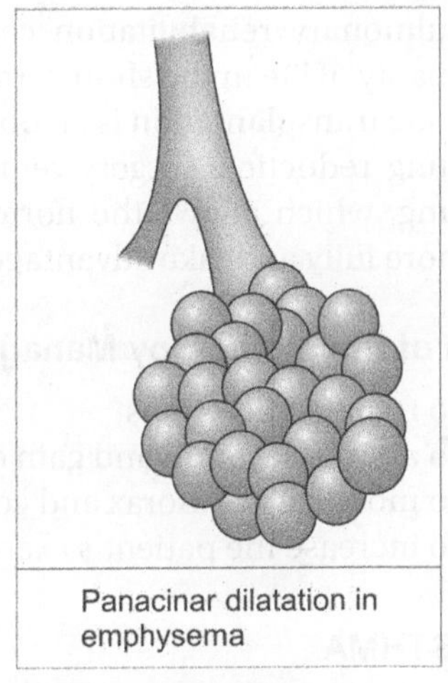

Panacinar dilatation in emphysema

Fig. 7. 10: Two common type of emphysema

Risk Factor

- Cigarette smoking, tobacco consumption is the most common cause of emphysema
- Lack of alpha-1 antitrypsin.

Symptoms

- Reduced fresh oxygen—shortness of breath
- Chronic cough with or without sputum production
- Wheezing due to air entrapment
- Decreased ability to exercise because reduced availability of oxygen
- Anxiety due to reduced oxygenation and increased breathing rate
- Unintentional weight loss and chronic fatigue due to continuous increased breathing cost.

Diagnosis

Diagnosis includes physical examination, pulmonary function testing, chest X-ray, arterial blood gas analysis, chest CT.

Treatment

- Smoking cessation
- Bronchodilators—by inhalers, nebulizer
- Antibiotics to manage associated infections
- Prophylactic pneumonia vaccine
- Low-flow oxygen positive pressure support can be used during exertion, continuously, or at night
- Pulmonary rehabilitation can improve exercise tolerance and quality of life in the short-term
- Lung transplantation is an option for patients with severe disease
- Lung reduction surgery removes the damaged portions of the lung, which allows the normal portions of the lung to expand more fully and take advantage of increased aeration.

Aim of Physiotherapy Management in Chronic Bronchitis

- To remove secretions
- To assist relaxation and gain control of breathing
- To mobilize the thorax and co-ordinate respiratory movement
- To increase the patient's exercise tolerance.

ASTHMA

Asthma is a condition characterized by the airway constriction, secondary to inflammation and/or excessive mucus accumulation.

The episode(s) of airway constriction is almost always triggered by some triggering factors such as environmental stimulant (or allergen),cold air, warm air, perfume material, weather change, humid air, dust, stress and tension, cold, feathers, exercise or exertion, and many more factors. Seasonal variations and dust are two most common triggering factors. The triggering factor may vary from person to person, and the severity of airway constriction may vary from time to time.

Symptoms of Asthma

The event of airway inflammation results in narrowing of airways leading to following symptoms of asthma:

- The airway narrowing in such way that expiration is longer than inspiration
- Shortness of breath—due to the limited amount of gaseous exchange secondary to airway narrowing. This may also lead to the loss of ability to do some physical work and may compromise the ability to talk for the moment
- Wheezing occurs when the client attempts to breathe in and out across the narrowed air passages
- Pain in the chest secondary to excessive air entrapping in the lungs
- Cough—secondary to excessive accumulation of mucus or due to the deliberate attempt to clear the secretion across narrowed airway
- Hyperinflation of lungs secondary to the entrapment of air in lungs. The symptoms aggravate when lying down straight. The client prefers to sit bending slightly relaxed forward and avoids lying straight.

Causes and Risk Factors of Asthma

Nocturnal asthma: Usually asthma associated airway narrowing are most prominent during night time, this is called as nocturnal asthma. This occurs due to the reduction in body's temperature, cooling of airways, reduction in the sympathetic nervous system functioning.

Pathophysiology

The primary pathology of the asthma lies in the inflammatory narrowing of airways passages in cases of hyperreactive bronchi, usually secondary to some events triggered by specific factors.

The trigger factors leads to the inflammatory process in the airway passages, narrowing of airways due to associated mucus accumulation and the narrowing of the airways.

Diagnosis of Asthma

- Diagnose of asthma is difficult when the symptoms appear in mild severity, because now it could be confused with some other pathological states which could cause the airway narrowing. The careful documentation of the sign and symptoms has to be made. Also the events associated just prior or few hours prior the dyspneic phase must be documented to identify the possible triggering factors
- The systematic assessment includes the medical history and examination
- Chest radiological investigations to rule out other confounding pathologies
- Laboratory investigations to rule out the possible infections and the allergic reactions
- The client's ability to inspire and expire in terms of the volume of air and the rate of flow
- The spirometer records the rate and total volume of the exhalation of air from lungs
- Peak flow measures (Fig. 7.11) the maximum rate at which the air can be exhaled forcefully. It has a electronic or mechanical meter mounted on a small mouth piece through which the client attempts to blow out air for exhalation.

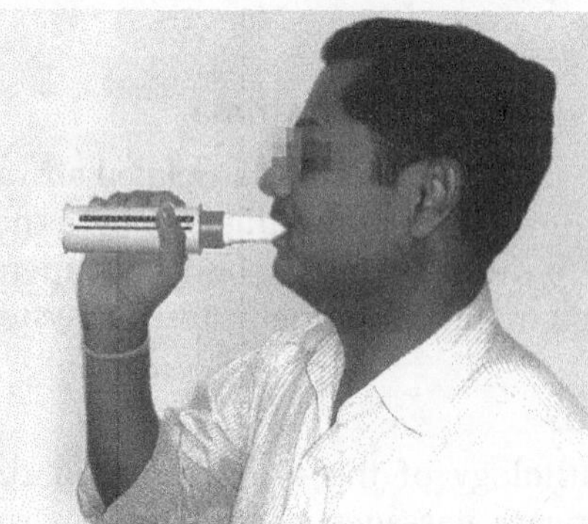

Fig. 7.11: Peak flow meter used to determine peak flow rate

Treatment of Asthma

Asthma treatment consists of trigger factor control, the medical management, physiotherapeutic management and the prophylactic management. Humans have always been surrounded by the environment which has enormous things which could act as trigger factor for provoking asthma. Thus the asthma management also depends on the control of the environment so as to prevent the direct exposure of the client to the allergen.

The possible list of allergens responsible for triggering event of airway constriction must be identified for the specific individual. The attempts must be done to minimize the exposure of the client to these trigger factors. During cleaning the houses must wear mask and must wipe the floor instead of removing dust with dry cloth; the dust must be removed to minimize entering into nostrils; must cover mattress, pillows with dust proof covers; must keep humidity low; must wear prophylactic masks during weather change.

The careful documentation of the pulmonary function is important to identify the lungs which are at higher risk of developing asthma attack.

Medication in Asthma

- Anti-inflammatory medicines help to reduce the inflammatory cells in the airways and prevent blood vessels from leaking fluid into the airway tissues. By reducing inflammation, they reduce the spontaneous spasm of the airway muscle. Anti-inflammatories are used as a preventive measure to lessen the risk of acute asthma attacks.
- Corticosteroids can be given by pill/tablet or liquid form.
- Bronchodilators work by increasing the diameter of the air passages and easing the flow of gases to and from the lungs.

Physiotherapy Management in Asthma

Aims of Physiotherapy in Asthma

- To relieve bronchospasm
- To promote relaxation
- To promote control of breathing
- To normalize breathing pattern
- To encourage co-ordination of respiratory movement
- To minimize air entrapment

- To encourage correct posture to maximize normal mechanics of breathing.
- Bronchospasm if persisting for long time, stops the normal breathing mechanics, and thus does not allow normal aeration. This causes accumulation of secretions, the deficient of oxygen in body and the excessive carbon dioxide accumulation in body.
- Due to the accumulation of secretions, the client has tendency to attempt cough to clear secretion but this further can aggravate the bronchospasm.
- The coughing, houghing, percussion techniques must not be intervened in such patients to clear off the secretions.
- The bronchospasm leads to the airway narrowing, thus the intervention to increase the airway lumen diameter is desirable. For the same reason the intermittent positive pressure breathing must be administered along with bronchodilator medicines.
- Due to the impaired mechanism of breathing the clients usually become anxietic, and this further impaired the breathing ability. To relieve this it is highly important that the client must stay relaxed, in comfortable position. The breathing needs to be promote via recruitment of the diaphragm and also must reduce the work of accessory group of muscles.
- Must encourage slow, rhythmic, breathing with awareness on the diaphragmatic pattern of breathing.
- Subject must remain in relaxed position (Fig. 7.12) which aids the excursion of the diaphragm. For this the forward leaning with forearms supported on thigh may be optimum.
- If any secretion is present they can't be removed by coughing, houghing, or percussion methods in asthmatic patients as this would further aggravate the bronchospasm.
- The secretion clearance must be attempted only when the adequate bronchodilation has occurred, the respiratory control is gained and the client is in state of expectorating them.
- During bronchospasm the bronchodilator medicine and mucolytic agents may be used to loosen the secretions. Once the secretions have been liquefied, the gentle chest vibration may be initiated during expiratory phase to further directing the secretions towards larger airways to be coughed out. As the amount of secretions clear off, the client's condition improves.
- As the condition of client improves, further exercises may be initiated to gain the breathing control. These exercises also focus

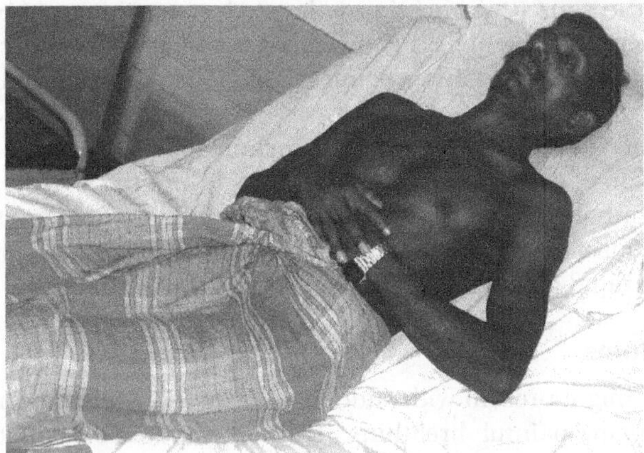

Fig. 7.12: Commonly used relaxed positions used for asthma management

more on the expiration to avoid any accumulation of air in the lungs, and also to keep airways open and patent for relatively long time.

- During breathing the diaphragm pattern is encouraged with keeping the upper chest and accessory muscles relaxed.
- One study found that the self management techniques along with bronchodilator medicines are more efficacious than the medicines alone to reduce the severity, duration, and to improve the peak expiratory flow rate. It put an emphasis that the patients of asthma over period of time develop their own management strategies to deal with the acute exacerbation of asthma. The same study also found that the trait anxiety related asthma cannot be controlled by external interventions (Vazquez and J. M. Buceta, 1993).

LUNG ABSCESS

Lung abscess is a condition in which the infection of lung tissue leads to the necrosis of this tissue and formation of cavity due to this necrotic damage. The necrotic infection material is contained with in the cavity. The size of cavity may be more than 2 cm.

Alcoholism, chronic lung infection, rupture of bullae of emphysema is the common causes of lung abcess. In majority of cases, the source of infection is located within lung parenchyma itself therefore the abcess is primary lung abcess in such cases. In remaining cases the source of infection is located at extrapulmonary site.

Other causes of the lung abscess include the regurgitation and the aspiration of gastric secretion or oral fluids into the airways, spread of the emboli and infection from the extrapulmonary regions.

The onset of formation of lung abscess is often gradual however it may be rapid in patients with other comorbid conditions.

Symptoms

patient might present with sudden onset fever, sweating, shivering, chest pain, painful breathing, sputum production, might have hemoptysis. In some cases the sign of oxygen deficit develop in body, such as lethargy, fatigue, chronic irritation. On examination, there is area of tenderness on the chest wall overlying the affected lobe of lung, the features of lung consolidation may occur as dullness on percussion.

X-ray may sometime reveal the localized areas with abnormal round cavity like appearance which seems to be circumscribed with the fluid film.

The abscess in lungs is most common in the apical segments of the lower lobe as these are gravity dependent when lying down.

Laboratory Studies

The hemogram analysis may reveal the presence of infection in the body. The hemogram reveals elevated ESR, C-reactive protein, the differential leucocytes counting (DLC) may reveal raised levels of lymphocytes in body.

The sputum examination is highly important study as this will reveal whether true infection is present in body or not. Also the sputum culture examination will reveal the severity and nature of the infection. The antibiotic sensitivity also reveals the suitable antibiotics for prescription. In cases where sputum samples cannot be collected, the bronchoscopic aspirating fluid can be used for culture examination.

Management is usually broad spectrum antibiotics. With the antibiotic usage, most of the cases of lung abscess resolve definitely. The cases which do not recover, may require the surgical procedures or lung lobe resection may be needed.

In cases of the chronically present lung abscess the secondary pathological conditions may also develop lyke bronchiectases, septicemia, empyema, pleurisy, brain abscess. The cavity remained after the clearance of the infection may act as site for accumulation of other infections. The chronic presence of abscess may also create pressure on the bronchi and may cause its structural alternation, which may hamper the clearance of the secretion from the lung.

Physiotherapy Management

To prevent the accumulation of secretions in lung the postural drainage is very important. The postural drainage must also be taught for the home advice.

If over period of time the size of lung abcess increases then deep breathing exercises should not be advised as because this would further lead to the aggravation of pain and the fatigue. When size of lung abscess diminishes only then the breathing exercises are advised.

BRONCHIECTASIS

Bronchiectasis is characterized by localized, irreversible dilatation of part of the bronchial tree. This occurs as sequelae of variety of pulmonary conditions including infectious diseases. The involved airways remain weak, can easily collapse. This narrow the airway lumen, blocks airway flow, causes secretion accumulation. The dilated areas act as a storehouse of sputum, which now can't be drained towards larger airways for being expectorated. The sputum provides optimum environment for infection, inflammatory damage to pulmonary tissue, loss of elasticity, dilatation of airways, and further damage of airways. Severe form of disease can lead to respiratory failure (Kolbe and Well, 1996). The dilation of the airway is permanent and irreversible therefore the secretion clearance mechanism is permanently lost. The foul smelling sputum produced in significantly large quantity in the bronchiectasis, with the impaired secretion clearance mechanism and the altered malsufficient breathing efficiency.

Pathogenesis

On basis of bronchospasm evaluation, the following types of bronchiectasis are found (Mootoosamy, et al. 1985)

- Cylindrical type: The bronchi have regular outline
- Varicose bronchiectasis: Bronchial tree is beaded, with alternate areas of dilation and constriction in bronchial walls
- Saccular bronchiectasis: Irreversible ballooning of bronchi.

The other causes of bronchiectasis could be the poor mobility of cilia in lungs, chronic lung infections, alpha-1-antitrypsin decieiency, poor immune mechanisms of the body, chronic immune responses of body.

Diagnosis

Carefully documented clinical history, auscultation and the radiological investigations such as CT scans are main stay of diagnosis. The sputum culture and sensitivity examination may reveal the associated infection. CT scan is helpful to locate extent, site, type and lobar distribution of the bronchiectasis (Reiff et al. 1995).

Treatment

The foul smelling sputum produced in significantly large quantity in the bronchiectasis, with the impaired secretion clearance mechanism and the altered malsufficient breathing efficiency. The produced sputum has to be necessarily expectorated with the postural drainage techniques. Usually coughing maneuvers remain non-preferred method of dislodging secretions because repeated attempt of coughing further lead to bronchospasm and the respiratory muscle fatigue.

Preventive aspect of management depends of prevention of bronchial secretion formation and preventing the possible infections. Prophylactic use of antibiotics and early cure of any other infection is the preferred method of prevention aspect. The chest X-ray must be taken after suitable time frames to identify the development of the bronchiectasis in clients suffering from other pathological conditions of the pulmonary parenchyma.

The natural mechanism of the airway clearance in lungs consists of the ciliary movement, which gets impaired in bronchiectasis. Postural drainage has to be carried out by patient on regular basis. The frequency and the duration of assuming postural drainage position depends on the severity of the problem and the amount of sputum production. The bronchodilators and the mucolytic medicines can also be prescribed for the loosening of secretions and facilitating their removal. In cases of 'dry bronchiectasis' the postural drainage is not prescribed. In refractory cases, the surgical removal of the obstructing cause of bronchiectasis is advised. In some specific portion of lung lobe is involved, then surgical removal of the affected part of lung is recommended. In infection prone patients, the prophylactic vaccination must be given for pneumonia and influenza.

Now beside postural drainage techniques the positive pressure techniques such as flutter device and ACBT (active cycle of breathing techniques) have also been employed and found to be effective for secretion clearance. However, the compliance towards exercise regime is found to be better with flutter device while compared to the ACBT technique (Thompson, et al. 2002).

CYSTIC FIBROSIS

This condition is characterized by the high concentration of sodium ions in exocrinal glandular secretions including sweat, pancreatic juices. The recurrent lung infections also occur in this condition, which in turn may lead to lung abscess, bronchiectasis, pneumonia etc. This can be a fatal condition, and the survival depends on the immunity of the body and the prevention/treatment of the pulmonary infection.

The diagnosis of the disease in relatively early stage has increased the timing of the survival, and reduced the morbidity associated with this disease. Once the diagnosis is made the prevention of pulmonary infection is encouraged with introduction of postural drainage.

Prevention of secretion accumulation is important to be attempted therefore the postural drainage is advised even for home advise, to at least delay the secretion accumulation. The different positions are taught to clear the secretions from all the lobes of the lung. The lower lobes and the middle lobes of lungs must be given special emphasis due to higher risk of developing secretion accumulation. Also the humidification and the steaming will help to loosen the thickened secretions and facilitate its clearance.

The mandatory postural drainages for twice or thrice a day are recommended (Mortensen, et al. 1991; Rossman, 1982). Breathing exercise are important component of daily routine activity. Chest expansion exercises, deep breathing exercises must be done regularly. Special emphasis on the basal expansion is done to avoid the higher tendency of the apical lobes to expand.

Bronchodilators, IPPB, nebulization, repeated steaming when done after postural drainage helps in clearance of the secretions.

PULMONARY TUBERCULOSIS

Pulmonary tuberculosis has become less common since the improvement of public health standards and treatment by effective chemotherapy. Physiotherapy is rarely requested for this condition, but it is, sometimes, necessary to treat associated complications.

The first infection with the tubercle bacillus is known as primary tuberculosis. A small pneumonic lesion may occur in any part of the lung and the nearest lymph glands become enlarged. The lesion usually heals by fibrosis and calcification and subsequently causes no problem; occasionally it spreads through the lobe and may then expansion exercises are required.

In infants and young children, the enlarged hilar lymph nodes may compress a bronchus and cause segmental collapse. Prolonged compression may lead to permanent bronchiectasis as in the 'middle lobe syndrome'. Another cause of segmental collapse may be discharge of caseous material from the affected lymph gland into the bronchus.

Physiotherapy Management

Physiotherapy may be requested to attempt re-expansion of a collapsed middle lobe. The result may be disappointing but it is worth persevering with breathing exercises, postural drainage and vibrations as re-expansion sometimes occurs.

Post-primary tuberculosis is a re-infection after the prjmary lesion. The infection usually occurs in the upper lobes or apical segments of the lower lobes. A small area of tuberculous bronchopneumonia appears at first, and this spreads by direct infection to neighbouring lung tissue. Caseation follows, and the necrotic center of the lesion is discharged into a bronchus, leaving a cavity. The patient coughs up infective sputum, some of which may be inhaled into other areas of lung, producing new tuberculous lesions. Hemoptysis occurs if there is erosion of blood vessels.

Peripheral lesions may cause pleurisy leading to tuberculous effusion or empyema. In these cases, physiotherapy is important to prevent chest deformity and loss of respiratory function by pleural thickening. There is no risk of physiotherapy causing spread of the disease once medical treatment has been established.

In contrast to acute tuberculosis with infiltration and cavitation, a chronic fibrocaseous condition may develop. Gross fibrous contraction of the upper lobes with compensatory emphysema of the lower lobes results in dyspnea and diminished respiratory reserve.

Breathing control and assistance with removal of secretions, during periods of superimposed chest infection, may be helpful. IPPB may be contraindicated if cavitation has taken place.

A tuberculoma is a cavity with thick walls containing inspissated material which appears radiologically as a rounded opacity. It may be removed surgically since it is sometimes difficult to differentiate tuberculoma from carcinoma.

Tuberculous bronchiectasis may be a complication of either primary or post-primary tuberculosis. Postural drainage may be given, but percussion will be contraindicated if there is a large cavity, or hemoptysis is occurring. The physiotherapist should stand behind the patient when he is coughing. Treatment is carried out two or three times daily according to the quantity of sputum.

PNEUMONIA

Pneumonia is the pathological condition of lungs which is characterized by inflammatory consolidation and exudation of lung parenchyma. Depending on location this may be called as lobar pneumonia (common in adults) or lobular pneumonia (common in children).

The pneumonia can be caused by large number of causative factors including—bacterial infection (*Diplococcus pneumoniae*), viral infections, herpes simplex virus infection (Whitley and Roizman, 2001), fungal infections, chemical irritants, idiopathic factors, hospital related infections (Rowe and Cheadle, 2000), comorbid conditions. The hospital acquired infection is also a common cause of pneumonia.

The clinical features of pneumonia include fever, chills, pleuritic pain, chest pain, breathlessness, tachypnea, fast pulse (more than 100 beats per minute), and decreased breathing sounds as heard on auscultation of chest. The infection of the pulmonary tissue causes the inflammatory involvement of tissue and the accumulation of fluids within lung region. Due to this the painful cough, painful breathing occurs. During increase in the intrathoracic pressure like coughing and deep breathing the pain aggravates more.

Cough may be less, filled with mucoid sputum, blood stained rusty appearance. Area of consolidation appears on radiography. In suspected cases, the X-ray of lung shows consolidation, which can further be confirmed by reduced breath sound and the percussion dull node. The virus associated pneumonia is associated with diffused interstitial edema (Ramsey, et al. 1992). The breathing exercises are encouraged, with special emphasis on the increasing air movement through the affected portion of lung. Since in initial stages, the consolidation is more clear compared to the secretions therefore percussion maneuver, chest shaking method must not be used as these methods would be painful and may further cause spasm and reduce the breathing. For the same reason coughing maneuver must not be encouraged as this would repeatedly increase the lung parenchymal pressure and further aggravate the consolidation.

When consolidation resolves, the sputum is formed in significant quantity. Gradually as condition of patient improves, consolidation resolves, associated pain diminishes the physiotherapeutic interventions to aid the secretion removal may be started. This includes percussion methods, coughing, houghing, etc.

PHYSIOTHERAPY MANAGEMENT FOR RESPIRATORY CONDITIONS

Physiotherapy is an integral part of the management of patients in respiratory intensive care units (Enrico and Ambrosino, 2005). Physiotherapy is a vital component for the management of the patients with pulmonary conditions. Its role extends from the acute phase up to the full functional rehabilitation. Suitable physiotherapeutic intervention depends on the pathological state of the client, severity of involvement, general condition of the client, associated comorbid conditions.

Aims of the physiotherapeutic interventions in respiratory conditions are as follows:

- To keep the airways clean
- To reduce the anxiety
- To relieve bronchospasm

- To establish the control of breathing pattern, frequency and depth by the patient
- To minimize the formation of secretions
- To minimize the accumulation of secretions in patients
- To encourage correct posture
- To normalize mechanics of breathing
- To normalize coordination of respiratory movement.

The most important physiotherapeutic aim in the acutely ill patients is to enhance patient's overall patient's functional capacity and to restore his/her respiratory and physical independence, thus decreasing the risks of bed rest associated complications (Enrico and Ambrosino, 2005). The important aims also include to decrease the patient's dependency on the ventilator, to improve residual function, to prevent the need for new hospitalizations and to improve the patient's quality of life (Stiller, 2000).

Physiotherapy is an essential part of the treatment regime and is instituted immediately. Purulent or mucopurulent sputum is present in considerable quantities causing obstruction of the airways. As there is no consolidation or pleural inflammation causing pleuritic pain, there is no contraindication to early physiotherapy.

It must always be borne in mind that the most of the patients who are admitted in intensive care unit (ICU), are generally victim with exacerbation of chronic obstructive pulmonary disease (COPD), or an acute medical or surgical event, superimposed on some other underlying chronic lung disease. Majority of these patients need the ventilator support in form of mechanical ventilation. Most of these patients are given sedation to minimize the discomfort associated with endotracheal, orotracheal intubation (ACCP task force guideline, 2001). This leads to the impairment of the natural airway clearance mechanisms, suppression of cough reflex, impaired ciliary movements (Sackner, et al. 1973).

The various techniques used by physiotherapist to deal with the patients of respiratory complications include:

- Posturing
  - Limb positioning
  - Postural drainage
- Mobilization techniques (Enrico and Ambrosino, 2005)
  - Passive and active limb exercises
  - Continuous rotation two hourly
- Chest physiotherapy (Enrico and Ambrosino, 2005)

- Airway clearance techniques
- Vibration: It is mechanical or manual, fine shaking movements of chest wall, to direct the secretions from periphery to large airways (Parker, 1993)
- Percussion techniques
- Manual hyperinflation
- Postural drainage (Fig. 7.16)
- Assisted coughing

• Techniques to dislodge the thickened secretions
  - Percussion techniques (Pryor, 1992)
  - ACBT (active cycle of breathing technique)
  - Steaming
  - Nebulization-with bronchodilators, mucolytic agents (the medically prescribed medicines). This includes the drug delivery for the purpose of facilitating the inhalation (Fig. 7.13). During this, the pressure is applied on liquid drug which due to pressure gets transformed to mist and can easily be inspired.
  - Aerosol therapy the portable hand held device for friendly use by the patient for delivering the desired drug to respiratory tract.

• Techniques to clear the secretions
  - *Coughing*: The client performs deep inspiration (to get high lung volume), holds breath in inspirited position, then tightens abdominal muscles and finally performs coughing against

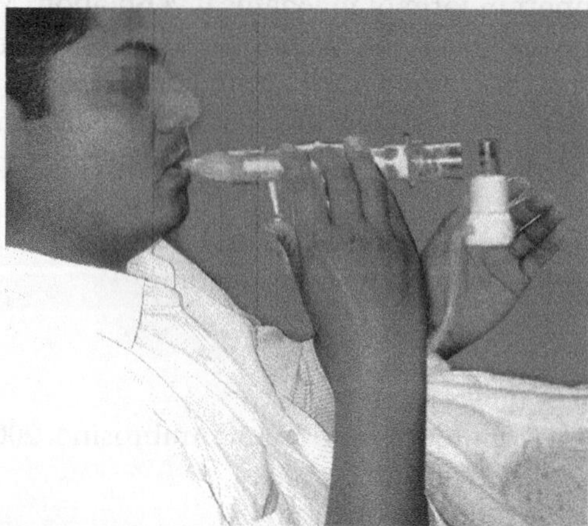

Fig. 7.13: Use of nebulization

closed effort. As air is forced out of lungs, the secretions also move upward along with.
- *Huffing*: The client does mid inspiration (mid lung volume), holds breath in the mid inspiratory position, tightens abdominal muscles, and finally opens mouth to forcefully huff out the air against open glottis.
- *Suction*: The negative pressure device is attached to the catheter which passes through endotracheal, or tracheostomy or mouth into the airways (Fig. 7.14). When the secretions have reach upward in large airways but client can not expectorate them, then the negative pressure of the suction will help to remove these secretions.

- Muscle re-training
  - Relaxation exercises (Fig. 7.15) to reduce anxiety, to reduce shortness of breath
  - Gain respiratory control
  - Inspiratory muscle training
  - Diaphragmatic resistance training
  - Diaphragmatic facilitation
  - Incentive spirometry method
- Respiratory muscle training (Enrico and Ambrosino, 2005)
- Active cycle of breathing (ACBT)
- Intercostals facilitaton
  - PNF (proprioceptive neuromuscular facilitation) techniques of the intercostals muscles
  - Discouraging the labored breathing
  - Facilitation of diaphragmatic and intercostal activity.

If these measures are not effective, IPPB is used to assist ventilation and clearing of secretions.

Posturing/Positioning

In cases, where patient is unconscious or the voluntary attempts to clear the secretions is absent, the positioning/posturing are most commonly used to direct the secretions towards larger airways to stimulate their clearance. As the secretions reach the larger airways, they can be cleared off form there by the help of suctioning procedure.

The postural techniques aim to (Dean, 1994; Enrico and Ambrosino, 2005):

- Improve ventilation/perfusion ratio
- Improve lung volumes and gaseous exchange

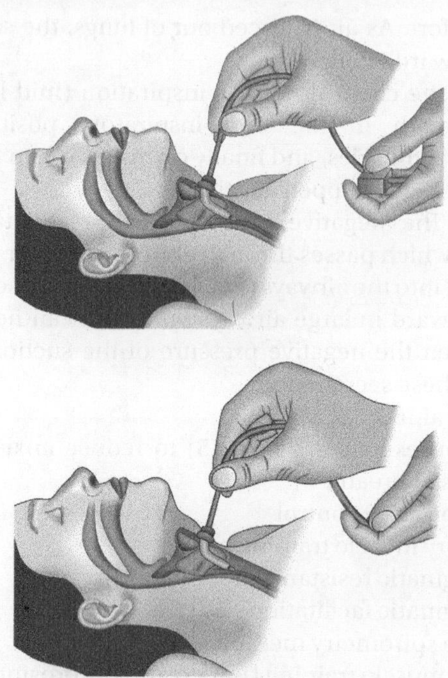

Fig. 7.14: The suctioning procedure via tracheostomy tube

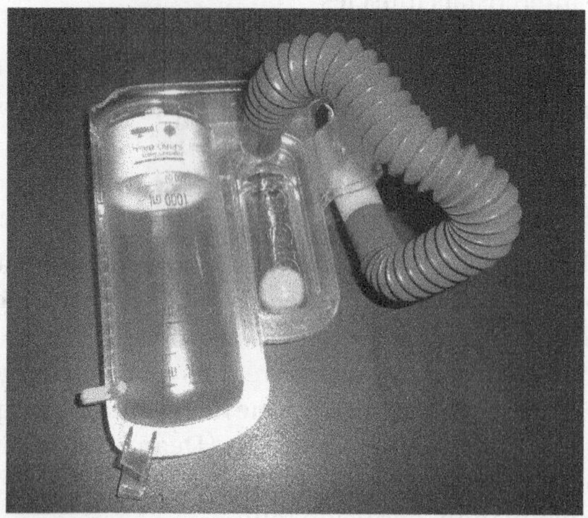

Fig 7.15: Incentive spirometer for training of respiratory muscles

- Increase mucociliary clearance
- Reduce work of breathing
- Reduce load on heart.

The common positioning include:

- Upright positioning: To improve lung volume
- Prone positioning (Jolliet, et al. 1998): To improve ventilation/ perfusion matching and to redistribute edema. In patients of acute respiratory distress syndrome, the prone positioning improves oxygenation by about 57–92% (Mure, et al. 1997)
- Side lying with the affected side on upper side to improve ventilation of this affected segment of lungs (Prokocimer, et al. 1983)
- Semirecumbent positioning to reduce the gastric contents pulmonary aspiration (Ibanez, et al. 1992)
- Beside this the specific positioning are used (Fig. 7.16) in form of postural drainage (PD) to clear the secretions from specific portion of lungs.

Limb Exercises

In bedridden patients, the cardiovascular, and cardiopulmonary systems undergo deconditioning (Casabury, 1996) which in turn lead to the reduced capacity to meet the stresses placed on these systems during physical exertion. To minimize the detrimental effects of this deconditioning, the limb exercises are implemented in such bed ridden or limited mobility patients. The beneficial influences (Dean, 1994) include the improved blood circulation throughout body, improve ventilation and the pulmonary mechanics, improved oxygen consumption in body (Norrenberg, et al. 1995); redistribution of fluid from periphery, reduced risk of emboli or adhesion formation. The active exercises are most preferred method to reduce adverse effects of deconditioning. These interventions may include active movements in bed, active or active-assisted or passive movements of ankle, knee, upper extremity; sitting, transfer from bed to chair and then return, sitting, standing, walking. The progression in intensity and volume can be made as the improvement progresses.

REMOVAL OF SECRETIONS

In patients with bronchitis the primary problems to be considered by physiotherapist are:

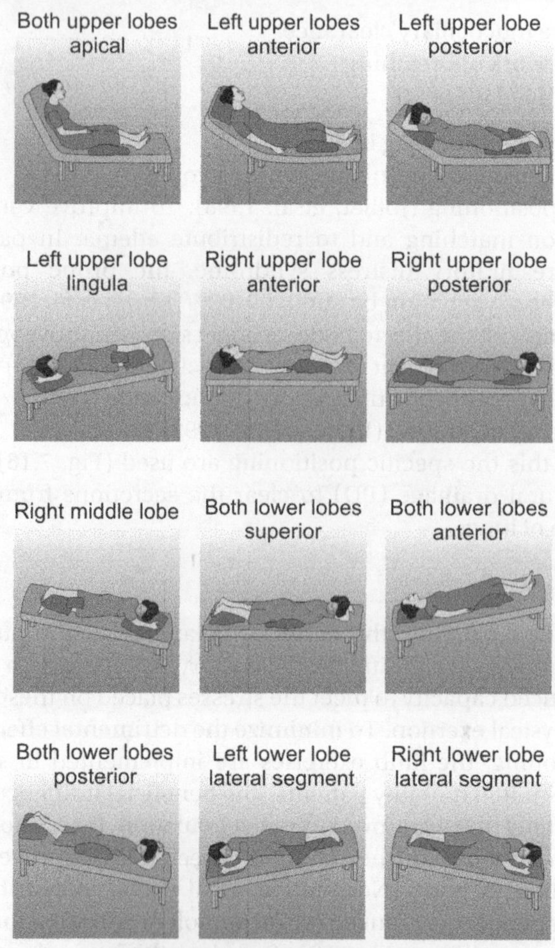

Fig. 7.16: Different positions for the postural drainage of different lobes of lungs

- Increased sputum production
- Respiratory muscle fatigue due to repeated coughing
- The altered breathing pattern
- The chest pain due to repeated coughing which increases the intrathoracic pressure.

The coughing maneuver is not preferred, therefore postural drainage is recommended along with gentle vibrations to aid the clearance of secretion from lungs. Postural drainage may be done using specific postures for targeting specifically the affected portion of lung. The frequency of postural drainage may vary depending on the severity of the involvement. In case of the infection or significant inflammation the amount of sputum production is large, therefore longer duration of the postural drainage positioning may be advised.

In case of thick tenacious secretions the steam inhalation, mucolytic agents via nebulization may be used to loosen up the secretions and to facilitate their clearance.

As the condition of client improves, the deep breathing exercises are advised to facilitate the aeration of the lung tissues and promote the mobilization of secretions.

If patients are on higher dosage of corticosteroid therapy for prolonged time the percussion methods may lead to ribs fracture and lead to higher risk of bullae rupture. If airways are narrowed severely then the bronchodilator medicine may be advised before any other physiotherapeutic interventions. In uncounscious patients or those who are unable to maintain the respiration adequately the artificial ventilation may be provided by IPPB (intermittent positive pressure breathing). Carefully implemented postural drainage may also aid the secretion clearance.

Relaxation and Control of Breathing

During severe attack the client has tendency to keep the lungs inflated by sustaining the inspirated positioning of chest. This reduces the excursion of diaphragm, increases loading of accessory group of muscles. The patient has general attitude of becoming anxious. The faulty breathing pattern further aggravates the condition of the client. The primary role of physiotherapy in this phase is to gain the control of breathing pattern. This may be done by assurance, relaxation exercises, ventilatory support.

Emphysematous patients do short uncontrolled inspiration using accessory muscles, followed by prolonged forceful expiration which significantly increases introthoracic pressure. This increased pressure, in turn, damages the weakened airways. This uncontrolled pattern of breathing is an exhausting and uneconomical method of ventilation, which the physiotherapist should attempt to reverse.

Some emphysematous patients spontaneously develop a technique of 'pursed lip' breathing. Such patients breathe out through the mouth with the lips held together loosely in a pursed position. By increasing the pressure in the pharynx and upper airways, the damaged collapsible airways are kept patent a little longer, and probably the patient feels relief from the resultant slightly increased tidal volume and slower respiratory rate. This method of breathing should not be discouraged, provided that it is carried out correctly in a relaxed manner. If one attempts to teach this form of breathing to a patient who has not developed it spontaneously, there is a great danger of expiration becoming forced, thus defeating the purpose of the technique. Unless this pattern is already established, it should be omitted from the treatment program.

All patients with obstructive airways disease are taught to breathe with an active inspiratory phase using the diaphragm, and a passive relaxed expiratory phase. If the patient can control his breathing, it can be of great benefit during attacks of dyspnea. He is instructed to adopt a relaxed position. All designed to combine the maximum relaxation of the upper chest, with freedom of movement of the lower chest. At this stage the rate of breathing is not important but control of the upper chest is essential. The patient should be encouraged to breathe gently with the lower chest without prolonging expiration until he begins to breathe in a more coordinated manner. Once this has been achieved, an effort should be made to slow down his respiratory rate and increase the depth of respiration. The patient may prefer to breathe with his mouth open during an attack of dyspnea. The position can be adapted to different situations in everyday life.

High Side-lying

The patient lies on one side, slightly rolled forward, with a slope of three or four pillows to raise the shoulders, and an extra pillow placed to fill the gap between the waist and axilla to prevent him sliding down the bed and to maintain a straight thoracic spine. The knees are slightly bent and the top leg placed in front of the lower one. This position is helpful for patients in acute respiratory distress, or at night for those suffering from orthopnea.

Forward Lean Sitting

Certain patients who prefer not to stay in bed find this position comfortable. Two or three pillows are placed on a table and the patient can relax with the upper chest and head resting against them. Care should be taken that the patient maintains a straight thoracic and lumbar spine as otherwise this would tend to inhibit diaphragmatic movement.

Relaxed Sitting

This is an extremely useful position and can be taken up unobtrusively in public places.

Many patients are inclined to grip their knees and raise their shoulders when in distress, but if they can sit leaning forward with the forearms resting on the thighs, and the wrists relaxed, they will recover more quickly. Care must be taken to ensure that the lumbar spine is not flexed, as this could impede free forward movement of the abdominal wall.

Forward Lean Standing

If they are unable to sit down distressed patients are inclined to grasp the nearest available object and hold themselves in a tense position; for instance they hold on to the bannisters after climbing a flight of stairs. They should be encouraged to lean forward.

Relaxed Standing

The distressed patient may also help himself by leaning back against the wall or a right support. The feet should be approximately twelve inches from the wall, the shoulders relaxed and arms hanging loosely by the sides.

Control of Breathing during Exercise

When the patient is able to control his breathing in these relaxed positions he should practice while sitting and standing upright without support. Progression can then be made to control of breathing while walking on the level, on stairs, and on hills. Many patients tend to hold their breath during exercise. Breathing in rhythm with their steps can be helpful; for example, breathing out for two steps and in for one step, or out for three steps and in for two steps. A breathing pattern must be worked out for each individual patient.

Some patients tend to become distressed when bending forward (e.g. to tie shoe laces).

Many of them breathe in before bending down, and thus experience discomfort due to the upward pressure of the abdominal contents against the flattened diaphragm.

This discomfort is alleviated to certain extent if breathing out is encouraged whilst bending down; breathing in takes place during the return to an upright position.

Although pulmonary function tests do not show any significant improvement in patients who have been taught controlled breathing, they appear to derive benefit from the fact that they are breathing in a more economical manner. By eliminating superfluous muscular activity during respiration, the work breathing is reduced.

Mobilization of the Thorax and Co-ordination of Respiratory Movement

Treatment is not progressed until the patient has mastered breathing control and relaxation of upper chest whether during attacks of dyspnea or during normal breathing.

Localized expansion is then started. This is taught unilaterally and can be progressed to belt exercises. Basal expansion is helpful in loosening secretions during postural drainage. By improving the mobility of the lower thoracic cage together with control of the upper chest, the patient should achieve a more normal coordinated pattern of breathing.

In patients with emphysema, the domes of the diaphragm are flattened or even inverted, abnormal position of the diaphragm can cause rib retraction on inspiration, but with perseverance a little lateral basal movement may eventually be achieved.

Increase of Exercise Tolerance

At one time, it was common practice in physiotherapy departments to hold breathing classes for groups of patients; but it is now generally accepted that adults benefit more from individual treatment.

The aim of physiotherapy for severely disabled patients is to increase their exercise tolerance to enable them to carry out useful daily activities. Patient should be encouraged to be as mobile and active as possible. Their exercise tolerance may be increased by improving control of breathing, while gradually increasing the distance walked both on the level and on slopes and stairs.

A few patients are so handicapped that they may need portable oxygen therapy, and in some cases the assistance of a high walking-frame to enable them to get about but that gradually increasing the activities of daily living is more functionally beneficial.

Home Instruction

There is evidence that the improvement in the patient's exercise tolerance with a program of graduated activities is due to reduced oxygen consumption during exercise. Although the precise mechanisms by which this occurs are as yet unclear. A number of research papers have been written on the effects of exercise (bicycle, treadmill and stairs) whilst the patient is using portable oxygen. The consensus of opinion would seem to be that the reduced dyspnea, and increase in speed and distance walked is probably related to the opening up of the pulmonary capillary bed (due to reduced pulmonary vascular resistance) and improved oxygen uptake. It is our experience that the use of a bicycle and treadmill as a means of treatment are not particularly advantageous in improving the exercise tolerance in the severely disabled patient.

It is essential that all patients with chronic obstructive airways disease carry out physiotherapy at home. Prolonged outpatient treatment is usually unnecessary if careful instructions have been given.

BIBLIOGRAPHY

1. ACCP, AARC, ACCCM task force. Evidence based guidelines for weaning and discontinuing ventilatory support. Chest. 2001;120:375s-95s.
2. Andrea B, Rosaria L, Stefania R, Laura G, Roberto A. Chest physical therapy in patients with acute exacerbation of chronic bronchitis: effectiveness of three methods. Arch Phys Med Rehabil. 2000;81: 558-60.
3. Bockenhauer SE, Chen H, Kell NJ, MFA Weedon J. Measuring thoracic excursion: reliability of the cloth tape measure technique. Journal of American Academy of Osteopathic Association. 2007;107(5):191-6.
4. Campbell AH, O'Connell JM, Wilson F. The effect of chest physiotherapy upon the FEV1 in chronic bronchitis. Med J Aust. 1995;1(2):33-5.

5. Casaburi R. Deconditioning. In: Fishman AP (Eds). Pulmonary Rehabilitation. New York: Marcel Dekker. 1996;213-30.
6. Cassart M, Estenne M. The respiratory muscles in emphysema: The effects of thoracic distension. Rev Mal Respir. 2000;17(2):449-57.
7. Dean E. Oxygen transport: a physiologically-based conceptual framework for the practice of cardiopulmonary physiotherapy. Physiotherapy. 1994;80:347-55.
8. Enrico C, Ambrosino N. Early physiotherapy in the respiratory intensive care unit. Respiratory Medicine. 2005;99:1096-1104.
9. Gartner Leslie P, James L Hiatt. Color Textbook of Histology. 2001;2.
10. Ibanez J, Penafiel A, Raurich JM, Marse P, Jorda R, Mata F. Gastroesophageal reflux in intubated patients receiving enteral nutrition: effect of supine and semirecumbent positions. J Parenter Enteral Nutr. 1992;16:419-22.
11. Jolliet P, Bulpa P, Chevrolet JC. Effects of the prone position on gas exchange and hemodynamics in severe acute respiratory distress syndrome. Crit Care Med. 1998;26:1977-85.
12. Kolbe J, Wells AU. Bronchiectasis: a neglected cause of respiratory morbidity and mortality. Respirology. 1996;1(4):221-5.
13. May DB, Munt PN. Physiologie effects of chest percussion and postural drainage in patients with stable chronic bronchitis. Chest. 1979;75: 29-32.
14. Miyagi S, Irei M, Kyan Y. Physical signs and lung function tests in patients with chronic obstructive pulmonary disease (COPD).Rinsho Byori. 1990;38(4):415-9.
15. Mootoosamy IM, Reznek RH, Osman J, Rees RS, Green M. Assessment of bronchiectasis by computed omography. Thorax. 1985;40:920-4.
16. Mortensen J, Falk M, Groth S, Jensen C. The effects of postural drainage and positive expiratory pressure physiotherapy on tracheobronchial clearance in cystic fibrosis. Chest. 1991;100:1350-7.
17. Mure M, Martling C-R, Lindahl SGE. Dramatic effect on oxygenation in patients with severe acute lung insufficiency treated in the prone position. Crit Care Med. 1997;25:1539-44.
18. Norrenberg M, De Backer D, Moraine JJ. Oxygen consumption can increase during passive leg mobilization. Intensive Care Med. 1995;21:S177.
19. Parker A. Neonatal problems and the neonatal unit. In PM Eckersley, Elements of Pediatric Physiotherapy. 1993;1024-9.
20. Prokocimer P, Garbino J, Wolff M, Regnier B. Influence of posture on gas exchange in artificially ventilated patients with focal lung disease. Intensive Care Med. 1983;9:69-72.
21. Pryor J. Mucociliary clearance. In: Ellis E, Alison J (eds). Key Issues in Cardiorespiratory Physiotherapy. Oxford, UK: 1992. Butterworth-Heinemann. 1992.p.105-30.

22. Rabe KF, Hurd S, Anzueto A, et al. "Global strategy for the diagnosis, management, and prevention of chronic obstructive pulmonary Disease: GOLD Executive Summary". Am J Respir Crit Care Med. 2007;176(6):532-55.
23. Ramsey PG, Fife KH, Hackman RC, Meyers JD, Corey L. Herpes simplex virus pneumonia : clinical, virologic, and pathologic features in 20 patients. Ann Intern Med. 1982;97(6):813-20.
24. Reiff DB, Wells AU, Carr DH, Cole PJ, Hansell DM. CT findings in bronchiectasis: limited value in distinguishing between idiopathic and specific types. American Journal of Roentgenology. 1995;165:261-7.
25. Rossman CM, Waldes R, Sampson D, Newhouse MT. Effect of chest physiotherapy on the removal of mucus in patients with cystic fibrosis. Am Rev Respir Dis. 1982;126:131-5.
26. Rowe S, Cheadle WG. Complications of nosocomial pneumonia in the surgical patient. The American Journal of Surgery Bottom of Form. 2000;179(2):63-8.
27. Rundsch S: Pathophysiology of cor pulmonale. Med Prax. 1993;82(4): 95-8.
28. Sackner MA, Landa J, Greeneltch JF, Robinson MJ. Pathogenesis and prevention of tracheobronchial damage associated with suctioning process. Chest. 1973;64(3):284-90.
29. Stiller K. Physiotherapy in intensive care: towards an evidence-based practice. Chest. 2000;118:1801-13.
30. Swift GL, Rainer T, Saran R, Cambell IA, Prescott RJ. Use of Flutter VRP 1 in the management of patients with steroid-dependent asthma. Respiration. 1994;61:126-9.
31. Thompson CS, Harrison S, Ashley J, Day K, Smith DL. Randomised crossover study of the Flutter device and the active cycle of breathing technique in non-cystic fibrosis bronchiectasis. Thorax. 2002;57:446-8.
32. Vazquez MI, Buceta JM. Effectiveness of self-management programs and relaxation training in the treatment of bronchial asthma: relationships with trait anxiety and emotional attack triggers. Journal of Psychosomatic Research. 1993;37(1):71-81.
33. Whitley Rand Roizman B. Herpes simplex virus infections. The Lancet. 2001;357(9267):1513-8.
34. Wilson TA, Rehder K, Krayer S, Hoffman EA, Whitney CG, Rodarte JR. Geometry and respiratory displacement of human ribs. J Appl Physiol. 1987;62(5):1872-7.

CHAPTER

8

Cardiovascular Conditions

ANATOMY AND PHYSIOLOGY OF CARDIOVASCULAR SYSTEM

The Heart

The heart is the three layered, four chambered vital organ of the body, located within thoracic cavity, and enclosed by a sac known as the pericardium. The three layers from out to inward are named as epicardium, myocardium and endocardium.

The innermost cavity of the heart is divided in four chambers (Fig. 8.1), including two cavities called atria for receiving blood by heart and two cavities called ventricles for pumping out the blood by the heart. After the birth there is no direct communication between the right and left chambers of heart. The right atrium is separated

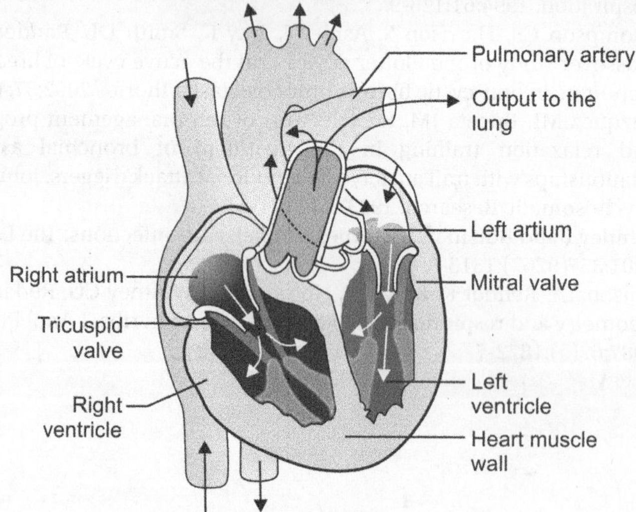

Fig. 8.1: The chambers of heart

from right ventricle by a tricuspid valve, having three cusps. The left atrium is separated from the left ventricle by a bicuspid valve having two cusps. This bicuspid valve is also called as mitral valve.

Atria are the blood receiving chambers of heart, which receive blood from the blood vessels termed as veins. Ventricles are blood exiting chambers of heart which push blood out of heart into blood vessels termed as arteries.

The right atrium receives deoxygenated blood from the body by two large veins called as superior vena cava and inferior vena cava. This blood is further directed via tricuspid valve into the right ventricles. From the right ventricle, this deoxygenated blood is pumped into the pulmonary artery to be sent to lungs for oxygenation. The valve between right ventricle and pulmonary artery is called as semilunar valve, which prevents backflow of blood from pulmonary artery into right ventricle.

From lungs, the fresh and oxygenated blood is sent into left atrium by pulmonary veins, which is then pushed through bicuspid valve into the left ventricle of heart. From here the blood is further pumped into the major arterial vessel of body called as aorta. The aorta is responsible for dispersing the blood into whole body for the utilization of oxygen and nutrients. The valve between left ventricle and aorta is called as aortic valve.

The left side of heart contains pure and oxygenated blood while the right side of heart contains deoxygenated blood. Thus the right and left side of heart work as two different units. However, both atria contract at same time and both ventricles also contract at same time.

Blood Supply of Heart

Heart is the pumping organ of body which is responsible for supplying the fresh blood to all organs of body. This pumping action of heart is due to its specialized muscles, called as myocardium. The initiation of pumping action is emerged at the SA (sino-atrial node), which is located at inner aspect of upper part of right atrium. The muscular efforts to perform pumping action need the regular supply of oxygen and nutrients and fresh blood supply. This is provided to heart by right and left coronary arteries, branches of the ascending aorta. These arteries supply blood to the walls of the myocardium. After its utilization, the used blood from the heart muscles enter into cardiac veins called as coronary veins, which further drain into coronary sinus opening into right atrium (Fig. 8.2).

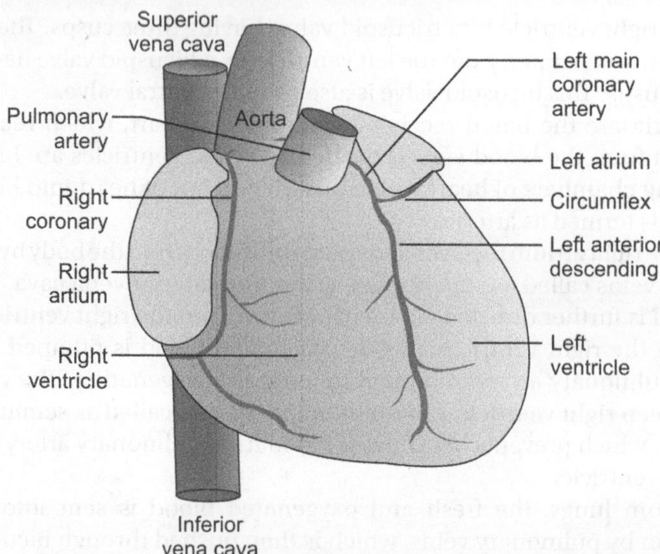

Fig. 8.2: The coronary circulation, the blood supply of heart

Blood Vessels

Beside heart, the cardiovascular system consists of blood vessels (arteries, veins, capilleries) which are conducting channels responsible for transporting and distributing blood in body tissues and organs. The vascular system is located in body in form of two closed systems—the pulmonary system and peripheral system. The pulmonary system transports blood from the right ventricle to the lungs and back to the left atrium. The peripheral system transports blood from the left ventricle to the tissues in all parts of the body and then returns the blood to the right atrium (Flow chart 8.1).

Blood vessels further can be divided into arteries and veins. Arteries are responsible for carrying blood away and out from heart. The veins are responsible for bringing blood towards heart.

Arteries (Table 8.1)

- These are vessels responsible for carrying blood away from heart. The pulmonary artery contains deoxygenated blood which is carried by it from the right ventricle of heart to the lungs for

Flow chart 8.1: The path of blood flow in the body

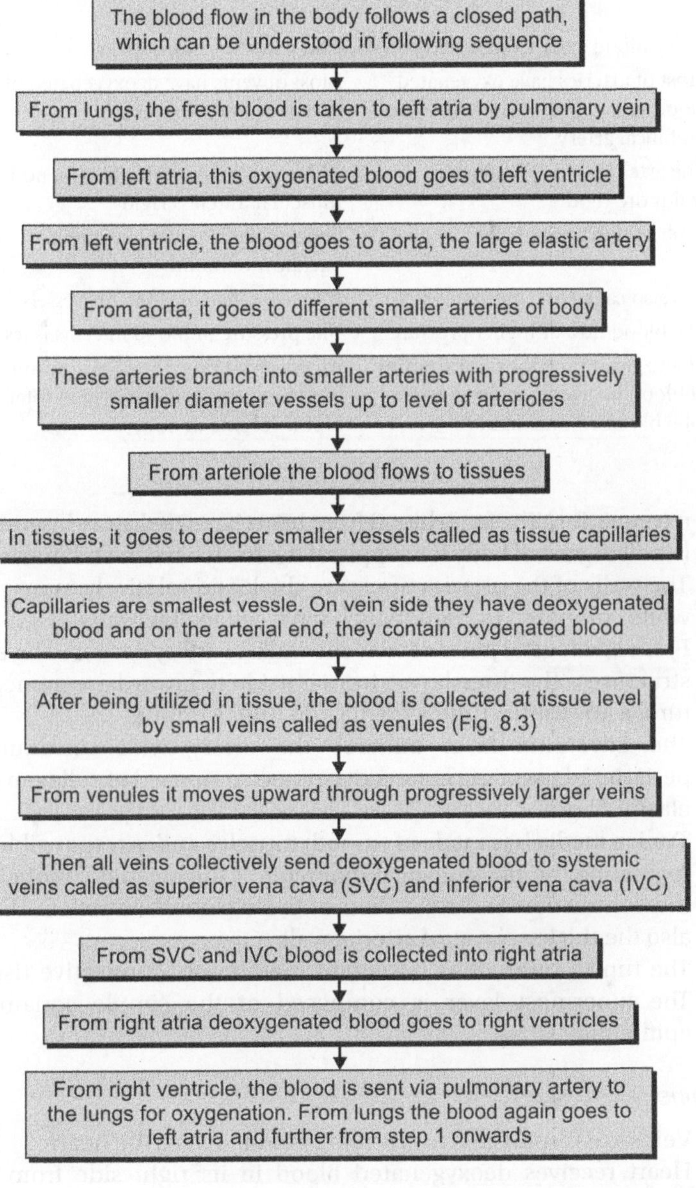

TABLE 8.1 Comparison of arteries and veins

Arteries	*Veins*
Carry blood away from heart	Carry blood towards heart
Most of arteries have oxygenated blood except pulmonary artery and umbilical artery	Most of veins have deoxygenated blood except pulmonary veins
The arterial wall is thick, muscular and more rigid	The vein wall is relatively thin, non-muscular and less rigid
Arteries don't have valves	Veins contain valves to prevent backflow of blood
It is also called as conducting vessels	It is also called as reservoir vessels
The blood flow at higher pressure	The pressure of blood in veins is less
At any given time the total amount of blood in arteries is up to 10% of total blood volume in body	At any given time the total amount of blood in veins is up to 70% of total blood volume in body

oxygenation. The fresh blood from heart is carried away by aorta to the all organs of body for supply of the fresh oxygen and nutrients.

- The walls of the arteries are more thick and relatively more rigid while compared to veins, which have collapsible walls.
- From hisological point of view the walls of artery has three layered structures. The three layers from outside to inward are named as tunica adventitia, tunica media and tunica intima.
- The adventitia layer adheres the artery with surrounding periarterial tissue via connective tissue composed of collagen and elastin fibers.
- Tunica media has made of smooth muscles and is responsible for regulating the physiological diameter of the arterial channel, by the contraction and relaxation of these smooth muscles. This is also the thickest layer of arterial wall.
- The tunica intima has basement membrane, connective tissue. The innermost layer is composed of the simple squamous epithelium.

Veins

- Veins are responsible for carrying blood toward the heart.
- Heart receives deoxygenated blood in its right side from the superior vena cava and inferior vena cava

- Heart receives fresh oxygenated blood in its left chamber via pulmonary veins which brings fresh oxygenated blood from lungs
- In contrast from arteries the walls of veins of heart has valves to prevent the back flow of blood
- Also the walls of veins are thin due to little amount of muscles and connective tissue, thus it has less blood pressure compared to arteries and less rigidity. Due to thin wall and less rigidity it has more blood storage capacity and thus also called as reservoir vessels.

Capillaries (Fig. 8.3)

- Capillaries, the smallest and most numerous of the blood vessels
- They form the bridging to bring about the material exchange between arteries and veins
- Also cause the exchange of gases, nutrients, metabolic waste products, oxygen between tissues and blood
- Amount of capillaries is directly proportional to the metabolic activity of body tissue.

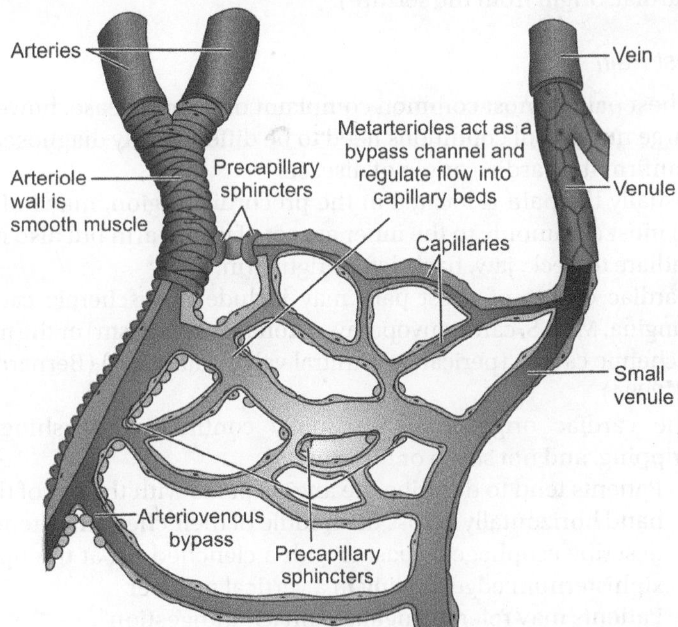

Fig. 8.3: The exchange between artery and vein via capillaries

CARDIOVASCULAR HISTORY AND EXAMINATION

History

Common chief complaints:

- Chest pain—might be sudden onset
- Tightness in chest associated with reduced coronary circulation
- Palpitation due to faster heart rate
- Dyspnea due to reduced oxygen in body
- Blackouts, syncope or dizziness due to reduced blood supply to the brain and vital organs of body
- Palpitation and chest pain which increases with activity and exertion
- Chest pain radiating to the left axillary aspect of upper arm
- Excessive swelling in the peripheral part of the body
- History or known case of peripheral vascular disease, cramps or cyanosis of the dependent part of the body
- Does the client have any history of loss of consciousness? If yes then what was the frequency and duration of consciousness? Does he/she have retrograde amnesia? (need to differentiate the cardiac origin from the seizure).

Chest Pain

- Chest pain is most common complaint of heart disease, however large number of conditions need to be differentially diagnosed to confirm the cardiac origin of disease
- Usually the pain is located in the precordial region, may radiate to most commonly to the inner aspect of upper arm but also may radiate to neck, jaw, back, left or right arm.
- Cardiac causes of chest pain may include the ischemic causes (angina, MI, AS, cardiomyopathy, coronary vasospasm) or the non-ischemic causes (pericarditis, mitral valve pathology) (Bernard, et al. 2004)
- The cardiac origin pain is usually continuous, crushing or gripping, and not sharp or interrupted.
  - Patients tend to describe the angina pains with the flat of their hand horizontally across the middle of their chest; they tend to describe esophageal spasms with a clenched fist at the upper xiphisternum edge moving in a vertical manner
  - Patients may refer to anginal pain as "indigestion".

- Usually the aggravating factors may include the physical exertion, exercises, stress
- The associated features may include vomiting, nausea, fever, sweating, palpitation, dizziness.

Breathlessness

- Breathlessness is another common complaint associated with heart disease.
- It may have non-cardiac origin especially if it is associated with rhonchi, wheezing. If associated with cardiac cause, the dyspnea aggravates on exertion. The severity of cardiac insufficiency is determined with the amount of physical activity that the client can bear before representing the symptoms of cardiac failure.
- Does the client presents with the features of sweating, cough, asthma, hemoptysis?
- Does the client presents the features of altered sensorium or disorientation.

Palpitations

- Palpitation is the subjective feeling of throbbing or thumping
- The best way to know about the nature of the palpitation is by asking the client to tap on the table the rate, frequency, intensity and regularity of the palpitation. If beat is irregular, it may represent dysrhythmia. The long duration of irregularity indicate atrial dysrhythmia. The small duration of irregularity may indicate coronary vasospasm, paroxysmal tachycardia, or early stage of the cardiac pathology.

Medical History

- The medical history of the drugs must be carefully documented
- Family history may be noted as cardiac pathologies might be having familial predisposition. This is more extensively documented if the symptoms of cardiac pathology appear before the age of 60 year.

Observation

- General features like body build, accessory muscles usage, gasps for breathing?
- The skin color and mucos membrane color for the appearance of pallor, jaundice, sweatiness and clamminess

- Look out for evidence of cyanosis on finger, nail bed, lips, eye sclera
- Evidence of finger clubbing, nail brittleness, skin hemorrhage
- Observe for presence of evidence for peripheral or local or generalized edema.

Auscultation

- For dept, rhythm of breathing
- Auscultate for presence of any additional heart sounds.

Pulse Palpation

Check blood pressure using brachial artery and popliteal artery. The systolic and diastolic blood pressure must be clearly documented.

Chest Examination

- Observe chest wall deformity, the equal expansion of chest wall
- Palpate over chest wall to record any thrill
- Auscultate chest wall for adventitious sound or murmur

Various Investigations Used for Cardiovascular Conditions

Chest X-ray

- Helps to judge the size of heart and chambers
- Helps to see the orientation of heart apex
- Helps to evaluate the prominency of pulmonary vasculature
- On full inspiration, the ratio of heart diameter to the chest diameter must not be more than half in a normal case
- Expiratory films may falsely give the impression of cardiomegaly and pulmonary congestion. Supine films may also give a similar appearance.

Electrocardiography (ECG)

- Helps to indicate the performance of the cardiac conduction
- Alteration can indicate the block of conduction of heart contraction impulses
- The ischemia, cardiac arrest, arrhythmia can be determined by this
- If ECG changes are within normal limit, then ECG testing can be done under stressful conditions including the graded treadmill test

- Specific parameter, shape, duration and amplitude of specific portions of the wave are studied and interpreted to determine the nature of cardiac pathology
- When specific pattern or abnormal wave is not noticeable during testing, then halter ECG is used where a portable ECG recorder is tied on thorax wall for 24 hours to record the timing, nature and associated causes of abnormal wave.

Ultrasound

- Patients in whom peripheral venous access cannot be gained with traditional insert and trial techniques pose a challenge to emergency departments across the world. Alternative access sites include central lines and deeper peripheral veins. Increased use of ultrasound machines makes ultrasound-guided peripheral venous access an increasingly popular option (Abboud and Kendal, 2004; Goldstein, 2006). It also helps to minimize the risks associated with the repeated venous or arterial puncture while searching the vascular access by otherwise traditional methods (Goldstein, 2006).
- Ultrasound technique is employed in echocardiography and Doppler examination to reveal anatomical abnormalities as well as flow disturbances through vessles, narrowed valves, cardiac chambers filling and functioning, identification of the abnormal dilatation of the vasculature (aneurysm), identifying the location and amount of the fluid accumulation in deeper tissues
- Ultrasound imaging is also useful to locate the pericardial effusion and used to guide its removal with 'tapping' if necessary.

Echocardiography

- Also known as TTE (transthoracic echocardiography) or simply as ECHO.
- It is highly useful, non-invasive and the risk free investigative procedure for knowing the cardiac functioning
- Echocardiography is useful for determining:-
  - The motion of heart wall
  - The chamber size
  - Thickness of heart wall chambers
  - Ejection fraction and stroke volume
  - The functioning, opening and closing of the heart valves—any evidence of regurgitation

- Congenital defects of heart
- The presence of the emboli or thrombosis
- The diameter of aorta root.

Isotope Scanning

Technetium scan is a noninvasive nuclear scan that uses a radioactive isotope called technetium Tc-99m stannous pyrophosphate to evaluate:

- Blood flow after a heart attack
- Helps to confirm the heart attack even if the heart attack associated symptoms and pain were absent
- Areas of reduced blood supply can be identified by its appearance as the reduced uptake of the isotope amount in the area of diminished blood supply
- Helps to know size and location of heart attack
- It is more useful when ECG and cardiac enzyme studies do not provide definitive results—after heart surgery, for example, or when chest pain occurred more than 48 hours before the patient was examined
- It is also used to evaluate the heart before and after heart surgery
- Also helps to identify the "hot spot areas" which provide higher risk of calcium deposition and plaque formation
- It gives better quality imaging than the thallium imaging because of smaller lifetime and the possibility of injecting in higher amount
- Test may be repeated over weeks to see the progression or resolution of the heart pathology.

The isotope is injected into a vein, via blood it reaches heart and is absorbed by healthy tissue at a known rate during a certain time period. The radionuclide detector is used to pick up the gamma rays emitted by the isotope. Another advantage is lesser radiation risk because of quick removal from the body. The exposure volume to radiation is not more than a simple chest X-ray.

Computed Tomography (CT)

- CT scan has advantages such as:
  - CT scan gives a detailed three dimensional view of heart and the surrounding blood vessels.
  - CT scan takes images of heart in form of slices across any plane or axis, so as to give its detailed structure analysis

- Helpful to identify areas of arterial narrowing and myocardial ischemia thus helpful in better way to identify coronary artery disease
- It is helpful to identify plaques in the coronary artery
- It is helpful to diagnose thoracic aneurysm, tumors, effusions, ischemia, amount of calcium deposition in the coronary arteries.

- It has some disadvantages too:
  - It exposes the client to higher amount of radiations
  - Though it can identify coronary artery plaque, it cannot tell whether or not the plaque is compromising the blood supply to underlying heart tissue. Thus to identify this detailed study with angiographic imaging, PET (positron emission tomography) and MRI are required.

Magnetic Resonance Imaging (MRI)

- MRI can be used to examine the heart in multiple planes and is able to differentiate many pathological states such as pericardial effusions, cardiomyopathy, pathology of heart chamber, valve diseases, aneurysm, stenosis, dissecting point, emboli, etc.
- Coronary magnetic resonance angiography has an accuracy of about 72 percent in diagnosing coronary artery disease (Kim, et al. 2001).

Venography (Peterson, et al. 2010)

Venography is also called as phlebography and it involves the taking X-rays of veins after enhancing their appearance upon injecting a special dye into veins. Before development of Doppler and ultrasonography, it was highly useful for diagnosing deep vein thrombosis and chronic venous insufficiency. It also can identify that for how long are veins not working, as chrnoic vein problem would be having clots while the recently malfunctioning veins will not have clots.

Angiography

Coronary angiography is considered to be the diagnostic gold standard for CHD patients. It is almost always indicated in the patients presenting with the abnormal control of their symptom. In such patients this investigation along with some stress testing shows abnormal findings including significant ST segment shift on the ECG, significant left ventricular wall-motion abnormalities on echocardiography or substantial defects on myocardial perfusion imaging. Occasionally, angiography may be required for patients who have atypical chest pain or inconclusive exercise tolerance tests (David Barrett, 2006).

In this investigation the vascular access is done by a percutaneous approach through femoral artery, and less commonly radial, axillary, popliteal or brachial artery. The major vessels of body can be studied using this method. Further contrast dye injections can be used to enhance clarity. The actual structure or the presence of any foreign material such as atherosclerotic plaque, hematoma, blooding points, thrombi, aneurysm, and frail region of vessels can be actually visualized.

Beside these investigative procedures, the various physical performance testing can be done including graded exercise tolerance testing (GXT), aerobic capacity testing, 6 minute walk testing.

Biochemical Markers of Heart Disease (Karras and Kane, 2001)

- The biochemical markers are helpful in evaluation of acute myocardial infarction (AMI) where no other test is highly specific and sensitive to diagnose AMI within first 6 hours after onset of chest pain
- A screening test and serum of patients with abnormal total CK (Creatine kinase) values should undergo a CK-MB mass assay. Elevation (more than 5% of the total CK value) level of CK-MB is highly suggestive of AMI
- The cardiac troponins are highly useful as markers of acute coronary syndromes, rather than specifically of AMI
- After 6 to 8 hours of symptom duration has elapsed, the cardiac-specific markers are highly effective in diagnosing AMI.

HEART FAILURE

Heart failure refers to the state when heart can't pump the blood in sufficient amount as per the requirement in the body. The heart can't pump the enough blood into body, either due to limited filling, poor hear rate, less force of contraction. The heart failure can occur as right heart failure or left heart failure which refers to the poor pumping ability of right ventricle or left ventricle respectively. Thus in left heart failure, the body develops a state of deficiency of fresh blood supply. The vital and non-vital organs of body develop starvation of nutrients, oxygen while simultaneously suffering metabolite accumulation. In right heart failure, the blood cannot be emptied from right ventricles into the lungs, and thus blood accumulates in right side of heart. Since blood is not reaching in lungs, it can't be oxygenated, and the body develops oxygen deficiency indirectly.

Symptoms

The most common signs and symptoms are:

- Shortness of breath or difficulty in breathing due to the increased pulmonary congestion as now lungs have less space to receive fresh blood from the environment therefore less oxygenated blood goes to various organs
- Feeling tired due to the reduced supply of fresh oxygen and nutrients to the working organs of body
- Swelling in the ankles, feet, legs, and sometimes the abdomen due to the increased venous congestion and the reduced ability of the veins to get empty
- Exercise intolerance
- Sometime the episodes of syncope and dizziness may also develop
- Cough may also occur when the increased pulmonary congestion lead to irritation and impaired gaseous exchange, called as pulmonary edema.

The symptoms frequency, severity, intensity and associated problems increase with the progression of the heart failure. In initial stages the symptoms come into action after strenuous activity but with higher progression and severity of the disease even the simple activities such as walking or standing may lead to symptoms (see New York Heart Association criteria).

Swelling may occur in either the specific organs or it may occur in generalized manner. It occurs due to the increased buildup of fluid in body.

Limitation on Physical Activity

The severity of the cardiac failure is done on the basis of severity of the symptoms during various levels of physical activity. This grading is based on NYHA (New York heart association) criteria (1994) as follows:

- *Class 1*: No limits—ordinary physical activity does not cause undue tiredness or shortness of breath.

- *Class 2*: Slight or mild limits—comfortable at rest, but ordinary physical activity results in tiredness or shortness of breath.
- *Class 3*: Marked or noticeable limits—comfortable at rest, but less than ordinary physical activity causes tiredness or shortness of breath.
- *Class 4*: Severe limits—unable to carry on any physical activity without discomfort. Symptoms are also present at rest. If any physical activity is undertaken, discomfort increases.

Diagnosis

The suspicion of the heart failure arises when symptoms such as dyspnea, fatigue, chest pain, reduced energy, palpitation, fluid accumulation in the peripheral extremities occurs.

There is no single test to determine if the heart failure has occurred. The diagnosis lies on the clinical diagnosis, combined with the investigative procedures and biochemical marker studies.

Congestive cardiac failure means a clinical syndrome due to heart disease, resulting in congestion in the peripheral circulation with or without congestion of the lungs.

Medical and Family History

The clients having positive history of heart failure or heart related pathology among their family member are probably at higher risk of developing cardiac pathology.

- The genetic factors have been found to be related to determine the risk of cardiovascular mortality. The frequency of myocardial infarction to be two to four times higher in first-degree relatives of patients
- With myocardial infarction than among first-degree relatives of healthy control subjects (Kate, et al. 1982).
- About fivefold excess risk of cardiovascular death is found in younger men (not in younger women) with positive family histories of heart disease, independent of all major heart disease risk factors (Barrett and Khaw, 1984).

Tests

In cases that have been suspected of suffering heart failure on basis of complaints and clinical testing, the investigative interventions are done to confirm or rule out the diagnosis.

- *Chest X-ray*: This is the preliminary testing to see if any enlargement of heart or lung has occurred. It may also show the fluid accumulation, the amount of the lung expansion, the orientation of the heart, shape of the heart, or the prominency of the pulmonary vasculature.
- *ECG (electrocardiogram)*: It is used to measure rate, regularity of the heart beat, pattern of the different components of the cardiac cycle. However, it is not significantly useful because in most of the cases the alterations in the ECG are temporary, and usually apparent either when ECG is taken immediately after attack or in severe cases. It may also reveal the arrhythmia, irregular beats or missed beats of heart.
- When the irregularity of heart beat or any other abnormality is not found on ECG testing, then a Holter moniter is attached to the thorax wall with its electrode placed on positions of the normal ECG electrodes. This is worn 24 hours a day and gives continuous recording of the heart rhythm and heart beat during daily routine activity. Thus it helps to know the activity which were responsible for leading to the symptoms of the heart failure.
- Technetium scans to locate the areas which have suffered the ischemia.
- The CT scan and PET (positron emission tomography) also helps to take the images of heart through many axis and also the moving pictures of the blood passing through heart chambers.
- *Coronary angiography*: The contrasting dye is injected in the coronary artery, and the images are taken or the echocardiography is done to trace the flow of blood through the heart muscles, the functioning of chambers and the pumping functioning of the heart.
- The echocardiography is also useful for determining the motion of heart wall, the chamber size, thickness of heart wall chambers, ejection fraction and stroke volume.
- *Cardiac catheterization*: The think, flexible tube with camera attached, is inserted into body via femoreal artery to reach upto coronary artery. This allows directly visualization of the arteries, see any blockage, checking pressure and blood flow in heart chambers, collecting blood sample from heart.
- *Stress tests*: Client is subjected to different grades of physical exertion so as to make heart work harder. It helps to know how well are the heart muscles working. The testing is done under this stressful condition of the heart so as to record the responses and

to know if any signs of cardiac insufficiency occur. Various stress tests employed include blood pressure changes; ECG testing; ECHO; heart scanning.

- The other causes of heart failure may also be needed to rule out. This includes the hormonal testing, and thyroid function testing because hyper or hypo functioning of thyroid can lead to heart failure.

Causes

Heart failure can occur due to the following causes:-

- When cardiac output is low
  - Poor/slow/less forceful contraction of heart muscles
  - Reduced stroke volume
  - Incomplete filling of heart walls
  - Heart muscles fatigue
  - Slow rate of heart beat
  - Hypovolemic shock.
- It may also occur when the demand of oxygen, nutrients and fresh blood supply in the body increases beyond the capacity of the heart
  - Anemia
  - Thyrotoxicosis
  - Beri beri
  - Acute fever
  - Septic shock.
- Weakening of the heart muscles such as due to
  - Failure of the contraction to occur at all (heart arrest)
  - Ischemic damage to cardiac muscles
  - Myocardial infarction
  - Cardiac enlargement
- *The leading causes of heart failure include*: Coronary artery diseases (CAD), hypertension (HTN), diabetes mellitus (DM), myocardiac infarction, hypovolemia (blood loss, septic shock, pelvic bone fracture, severe dehydration)
- Metabolic abnormality, high dosages of antidepression medicines also may lead to cardiac failure.

Classification of the Heart Failure

Heart failure may be classified as:

- Compensated versus uncompensated heart failure
- Right heart failure versus left heart failure (Table 8.2)

TABLE 8.2 Comparison of right versus left heart failure

	Left heart failure	*Right heart failure*
Cause	Can occur due to failure of left atria, left ventricle or both	Right heart failure can occur due to failure of right atria, right ventricle or both
Complication	Failure of left heart, causes failure to empty the pulmonary vein, thus backward increase in pressure to cause pulmonary congestion	Right heart cannot be emptied—superior and inferior vena cava cannot be emptied—blood keep on accumulating in systemic veins—increased congestions in systemic capillaries and veins
Symptoms	Poor gas exchange in lungs dyspnea, orthopnea (breathlessness on lying flat) poor supply of fresh blood to body increased fatigue, exercise intolerance, confusion, dizziness, easy fatigue, reduced peripheral pulses at rest	Excessive fluid accumulation in body—peripheral or/and general oedema—initially edema is most prominent in gravity dependent part of body (ankles, lower legs, sacral region)
Signs	Pulmonary congestion—tachypnea, respiratory distress; rales; pulmonary edema Cyanosis due to the poor blood supply to extremity apex beat due to left ventricle hypertrophy adventitous heart sound due to increased blood in heart mitral regurgitation because excessive blood in left ventricle impedes reception of blood from left atria	Fluid accumulation in abdomen causes ascitis; in liver causes hepatomegaly; in urinary bladder causes nocturia when blood return to heart is increased in lying position. Hepatomegaly—failure of liver function—poor detoxification in body; poor formation of clotting factors—coagulopathy. Engorged superior vena cava—prominent jugular vein—positive hepatojugular reflux

- Chronic heart failure versus acute heart failure
- Systolic dysfunction versus diastolic dysfunction heart failure

Right versus Left Heart Failure

Right and left side failure rarely do exist in isolation thus most patients represent features of body side failure.

The most common cause of right-sided heart failure is left-sided heart failure.

Acute versus Chronic Heart Failure

Acute heart failure is the rapid onset cardiac insufficiency while the chronic means the cardiac insufficiency which develops over long duration.

Compensated versus Uncompensated Heart Failure

- Compensated heart failure is the condition in which the compensatory mechanism play role to avoid the need of surgery. For example in case of reduced stroke volume the heart rate may increase to maintain the necessary cardiac output.
- Acute decompensated heart failure include episodes in which compensatory mechanisms fail to abort the immediate need of hospitalization or surgery

Chronic Heart Failure (CHF)

It is a complex clinical syndrome that can result from any structural or functional cardiac or non-cardiac disorder that impairs the ability of the heart to respond to physiological demands for increased cardiac output. Chronic heart failure is characterized by symptoms such as exertional breathlessness and fatigue, and signs of fluid retention as well assigns associated with the underlying cardiac disorder (SIGN guidelines, 2007).

Treatment

Medical Management

The medical line dealing with the heart failure depends on the cause, nature and severity of heart failure. Following medicines are most commonly prescribed for the patients suffering from heart failure.

- ACE inhibitors and nitrate medicines cause vasodilation to reduce the amount of work needed to pump the blood through narrow blood vessels
- Beta blockers reduce the force and speed of heart contraction, thus they reduce cardiac work
- Diuretics: They increase the volume and frequency of urination, thus reduce the blood volume and blood pressure

- Inotropic medicines reduce the force of heart contraction and reduce the speed of heart beating.

Surgery

- In cases of the bradycardia, arrhythmia the pacemaker may be inserted to regulate and correct the heart rhythm or the biventricular pacemaker may be inserted to coordinate the contraction of right and left ventricles in patients with heart failure.
- In case of the partial or incomplete blockage of the coronary arteries, the balloon angioplasty may be done where a catheter is introduced into the partially block artery, and then the attached balloon is inflated to rechanalise the blood flow across this obstructed vessel.
- Alternatively in case of repeatedly collapsible vessels the coronary stenting may be done where a wired mesh metal tube "stent" is introduced into obstructed vessels to keep them open.
- In cases of complete obstruction of the coronary artery, the arterial bypass grafting might be done to bypass the irreversibly damaged blood vessels, and using the new vessels to establish the blood flow to the affected regions of heart.
- In more severe cases the heart transplant may be an option subjected to the availability of the heart.

Physiotherapy Management

Physiotherapist must pay attention to the symptoms of the dyspnea and edema.

To achieve the increase in exercise tolerance is an important goal which is important to improve the quality of life (QOL). Also the changes in the symptoms of progression or resolution must be carefully documented as they may show the variation in the heart failure (Dracup, et al. 1994; Jaarsma, et al. 1999). Those who are able to care for themselves effectively will have fewer problems leading them to get hospitalized or visit emergency department (Happ, et al. 1997).

Lifestyle Modifications

In order to execute lifestyle modifications, enhance self care abilities, reducing risk of hospitalization and to increase functional outcome, the patients education is vital (Stockdale, et al. 1981; Dracup, et al. 1984).

Adjustment of lifestyle can be suggested by (Jaarsma, et al. 1999):

- Adhering to complex medication regimen
- Regulating the diet and fluid intake
- Adapting their activities
- Strategies to manage blood pressure. Avoid the excessive fluid intake or excessive salt intake or alcohol consumption
- Alcohol is myocardiac depressant (Norway, 1968) and the long-term alcohol consumption causes dilated cardiomyopathy
- Up to 6 mg/day salt can be consumed daily as safe limit for patients of chronic cardiac failure (SIGN guidelines, 2004)
- One RCT found that following 6 months, individually prescribed salt and fluid restricted diet, patients with mild to moderate heart failure showed clinical improvements with a greater absence of edema and fatigue, resulting in a significant improvement in New York heart association (NYHA) category and quality of life when compared to general advice (Alveos, et al. 2004).
- Weight management and regulation is important aspect for dealing with cardiac diseases. The client must keep a note of the body weight. Any increase in weight increases risk of progression of disease, while the fall in weight may indicate the increased energy needs. Thus daily or weekly regulation of diet intake must be regulated.

Exercises

- Exercises are vital to maintain the cardiovascular status of the client suffering from heart failure. Beneficial effects on exercise capacity and many of the physiologic processes involved in the development of, as well as, primary prevention of coronary artery disease
- The exercises that are most commonly prescribed, include aerobic activities, swimming, light to brisk walking, treadmill walking,
- The client must be educated about the limits as well as volume of physical activity as per the severity of cardiac failure and the medical fitness tests. Staying active is important, however there is some minimum amount of activity needed to get beneficial effects, and also the higher limits of exercises need not to be crossed as it would increase the risk. Appropriate volume of exercises with proper rest period in between to allow recovery.
- Current public health recommendations state that all people over 2 years of age should accumulate 30 minutes of moderate-intensity endurance-type physical activity on most (preferably

all) days of the week. Additionally, the American College of Sports Medicine (ACSM) recommends that at least two sessions each week incorporate resistance or strength training involving the major muscle groups (Pollock, et al. 1998)

- While designing the training regime for the patient of heart failure, the physiological limitations and the severity of pathology must be kept in mind.

The Physiotherapy management is also highly vital during the preoperative and postoperative phases of the cardiothoracic surgeries, including heart transplantation, coronary artery bypass grafting.

VARICOSE VEINS

Varicose veins (Fig. 8.4) are swollen, enlarged and tortuous veins that impair the return of the blood from periphery backward towards heart and thus become prominent due to venous stagnation. These are visible just under the surface of the skin.

They are most commonly seen (but not limited to) legs.

Related Vein Problems

Other types of vein related problems may exist either in isolation or along with varicose veins:

- Spider veins
  - Occur due to the dilatation of the capillaries, the smallest blood vessels of body

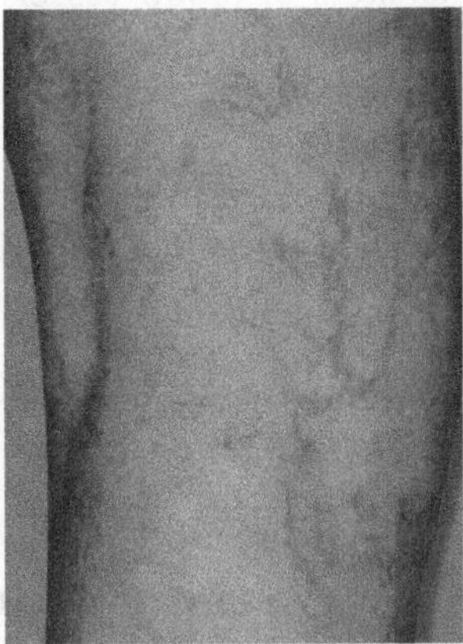

Fig. 8.4: Spider vein in the posterior aspect of knee (*For color version, see Plate 8*)

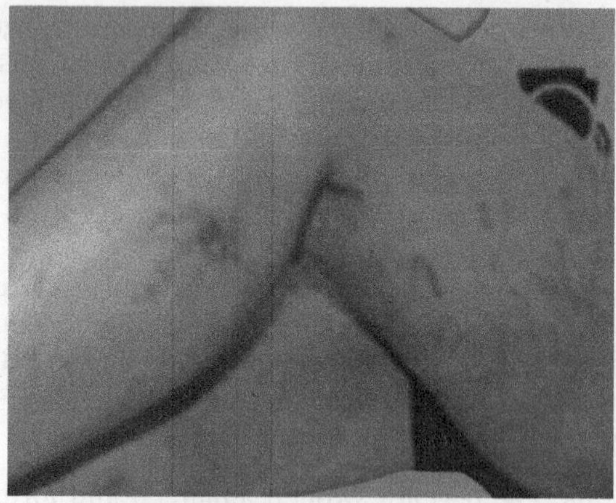

Fig. 8.5: Telangiectasias (*For color version, see Plate 8*)

- Are common around knees, face, around ankle and proximal calf muscle. Resemble a spider web or tree branch in appearance (Fig. 8.4)
- Their color may appear blue or red or light brownish
- These don't communicate with the underlying deeper veins and don't need medical or surgical interventions
- If they are not progressive, they may not need even any elastic stocking supports

- Telangiectasias (Fig. 8.5)
  - They are small clusters of blood vessels that look similar to spider veins however are red in color
  - They are red in color and are commonly found on the upper body, including the face
- Reticular veins (Weiss and Weiss, 1993)
  - They are flat (not bulged like spider veins) blue veins commonly seen behind the knees
- Hemorrhoids
  - They are varicose veins in blood vessels in and around the anus, which are responsible for leakage of blood with stool, especially in cases of dry feces
- Varicocele
  - This is the varicose vein in the scrotum (the skin over the testicles)
  - It may lead to infertility.

Symptoms

Common features of varicose veins include:

- Enlarged veins that are visible on skin
- Different degree of swelling in lower leg, around ankles and feet
- Painful, achy or "heavy" legs due to venous stagnation
- Throbbing or cramping in your legs due to starvation of fresh blood and nutrient supply
- Itching of the overlying skin, especially in the lower leg and ankle
- Discoloration of your skin surrounding the varicose veins
- In severe cases may lead to breakage of overlying skin or the skin ulceration.

Complications

The complications include dermatitis, thrombophlebitis, venous ulceration, bleeding of varicose vein.

- Dermatitis is the itchy rash on the lower leg or ankle due to the varicose veins in the legs. It can sometimes cause bleeding or a skin ulcer to develop if scratched or irritated
- Thrombophlebitis includes blood clot (thrombosis) formation in veins
- Thrombophlebitis may be superficial when clot formation occurs in superficial veins due to infection or skin irritation, and only small local area is affected
- In case of deep type of thrombophlebitis the thrombosis/blood clot develops in veins deeper in the body. It can be life threatening if the clot breaks off and travels to the lungs, which is called pulmonary embolism (Rabhi, et al. 2000), or upto the brain in case of cerebral embolism
- The deep type of thrombophlebitis does not occur in varicose veins but in cases of immobility or fracture of the bones.

Features

- The most common symptom of varicose veins and edema is the substantial pain experienced, as well as night cramps, numbness, tingling, the legs may feel heavy, achy, and possibly be unsightly (Weiss and Weiss,1993).
- The skin around the varicose vein may also itch, throb, or feel like it is burning. Symptoms tend to worsen after long periods of standing and with each successive pregnancy.

Diagnosis

For diagnosis of the varicose veins mostly the physical examination and observations of the affected body part in elevated and gravity dependent positions, are sufficient.

To diagnose the deep vein thrombosis in the leg, the Homan test is conducted, where the calf muscle belly is squeezed. The intense pain will be reported if the underlying deep veins have thrombosis.

Diagnostic tests (commonly ultrasound Doppler) are needed to rule out other similar disorders or conditions. In rare cases the venography and angiogram may be needed to visualize the occluding lesion within lumen of the veins.

Causes

- Varicose veins develop when the valves become weakened, damaged, or don't work well
- When the walls of veins have increased permeability or weakness
- The risk factors which increase the vein wall weakness include aging, pregnancy (increase venous pressure), obesity (increased pressure on the veins), standing jobs (prolong standing favors gravity assisted pooling of blood)
- Other risk factors include venous obstruction, leg injury, arterio-venous malformation
- Varicose veins are more common in women than in men (Andrew, et al. 2005)
- Genetic link has been found (Andrew, et al. 2005).

Pathogenesis

- Veins of the gravity dependent part of the body (especially those lower limb) are responsible for pumping the blood upward to assist the return of blood towards heart. The veins also have valves to prevent the backward flow of the blood and to allow only upward directed flow
- Due to any reason if walls of the veins become, the valve loose normal functioning, wall lose their normal elasticity like a rubber band, then the lumen of veins becomes wider. Its diameter increases. The valves tips don't approximate each other, thus valves fail to close to occlude the lumen. Valves now can not prevent the back flow of blood flow. The blood stagnates within veins, veins further dilate and engorge. Their elastic nature is

further impaired, they twist around axis. This further aggravates venous stagnation. The veins permanently dilate out.

- Established risk factors (Dimmer, et al. 2005) include older age, female gender, pregnancy, family history of venous disease, obesity and occupations associated with orthostasis.

Treatment

- In majority of cases the varicose veins usually don't impose medical problems. However, they may impose need to receive treatment for associated pain, cosmetic problems, skin problems, blood clots, or other complications.
- Compression stockings (Curri et al, 1989) have been recommended to prevent the radially flaring of the veins, and also to increase the support to the walls of the vein. The elastic nature of stocking also helps to work in similar way to the muscle pump, and aids the venous return and improve microcirculation to the region. These are most preferred conservative management and also the necessary adjunct for pre and postoperative management of the vascular surgeries.
- The stockings are mostly custom made according to the individual specific dimensions. The stockings have pressure gradients having relatively higher pressure on the distal end of the extremity, and relatively reduced pressure as we move towards proximal portions of the limb. They are worn during the day and taken off at night. The stockings are available in different material according to the comfort and the material quality. Stockings must be used with precautions in case of associated arterial insufficiency too.
- Injection therapy (sclerotherapy) is recommended for patients with small and superficial varicose veins and spider veins. This involves the injection of irritant chemical such as hypertonic saline solution or a sclerosing agent (glycerine, polidocanol, chromate glycerine) is injected into the offending veins, causing them to scar, shrink and seal the lumen. Following the injections, compression bandages are applied to prevent blood from refilling the veins and to allow them to heal. This is the non-surgical approach and prevents the progression of the vein occlusion of the deeper veins. The associated risks involve brown spotting at the injection sites, formation of blood clots in superficial veins, an allergic reaction to the injected irritant or the formation of new spider veins. It is not used to treat large varicose veins because the

scarring of these veins may permanently compromise the venous return from the drained portion of the body. Multiple treatments may be required.

- Laser surgery involves the projecting low intensity laser beaming over the superficial vein so as to resolve the clot, and fading the blockage.
- Ambulatory phlebectomy is done under local anesthesia and involves making tiny skin punctures on the skin to remove the underlying superficial vein clot.
- Endoscope assisted surgery is typically done in case of venous ulceration and the obstruction of vein is directly removed surgically with endoscope help.

Physiotherapy Management

Physiotherapy Goals

- To prevent or minimize edema
  - Home exercise program is the best to teach the patient for reduction of edema
- To minimize venous stasis
  - Pressure-gradient support stockings may be helpful to minimize the venous stasis
  - During exercise and ambulation support garment may be used
  - Active exercise, such as walking, on a regular basis
  - Elevation of lower extremities
  - Long standing should be avoided
  - Elevate effected extremity above the level of the heart (30° to 45°) when resting or sleeping
  - During rest the patients having varicose veins are advised to lie on their left side instead of right. This will avoid direct compression of the inferior vena cava (which is located on right) thus controlling the venous engorgement.
- To increase venous return and reduce edema
  - Use pneumatic compression therapy in the affected limb elevated position for several hours a day
  - Manual massage (primarily effleurage) to drain edema. Massage stroke in a distal-to-proximal direction clearing the proximal nodes and areas of edema first, then the middle, and finally the distal areas

- Relaxation exercises and active ROM (range of motion—pumping exercises) of the distal muscles while involved limb is elevated
- Muscle pumping exercises of the lower calf, muscles are done to promote venous return (Bamigboye and Smyth, 2008).

- To prevent ulcerations, wound infections and skin abression
  - Skin hygiene education
  - Keep the skin clean and supple; wash with disinfectant and use moisturizers however fragrance solutions are avoided
  - Avoid infections; pay immediate attention to a skin abrasion or cut, an insect bite, a blister, or a burn
  - The proper fitting shoes are recommended. The shoes longer than one's feet size are to be avoided as they may lead to frictional injury. The tight shoes may aggravate compressions
  - The sock must have loose upper brim as tight upper brim impairs venous return
  - Avoid contact with harsh detergents and chemicals
  - Use caution when cutting nails. Electric razors are recommended compared to blades and razor
  - Avoid hot baths, whirlpools, and saunas that elevate the body's core temperature.

RAYNAUD'S DISEASE

Raynaud's disease is rare disorders that are characterized by the brief episodes of vasospasm affecting the blood vessels of the fingers (more common) and toes. Due to this the temporary reduction in the blood flow occurs to these regions.

When the features occur without any know or related underlying causes, it is called as Raynaud's disease however when it occurs secondary to some associated pathological state; it is labeled as Raynaud's phenomenon.

Features

- The patients of Raynaud's disease are hyperesponsive to cold
- The cold temperature triggers the vasospasm attacks to temporarily impede the blood flow to the affected part(s), and the skin appears white followed by bluish (lack of oxygen). The affected areas can throb or feel numb and tingly, painful

- In people with Raynaud's, the response to cold is exaggerated and may be provoked by short exposure to cold such as taking something out of the freezer
- Later on as vasospasm ends, the blood flow is resumed and the skin turns red
- With severe Raynaud's (very rare condition), prolonged (20 minute cold exposure, to temperature less than 60 degree Fahrenheit) or repeated episodes can cause sores or tissue death (gangrene), and major tissue damage
- Attack mostly lasts about 15 minutes, and less commonly upto less than one minute or hours
- Attack can occur daily or weekly
- Sometimes attacks affect only one or two fingers or toes. Different areas may be affected at different times.

The two commonly identified triggering factors are cold and the stressful emotional stresses.

Diagnosis

Diagnosis of Raynaud's disease is based on a patient's history of experiencing color changes in their extremities in response to exposure to cold or emotional stress.

Cold exposure test may be used in clinic to reproduce the symptoms.

The temperature testing of finger is done where temperature sensors are attached to the fingers of the hand. The hand is then briefly exposed to the cold, usually by dunking it in ice water. If the patient likely has Raynaud's, it will take more than the normal time for the finger temperature to return to what it was at the start of the test.

Causes

- No definite factor is well established except cold exposure
- Vasculopathy or neuropathy affecting the action of blood vessels in the hands and feet
- Repetitive actions that damage the nerves that control blood vessels in the hands and feet
- Exposure to certain chemicals
- Use of vasoconstrictor medicines.

Risk Factors

- Scleroderma, systemic lupus erythematosus, scleroderma, Buerger's disease
- High risk jobs: Typing, playing the piano

Treatment

Raynaud disease has not clear known pathology therefore no definite treatment is available, yet the episodes of vasospasm may be deferred.

Precautions

- Warm clothing is recommended
- Avoid sudden exposure to cold and damp
- Attack may occur while standing near freezers and refrigerated sections of grocery stores
- Exercises are recommended to maintain the proper circulation to the distal portion of fingers and toes
- When the risk of attack is expected to happen brisk rubbing or warm water dip of hands and feet is recommended to increase circulation
- Must avoid the job which need repeated movements of the smaller joints of hand including piano, typing, vibratory tools, prolonged driving
- Avoid smoking, stressful environment, vasospasmodic medicines, tight clothings, tight shoe laces, tight socks.

Medical Management

- Vasodilators medicines to dilate the vessles if preventive measures fail. Calcium channel blockers are effective, particularly for Raynaud syndrome secondary to scleroderma. Medication may be limited to the colder months
- Medical treatment to the associated condition, which could be responsible for secondary Raynaud disease
- Amputation of gangrene affected finger or toe.

Physiotherapy Management

Physiotherapy Goals

- Teach the patient how to minimize or prevent potential impairments and correct impairments or functional limitations currently affecting functional capabilities.

- Self management of impairment—skin care, flexibility and mobility exercises
- Patient education
- Home exercise program
- Following preventive measures
- Technique to rapidly terminate the vasospasm phase
- Stress management technique—relaxation exercises, environmental modification, distraction, music therapy
- EMG biofeedback guided relaxation

- Communicate with health professionals from other disciplines appropriate for consultation with the patient
  - Medical or surgical management including medications to minimize vasospasm
  - Investigations to rule out other possible similar pathological conditions
- Improve exercise tolerance for ADL and decrease the incidence of intermittent claudication
  - Regular, graded aerobic conditioning program of walking or bicycling
  - Flexibility exercises to avoid any obstruction over the involved digital arteries
- Relieve pain at rest
  - Sleep with the legs in a dependent but supported position over the edge of the bed or with the head of the bed slightly elevated
- Prevent skin ulcerations
  - Proper care and protection of the skin, particularly the feet or hands
  - Proper nail care
  - Proper shoe selection and fit
  - Avoid use of support hose and restrictive clothing
  - Avoid exposure to extremes of temperature, both hot and cold
- Improve vasodilation in affected arteries.
- Prevent or minimize joint contractures and muscle atrophy, particularly if the patient is confined to bed.
  - Repetitive, active ROM against low loads and/or gentle stretching exercises
  - Proper positioning in bed to maintain joint and muscle extensibility
- Promote healing of any skin ulcerations that develop.
  - Wound management procedures for treating ischemic ulcers, including electrical stimulation and oxygen therapy

ATHEROSCLEROSIS

Atherosclerosis is the hardening and narrowing of the arteries secondary to the formation of the plaque on the arterial wall. Plaque causes the narrowing of arteries, diminishes amount of blood flow across it.

The composition of plaque may involve fat, cholesterol, calcium. The hard type of plaque thickens and hardens arterial wall. The soft plaque is unstable, may dislodge from wall, enters blood stream, may act as emboli to occlude the distant blood vessels. The occluded vessel impairs blood supply to organ, causing ischemia or organ damage.

The narrowing vessels lead to diminished blood supply and produce complications accordingly:

- Coronary artery obstruction causes heart attack and myocardial infarction
- Pulmonary embolism
- If blood supply to brain is impaired then stroke may occur
- When vessel narrow, its pressure rises, the brain vessels may rupture
- May impair renal functioning.

Symptoms and Diagnosis

Atherosclerosis usually does not cause symptoms until significant narrowing of vessel or the embolism has occurred. Diagnostic methods include:

- Ankle/brachial index: It compares the blood pressure in the lower extremity with that of the blood pressure in the arm
- Echocardiogram: It provides information about the size and shape, diameter and amount of the blood flow across any given vessel
- CT scan: It provides computer-generated images of the organ or vessels
- Angiography: It helps to look into lumen of arteries, find any obstructing lesion
- Stress test: It tests if the blood supply to heart has been affected due to the obstruction of the coronary vessel in atherosclerosis.

Causes

- Atherosclerosis is a slow and progressive disease
- Once a plaque adheres to the inner layer of arterial wall, it speeds up the process of further plaque formation

- Most common factor which initiates the plaque formation is low density lipoprotein (LDL), its deposition further accelerates the inflammatory changes, macrophage accumulation.

Treatment

The goal of the treatment is to restore as much blood flow as possible through the affected portion of the vascular system and to reduce the risk of a plaque rupture or emboli formation.

Medication

- Antiplatelets inhibit plaque growth
- Beta blockers block affect of sympathetic nervous system and reduce the workload of the heart
- Nitrates medicines cause vasodilation
- Cholesterol-reducing drugs (e.g. statins) lower the patient's level of fats (lipids) in the blood, such as cholesterol and triglycerides.
- Dietry modification: High LDL levels are associated with increased risk of heart attack and stroke. High density lipoprotein is increased in food while the LDL lipid is reduced from the diet.

Physiotherapy Management

The physiotherapeutic management of the atherosclerosis is done similar to the heart failure.

HYPOTENSION

Hypotension is the state when the blood pressure in the body falls abnormally below the considerably normal limits. Commonly also known as 'low blood pressure' it manifests when blood pressure falls (Wikipedia, 2010) below the 90/60 mm Hg. The normal blood pressure is a reading around 120/80 mm Hg (Chobanian, et al. 2003).

Symptoms

Orthostatic hypotension occurs when the fall in blood pressure occurs during the changing in posture to assume a position where the peripheral pooling of blood is facilitated by the force of gravity. This may occur while assuming the stand up position from sitting or lying down position. The more common causes involve dehydration, vomiting, excessive sweating, and prolonged immobilization in lying posture, pregnancy and excessive thermal exposure. The related medical causes can involve antihypertensive medicines ACE inhibitors, calcium channel blockers, psychiatric medicines. In most of the cases the symptoms of low BP last only for few seconds, and the symptoms disappear while returned back to sit or lying position, where the blood pressure returns to the normal level. In orthostatic hypertensive patients, the pathological causes such as anemia, endocrinal disorders, heart valve pathology has to be ruled out.

The severe hypotension may impair the blood perfusion to the brain tissues and other vital organs, and leads to life threatening emergency condition called as "shock". This condition occurs with significant blood loss, severe diarrhea, heavily sweating, anaphylactic reactions, kidney diseases, and excessive use of antihypertensive diuretic medicines, infections, external or internal hemorrhage. The autoregulatory mechanisms which work to maintain the blood pressure, fail to function and the drop in BP cannot be compensated. If the immediate emergency care is not given the multiple organ failure of vital organs of body may occur.

The lower blood pressure is not always pathological. Some people (like well conditioned athlete, people with higher aerobic capacity) may have low blood pressure all the time, however in these people there is no manifestation of signs or symptoms. However, the symptoms of low BP may appear only when the blood pressure falls significantly low. Therefore, the lower reading may be considered to be normal for them. Therefore, more accurately the person is labeled as hypotensive only if along with reduced blood pressure, the symptoms such as fainting, dizziness, cold extremities, poor orientation are manifested. With advancement in age, the little increase in the blood pressure occurs due to multiple factors including arteriosclerosis, atherosclerosis, reduced heart rate, comorbid pathological conditions.

Diagnosis

- The severe hypotension is not difficult to be diagnosed as the vitals of the patient are abnormally diminished, the consciousness is altered, extremities are cold, pulse is feeble, and the skin may appear yellow or white. The emergency care is important, the cause of the shock has to be eliminated, and the fluid has to be replenished so as to maintain appropriate blood pressure and the perfusion of vital organs.

- In case of the less severe form of hypotension, the clinical diagnosis is mainstay combined with the documented reduced blood pressure. The clinical feature includes complaint of dizziness, cold extremities, occasional complaints of palpitation
- The objective testing of hypotension involves:
  - Blood testing: The complete hemogram testing helps to identify the infective or other possible pathology linked with the fall in BP
  - The repeated episodes of fainting may require the ruling out of the seizures
  - The tilt table tests are helpful to put the patient in gravity dependent and neutral position. If during gravity dependent positions the features of hypotension appear and they disappear on bringing the client back to the neutral position, the diagnosis of orthostatic hypotension can be made.
- The study related to heart may need electrocardiogram to identify the ectopic beat, arrhythmia
- Echocardiogram (ECHO) test helps to provide the details about the functioning, shape of heart
- In case of unstable hypotension the detailed cardiovascular examination, investigation, stress test, MRI, venography, arteriography must be done.

Causes

- Hypotension may be due to the extracardiac or cardiac origin
- Hypotension is caused by conditions or events that interfere with the body's autoregulatory mechanisms to control blood pressure
- Sometime the excessive varicose veins may lead to excessive peripheral pooling of blood, reducing the total amount of blood in the circulatory channels. This also may lead to shock.

Treatment

- The medical treatment involves prescribing the medicines, which cause the retention of sodium ions in body, increase water retention and thus raise blood pressure. The plasma expanders may be helpful to maintain the blood volume
- Depending on the pathology the specific medications may be prescribed
- The commonly used medicines include caffeine, anti-inflammatory medicines, sodium supplements.

Physiotherapy Management

Physiotherapy Goals

- Educate the patients about the possible mechanisms and postures which could lead to the hypotensive state
  - Patient education—avoid prolonged standing after drinking warm fluids, tea, coffee
  - After episode of prolonged standing the client should lie down for few minutes with legs elevated above the level of heart so as to facilitate the centrally directed flow of blood
  - Self management skills for dealing with the hypotensive phase
- Prevent venous stasis
  - Minimize venous stasis
  - The elastic supportive stockings before the episode of prolonged standing or walking
  - The active exercises of ankle and foot to increase the venous return.
- Management of the causative factors of the hypotension. The causative factors such as infection, dehydration, varicose veins, and cardiac pathology must be managed accordingly by the multidisciplinary approach interventions. The facilitation of the venous return may be done by the stockings, mechanical compression devices, ROM exercises.

HYPERTENSION

Definitions

Hypertension refers to the state when the blood flows in the body at a pressure higher than the normal acceptable limits. On the basis of blood pressure the adult client can be classified into the normal, prehypertensive, stage I and stage II clients (Chobanian, et al. 2003). The Joint National Committee on Prevention, Detection, Evaluation, and Treatment of High Blood Pressure (JNC 7) classification (Table 8.3) of BP for adults aged 18 years or older is based on the mean of two or more properly measured seated BP readings on each of two or more office visits (Chobanian, et al. 2003).

There is an exception to the above definition of high blood pressure. A blood pressure of 130/80 mm Hg or higher is considered high blood pressure in people with diabetes and chronic kidney disease. Sometime it may happen that only systolic or only diastolic pressure may be higher without any increase in the other one. Only

TABLE 8.3 Joint National Committee on Prevention, Detection, Evaluation, and Treatment of High Blood Pressure (JNC 7) classification of BP for adults

BP nomenclature	*Systolic blood pressure, (mm Hg)*	*Diastolic blood pressure, (mm Hg)*
Normal	<120 mm Hg	And <80 mm Hg
Pre-hypertensive stage	120–139 mmHg	80–89 mm Hg
Stage I hypertensive	140–159 mm Hg	90–99 mm Hg
Stage II hypertensive	≥ 160 mm Hg	≥ 100 mm Hg

systolic blood pressure may be increased in cases of aged or the narrowing of blood arteries.

Symptoms and Diagnosis

High BP could be risky, and mostly undergo undetected unless the BP measurement is done for some other pathological state such as problems of heart, brain, kidney or pre-operative checkup. The continuously increased blood pressure may be risky as it can lead to the hardening of the blood vessels, leading them to be relatively more fragile and at the risk of developing small "hot spots" which could increase the risk of developing thrombosis and clots in blood.

The single most important and valid indicator for diagnosis the hypertension is its direct recording and documentation.

Complications associated with the hypertension include:

- Increased peripheral resistance, therefore the increased cardiac work
- The break in the innermost endothelial layer of the blood vessels causing dissecting hot spots which further increase the risk of thrombosis formation
- Damaged to the delicate arteries of the vital organs causing higher incidence of internal organ hemorrhage, organ failure or ischemia, brain stroke, retinopathy/retinal damage.

Causes

The idiopathic origin is the most common cause of the hypertension, and this is known to occur without any associated causative pathology. This is known as essential hypertension and in majority of cases this is not risky or harmful.

The hypertensive state secondary to some associated causative pathology is called as secondary hypertension. This is risky and may lead to large number of complications when present for the long time. In majority of cases this needs the medical interventions and lifestyle modifications along with the treatment of the causative pathology.

Sedentary lifestyle, higher salt intake, improper dietary habits, state of water retention, diabetes mellitus, increased blood thickness and viscosity are other common causes.

Treatment

Medications

- Diuretics: Flushes out excessive fluids, minerals and helps to curb down the blood pressure
- Alpha blockers and beta blockers cause vaodilation, reduce cardiac load
- Calcium channel blockers. Reduce the calcium ion action on heart and vessels wall.

Physiotherapy Management

Patient Education

Educate the patient about the risk factors, coping strategies, the importance of the exercises and healthy lifestyle.

Lifestyle Changes

- Smoking, alcohol consumption, high calory intake, obesity and weight gains are well established causative factors and therefore must be avoided to possible extent.
- Instead of regularly consuming the high calory diets, the high fiber diet and negative calory diets may also be prescribed.
- Weight control strategies. Dietary regulation, salt restriction, avoiding junk foods, may be practiced. The indulgence in regular exercises at moderate level of intensity also controls the weight to certain extent. Diets to be encouraged include fruits, whole wheat, green vegetables, low caloric, and high fiber items. The diet which is to be avoided includes low fiber diet, high amount of saturated fatty acids.
- Increase in the aerobic capacity of the patient helps to regulate the cardiac and pulmonary responses during the increased need.

This helps to curb down the anxiety and the rise in blood pressure. American College of Sports medicine recommends the thirty minutes of regular aerobic exercise participation on alternate days, at moderate level of intensity to enhance the cardiovascular fitness. Regular aerobic exercise optimizes body weight and body composition. If dietary caloric intake remains constant, exercise will produce slow weight loss (Irwin, et al. 2003). Intense exercises cause increase in energy expenditure and lipid oxidation process. Swimming appears to be less effective than land exercise for reducing body fat, reduced the joint loading and increasing bone mineral content.

- The dietary supplements included vitamins and minerals including sodium, calcium. Potassium, vitamin E, C and B complex helps to regulate blood pressure.
- Up to 6 g/day salt can be consumed daily as safe limit for patients of chronic cardiac failure (SIGN guidelines, 2004) however for the hypertensive patients this limit is 2 g/day (SIGN guidelines, 2004).
- Stress management methods, emotional control, risk factor management, lifestyle modification, associated problems management, regular fitness exercises.

DEEP VEIN THROMBOSIS

In case of the deep vein thrombosis (DVT) the blood clot is formed inside the deep veins of the body, which leads to partial or complete blockage of this vascular channel and impairs the blood return from the drained territory or commonly may break off to act as highly risky foreign body to occlude the blood vessels in lungs, heart, brain or any other organ.

The causative mechanism involves the reduced velocity of blood flow, its increased viscosity or the injury to inner wall of blood vessel, which increases the risk of blood stagnation. The blood may clot at the occluded place and form thrombosis. In cases of patients confined to bed, especially with a lower limb plaster cast, the early ambulation is highly demanded as in absence of early ambulation, the weight of cast acts to stagnate the blood locally and promoting the clot formation.

The higher risks of developing DVT involve prolonged bed rest, fractures, the atheromatous plaque formation, smoking (causes the blood vessel lumen narrowing), pregnancy, obesity, hypercoagulability of blood, blood vessel lining injury, the stagnated blood flow. The risk of developing DVT is higher in those who have long journey by the air flight (Scurr, et al. 2001). In case of post-surgical cases, the symptomless DVT may occur in about 30% patients if the prophylactic measures are not adopted (Collin, et al. 1988).

The thrombosed portion may either partially or completely break off from its formation site and may travel to distant site via blood. At whatever place it gets lodged, it would create trouble. If it gets entangled in pulmonary channel then it may lead to pulmonary embolism resulting in respiratory insufficiency or even death. It may also lead to cerebral blood flow obstruction and even stroke.

Symptoms

- Changes in skin color (redness) in one leg (Fig. 8.6)
- Increased warmth in one leg
- Leg pain in one leg
- Leg tenderness in one leg
- Swelling of one leg (Fig. 8.6).

Examination and Tests

The investigative procedure used for the assessment of the DVT include:

- The examination of the blood vessel and veins using Doppler imaging.

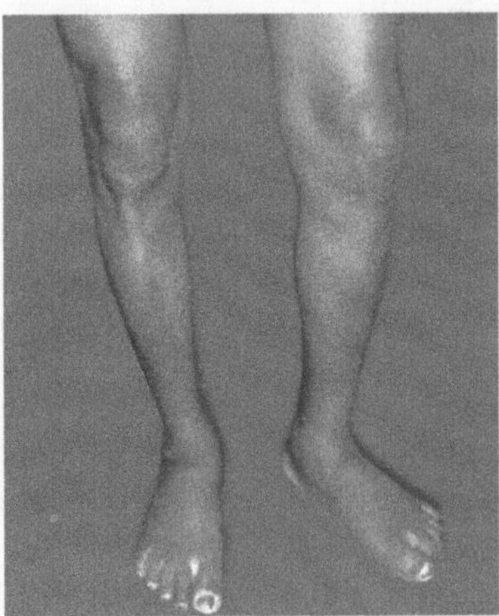

Fig. 8.6: Deep vein thrombosis of right leg with redness and swelling (*For color version, see Plate 9*)

- The clinically common test for diagnosis is Homan sign, which elicits abrupt sharp pain in calf or popliteal region when the ankle is dorsiflexed abruptly with knee in bend position (Shafer N, Duboff, 1980). This is most common test however its sensitivity and validity for diagnosis the DVT has been questioned.
- The clinical criteria have been used for the provisional diagnosis of the DVT on the basis of following criteria and score gained by the patient, known as Wells score (Scarvelis and Wells, 2006).
- It has been found that the clinical features and signs for diagnosis DVT are not reliable and false positive or false negative results do occur which can interfere with the accurate and timely treatment management technique, therefore it is recommened that instead of purely relying on clinical findings, the investigative procedures including venography must be done in all suspected patients (Hull, et al. 1981).

Wells score or criteria: (Possible score -2 to 8).

- Known case of cancer for upto last 6 months: 1 point
- Calf swelling >3 cm as comparison to other calf (measured about 10 cm below tibial tuberosity): 1 point
- Collateral superficial veins (non-varicose): 1 point
- Pitting edema (involving the involved leg: 1 point
- Swelling of entire leg: 1 point
- Pain along the distribution of deep venous system: 1 point
- Paralysis, paresis, or recent cast immobilization of lower extremities: 1 point
- Recently confinement to bed for > 3 days, or major surgery requiring regional or general anesthetic in past 4 weeks: 1 point
- Previous documented DVT: 1 point
- Alternative diagnosis at least as likely: Subtract 2 points.

***Note*:** Well score ≥ 2 possible DVT if supported with the investigative imaging of veins. Well score < 2, there is less chance of the DVT, however further investigative evaluation is needed to rule out.

Treatment

- In high risk patients or the bed confined patients, the compression graduated stockings are helpful for the prevention of the clot formation (Sachdeva, et al. 2010)
- In high risk patients the prophylactic use of anticoagulant medicines such as heparin (Kakkar, et al. 1982), aspirin is prescribed so as to prevent the increase in blood viscosity

- Those who have long journey by air flights are at significant risk of developing DVT therefore among such long flight travelers the prophylactic use of elastic compression stockings during long-haul air travel is recommended (Scurr, et al. 2001)
- Heparin is most commonly used medicine for the prophylactic purpose. Heparin has anticoagulant action due to its ability to active antithrombin III, which in turn inhibits several coagulation factors and thrombin (Kakkar, et al. 1982).
- In case where conservative methods fail, and thrombosis continued to progress the surgical interventions are used such as thrombolysis (Watson, 2004), thrombectomy.

Physiotherapy Management

Physiotherapy Goals

- *Preventive aspect*: The prevention is better than care in case of DVT. The preventive approach lies in medical based interventions as well as physiotherapeutic intervention. In case of bed confined patients the active ROM exercises of foot, elastic stockings (Sachdeva, et al. 2010), the early ambulation, active/resisted movement of the contralateral limbs.
- During acute inflammatory period
  - Bed rest is important to reduce the associated pain and also to reduce the risk of dislodging and migration of clot to the distant site
  - Elevation of the affected lower extremity, keeping the knee slightly flexed
  - While sitting for long time, must keep legs elevated above level of heart so as to prevent formation of clot, however if once the DVT has established that this positioning of leg is contraindicated as it can cause the migration of emboli from legs towards heart.
- As the acute symptoms reduce, the early ambulation is recommended to regain functional mobility. The compressive bandaging or graduated pressure support garments may be used while ambulation to further facilitate the venous return.
- To prevent the recurrence of the acute phase, the appropriate pharmacological management and the prevention strategy.
- If the thrombosis has formed, the pneumatic compression therapy and the passive mobilization is contraindicated.

EMBOLISM

Embolism is a wandering object which flows in the blood stream after dislodging form the source organ or blocked blood vessel, and then obstructs the blood vessel in the distant site to cause partial or complete blockage of the arterial blood vessels.

Various causes of the emboli do include air embolism, fat embolism from the bone marrow of the injured bones, septic causes, the dislodged thrombosis from the parent site, the injured fragments of the damaged muscles tissues. The thrombosis or the causative factor may travel either along the direction (anterograde flow) or against the direction (retrograde flow) of blood flow before getting stucked in the narrowed branch of artery or vein.

- In anterograde embolism, the emboli moves along with the direction of blood flow
- In retrograde embolism the emboli moves opposite to the direction of blood flow
- In paradoxical embolism the emboli crossed from veins to enter into the arterial blood system.

When they cause obstruction of the artery or vein, they totally or partially occlude the blood flow across it, and cause the oxygen depletion and diminished blood supply to the concerned organ. This leads to organ failure either temporarily or permanently.

Types of Embolism

- Depending on the nature of its constituent, the emboli may be named as gas embolism, fat embolism, thromboembolism, air embolism, amniotic fluid embolism. Thromboembolism is most common type of embolism and it arises from the fragments of the blood clot which blocks blood flow at some distant site.
- Depending on the location of blood vessels which are blocked by emboli, it can be named as cerebral emboli, pulmonary embolism, renal embolism.
- Depending on the nature of blood vessel blocked, it can be named as arterial or venous embolism.

Risk Factors

The patients who are at higher risk of developing the embolism include:

- Immobilization following the fracture, surgeries
- Fractures of the pelvic bone or long femur bone

- The higher blood viscosity (such as during dehydration or the dyselectrolytemia)
- Trauma to the deep veins such as the deep wound of calf muscles, the deep arterial or vein repairs
- The conditions which can lead to higher risk of developing the thrombosis such as valvular heart disease, infective endocarditis, myocardial infarction
- Menopausal women who are on hormone replacement therapy with combination of estrogen and progestin, are at higher risk of to develop deep vein thrombosis, which can lead to pulmonary embolism
- The other medical pathologies such as cancer, systemic infection, wound infections, intra-abdominal organ infection
- The deep water divers, and those who travel for long duration by airplane are at more higher risk of developing the embolism and deep vein thrombosis. During deep water diving the veins and blood vessels of body are at high pressure, but as the diver returns back to the surface, this pressure gets reduced and this rapid change in the pressure gradient increases the risk of dislodging the thrombosis from its parent site, or the pressure inside lungs makes the alveoli to burst and release air into the blood stream. During prolonged duration airplane travelling the pressure over the veins is very less, increases risk of embolism formation.

Diagnosis

Emboli formation mostly undergoes unnoticed unless it occludes some important blood vessel of the body and leads to the associated symptoms.

The history and the physical, clinical examination are main lines of the diagnosis of the emboli.

Clinical features related to the pathology of the organ, whose blood supply has been compromised, need to be carefully documented and asked for.

If coronary vessels are affected, the alterations on ECG and ECHO testing are noticeable along with the correlated clinical signs and symptoms.

Pulmonary embolism leads to sudden onset unexplained breathless, anxiety, chest pain, reduced oxygen levels in blood, decreased oxygen saturation, altered ABG (arterial blood gas) findings.

The occlusion of the renal vessels may lead to features of sudden onset renal failure.

Cerebral embolism leads to the stroke, altered consciousness and the features according to the involved region of brain.

The investigative procedures for the diagnosis of the emboli are not always reliable, however the CT scan, MRI scan, Doppler studies, blood gas analysis, chest X-ray, renal glomerular filteration rate, angiogram, catheterization are the methods most commonly employed.

Treatment

- Treatment for an embolism depends on the type of embolism, the organ affected, the extent of the obstruction to the organ.
- The significant obstruction of the blood vessels related to the vital organs needs immediate attention.
- The embolectomy is the surgical intervention used for those emboli which do not get resolved spontaneously.
- In cases where embolism is due to the thrombosis and surgery is not possible, then thrombolytic drug may be given along with an anticoagulant drug to prevent further clot formation.
- In high risk cases, the prophylactic use of heparin and other antigoagulants are prescribed. For this it is highly important to identify the high risk patient.

Physical Management

The preventive management to avoid the formation of the thrombosis or emboli is important.

This includes early ambulation, the treatment of the associated pathology, the management of thrombosis, etc.

The improved circulation is also important to prevent the formation of the thrombosis. For this, the active and passive range of motion exercises are recommended. The cases where dynamic movement is not possible, the isometric contractions may be used. In those cases where active contraction too is not possible, the mechanical compression devices may be used. It must, however, be noted that the active movements must be done very carefully, if the thrombosis dislodgment has been confirmed.

GANGRENE

Definition

Gangrene is a form of tissue death (necrosis) secondary to the lack of oxygen rich blood in tissue. It may affect almost any organ of the body including muscle, bone, nerves or skin. The blood supply to the organ and tissue is compromised, the tissue die due to the lack of fresh oxygen.

The rapidly increasing gangrene is an emergency condition which requires immediate attention, otherwise it may lead to the massive involvement of the body and the risk of life-threatening multiple organ failure. In case of the rapidly increasing gangrene the amputation of the involved bone may be urgently needed to avoid fatal involvement of the whole body.

The speed of the involvement of the body tissue depends on the type and the extent of the blood vessel involvement. The obstruction of the blood supply (dry gangrene) may be due to the arterial injury, post-traumatic events, infective involvement (called as wet gangrene), toxic involvement of the tissues.

Tissue death can progress quickly or slowly depending on the initial cause of the interruption in blood supply. In some cases, gangrene is triggered by a bacterial infection in a part of the body that is experiencing poor circulation. When the bacteria begin to grow, they release toxins that attack the tissue.

Classification

- Wet gangrene is due to the bacterial infection leading to the red, hot, damp appearance of the involvement of the tissue. Later on the tissue gets necrosed, the foul smelling black, blue oozing fluid appears. It is rapidly progressive form and needs immediate attention.
- Dry gangrene is due to reduced flow of blood through the arteries without infections. The tissues become dry, dead, atrophied, and necrosed. It appears black, breaky in nature and senseless.
- Gas gangrene is severe form of gangrene which results from the infection of clostridium perfringes. The infection causes gas bubble under skin, form blisters, purple discoloration of skin. It can sometimes lead to death within hours.

Cause

Impaired circulation arterial injuries, crush injuries, peripheral vascular disease, diabetic vasculopathy, thrombosis, emboli, crushing injury and trauma, failed blood supply in the operated wounds.

Signs and Symptoms

Signs and Symptoms of Gangrene

- Severe pain and swelling in the affected area
- Altered skin color to red or bronze as underlying tissues die
- Foul-smelling discharge from the wound
- In case of wet gangrene the associated infection can also be manifested

Diagnosis

- Diagnosis of the gangrene in majority of cases lies on the clinical findings. In majority of wet gangrene cases the rapidity of the progression is so fast that the investigative procedures can not be employed due to lack of time
- Tissue analysis may be used to examine the nature of the involved damage and the infective organ.

Treatment

- Hyperbaric oxygen therapy: Use of high-pressure oxygen to attack infection
- Amputation: If all other options fail, surgical removal of part or all of a gangrenous body part may be necessary.

Physiotherapy Management

Physiotherapy interventions are only used following amputation and antibiotic therapy. Otherwise physiotherapy of the gangrene affected area is contraindicated as there is risk of infection spreading to other parts.

In cases where the blood supply to the extremity or body part is compromised, the preventive strategies are used for avoiding the formation of the wound, ulcer and gangrene. This strategy may be useful to defer the need of amputation.

BUERGER DISEASE

Definition

Also known as thromboangiitis obliterans (TAO), Buerger disease is a rare type of peripheral arterial disease that involves inflammation of the smaller and midsize arteries in the extremities. This is recurring and progressive in nature (Olin, 1990).

More specifically, it may be defined as segmental occlusive inflammatory condition of the arteries and veins with thrombosis and recanalization of the affected vessel (Buerger, 1908 and 1924)

Pathogenesis

This is rare type of disease and involves the inflammatory process followed by the clotting and thrombosis in the small and medium size arteries. In less common forms, it may also involve the veins. Pathology involves the non-atherosclerotic inflammatory changes (Olin, et al. 1990). It is formed as result of vasculitis (inflammation of small arteries in extremities), blood clot formation and the scarring of vessels wall.

Signs and Symptoms

- Disease is progressive in nature which begins as pain in the small vessels of the hand, arm, leg and feet secondary to the reduced blood supply during some exerting activity (claudication)
- It rarely gives symptoms of the large vessel involvement unless it is associated with the vessel occlusive disease
- Numbness or tingling in the arms, legs, hands or feet
- Initially the symptoms are present only during exertion and activities, however as disease progresses the symptoms may persist even at the rest
- Ulcers on the toe or fingers of hands or feet (Olin, 2000)
- A white or bluish tinge to the skin on the hands or feet, similar to that seen in Raynaud syndrome
- Extremities that are cold to the touch.

Diagnosis

No laboratory test confirms the diagnosis of Buerger's disease. Instead, clinical finding, client history and smoking status are better clues. Buerger's disease occurs mostly due to the blood thrombosis and clots in the blood vessels. There are the angiogram of the peripheral blood vessels, which may be used for confirming the diagnosis.

Abnormal Allen's test along with presence of leg ulcer always must lead into the suspected case of TOA (Allen, 1924). In this catheter-based test, a special contrast dye is injected into the bloodstream to allow the doctor to obtain X-ray images of the blood vessels and assess how well they are functioning. It is common for physicians to test for blood clots in all extremities, even if symptoms occur in only one because the disease is typically widespread. Another test that may be useful is a Doppler ultrasound, which produces images of the blood vessels and the blood flow through them.

Following criteria have been laid down for diagnosing the Buerger's disease (Olin, 2002):

- The male or females typically under 45 years of age
- History of tobacco use
- Evidence of reduced circulation in the distal portion of limb. Sometime the unexplained ulcers, gangrene may occur
- Reduction of the circulation in the distal fortion of the limb can be objectively registered by the ultrasound, Doppler testing
- Absence of other causes of vasculopathy or the ulcers or diabetes mellitus
- Maintained circulation in the proximal portion of the limb
- Absence of any source of emboli from any other part of the body
- The echocardiography, Doppler study or arterial imaging studies fail to locate any other source of emboli or the arterial/venous occlusion.

Treatment and Prevention

There is no treatment for Buerger's disease, other to quit smoking immediately, after which patients can expect dramatic improvement if irreparable harm has not already occurred. In the meantime, physicians will also attempt to treat the pain, usually with aspirin or other painkillers.

If there is ulceration or dead tissue, then revascularization techniques may be performed to help restore adequate blood flow and prevent amputation. This procedure is rare, however, because the disease usually affects such a widespread area of the circulatory system.

To prevent tissue death, patients are encouraged to keep their hands and feet well protected in cold weather and to regularly exercise affected areas to improve circulation.

Because smoking is the chief cause of Buerger disease, the best way to prevent this progressive and untreatable condition is to quit smoking and avoid all second-hand smoke.

Physical Management

Physical interventions to improve peripheral blood flow while the patient is on bed rest may include warming the limb by reflex heating of the torso or opposite extremity or elevating the head of the bed slightly.

Contraindications

- Exercise—passive or active
- Prolonged positioning during bed rest, which could cause pressure on and potential breakdown of skin
- Local, direct heat on the involved extremity because of the potential for a burn to the ischemic tissue
- Use of support hose, which may increase peripheral resistance to blood flow
- Restrictive clothing that could compromise blood flow.

BIBLIOGRAPHY

1. Abboud PA, Kendall JL. Ultrasound guidance for vascular access. Emerg Med Clin North Am. 2004;22(3):749-73.
2. Allen EV. Thrombangitis obliterans: methods of diagnosis of chronic occlusive arterial lesions distal to the wrist with illustrative cases. American Journal of Medical Science 1929;178:237-44.
3. Alvelos M, Ferreira A, Bettencourt P, Serrao P, Pestana M, Cerqueira-Gomes M. The effect of dietary sodium restriction on neurohumoral activity and renal dopaminergic response in patients with heart failure. Eur J Heart Fail. 2004;6(5):593-9.
4. Andrew T, Spector T, Jeffery S. "Linkage to the FOXC2 region of chromosome 16 for varicose veins in otherwise healthy, unselected sibling pairs." J Med Genet. 2005;42(3):235-9.
5. Bamigboye AA, Smyth R. Interventions for varicose veins and leg oedema in pregnancy (Review). The Cochrane Library. 2008;4.
6. Barrett D, Gretton M, Quinn T. Cardiac Care: An Introduction for Healthcare Professionals. John Wiley and Sons, Ltd, 2006.

7. Bernard K, Holden MD, Hussain N. Chest pain: differentiating cardiac from non-cardiac causes. Hospital Physician. 2004;38:24-7.
8. Buerger L. Thromboangitis obliterans: a study of vascular lesions leading to presenile gangrene. American Journal of Medical Science. 1908;136:567-80.
9. Buerger L. The circulatory disturbance of the extremities: including gangrene, vasomotor and trophic disorders. Philadelphia, Saunders. 1924.
10. Chobanian AV, Bakris GL, Black HR. The seventh report of the Joint National Committee on prevention, detection, evaluation, and treatment of high blood pressure. The JNC 7 Report. JAMA. 2003;289:2560-72.
11. Collins R, Scrimgeour A, Yusuf S, Peto R. Reduction in fatal pulmonary embolism and venous thrombosis by perioperative administration of subcutaneous heparin. Overview of rêsults of randomized trials in general, orthopaedic, and urologic surgery. N Engl J Med. 1988;318:1162-73.
12. Conway N. Hemodynamic effects of ethyl alcohol in patients with coronary heart disease. Br Heart J. 1968;30(5):638-44.
13. Curri SB. Changes of cutaneous microcirculation from elasto-compression in chronic venous insufficiency. In: Davy A, Stemmer R (Eds): Phlebology '89, Montrouge, France, 1989, John Libbey Eurotext.
14. Dimmer JLB, John RR, Jennifer SE, David S. The epidemiology of chronic venous insufficiency and varicose veins. Annals of Epidemiology 2005;15(3):175-84.
15. Dracup K, Baker DW, Dunbar SB. Management of heart failure II: counseling, education and lifestyle modifications. JAMA. 1994;272:1442-6.
16. EC Barrett, K Khaw. Family history of heart attack as an independent predictor of death due to cardiovascular disease. Circulation. 1984;69:1065-9.
17. Goldstein JR. Ultrasound-guided peripheral venous access. Israeli Journal of Emergency Medicine. 2006;6(4):46-52.
18. Happ MB, Naylor MD, Roe-Prior P. Factors contributing to rehospitalization of elderly patients with heart failure. J Cardiovasc Nurs. 1997;11: 75-84.
19. Irwin ML, Yasui Y, Ulrich CM. Effect of exercise on total and intra-abdominal body fat in postmenopausal women: a randomized controlled trial. JAMA. 2003;289(3):323-30.
20. Jaarsma R, R Halfens, H Huijer Abu-Saad, K Dracup, T Gorgels, J van Ree, J Stappers. Effects of education and support on self-care and resource utilization in patients with heart failure. European Heart Journal. 1999;20:673-82.
21. Karras DJ, Kane DL. Serum markers in the emergency department diagnosis of acute myocardial infarction. Emerg Med Clin North Am. 2001;19(2):321-37.

22. Kate LP, Boman H, Daiger SP, Motulsky AG. Familial aggregation of coronary heart disease and its relation to known genetic risk factors. Am J Cardiol. 1982;50:945.
23. Kim WY, Danias PG, Stuber M, Flamm SC, Plein S, Nagel E, et al. Coronary magnetic resonance angiography for the detection of coronary stenoses. N Engl J Med. 2001;345:1863-9.
24. Olin JW. "Thromboangiitis obliterans (Buerger's disease)". N Engl J Med. 2000;343(12):864-9.
25. Olin JW, Young JR, Graor RA, Ruschhaupt WF, Bartholomew JR. The changing clinical spectrum of thrombangitis obliterans. Circulation 1990;82:3-8.
26. Patterson MS, Jagt RM, Khan M. Rotational coronary sinus venography and magnetic navigation to facilitate LV lead placement in cardiac resynchronization therapy. The Journal of Invasive Cardiology. 2010;22(2):27-9.
27. Pollock ML, Gasser GA, Butcher JD. The recommended quantity and quality of exercise for developing and maintaining cardiorespiratory and muscular fitness, and flexibility in adults. Med Sci Sports Exerc. 1998;30:975-91.
28. Hull R, Hirsh J, Sackett DL, Taylor DW, Carter C, Turpie AG, et al. Gent Clinical validity of a negative venogram in patients with clinically suspected venous thrombosis. Circulation. 1981;64:622-5.
29. Rhabi Y, Charras-Arthapignetic C, Gris JC, Ayoub J, Brun JF, Lopez FM. Lower limb vein enlargement and spontaneous blood flow echogenicity are normal sonographic findings during pregnancy. Journal of Clinical Ultrasound. 2000;28(8):407-13.
30. Sachdeva A, Dalton M, Amaragiri SV, Lees T. Elastic compression stockings for prevention of deep vein thrombosis. Cochrane Database of Systematic Reviews. 2010;7.
31. Scarvelis D, Wells P. Diagnosis and treatment of deep vein thrombosis. CMAJ. 2006;175(9):1087-92.
32. Scottish Intercollegiate Guidelines. Network (SIGN). Management of chronic heart failure- A national clinical guideline. 2007;95.
33. Scurr JH, Machin SJ, Sarah Bailey-King, Mackie IJ, McDonald S, Smith PDC. Frequency and prevention of symptomless deep-vein thrombosis in long-haul flights: a randomised trial. Lancet. 2001;357:1485-9.
34. Shafer N, Duboff S. Physical signs in the early diagnosis of thrombophlebitis. Angiology. 1980;22:18-30.
35. Stockdale Woolley R. The effects of education on self-care agency. Public Health Nurs. 1984;1:97-106.
36. The Criteria Committee of the New York Heart Association. Nomenclature and Criteria for Diagnosis of Diseases of the Heart and Great Vessels, 9th edn. Boston, Mass: Little, Brown and Co. 1994:253-6.
37. US Department of Health and Human Services. Physical Activities of Health: A Report of the Surgeon General, Atlanta, GA: US Department

of Health and Human Services, Center for Disease Control and Prevention, National Center for Chronic Disease Prevention and Health Promotion. 1996.
38. Kakkar VV, Djazaeri B, Fok J, Fletcher M, Scully MF, Westwick J. Low-molecular-weight heparin and prevention of postoperative deep vein thrombosis. British Medical Journal. 1982;284(6):375-9.
39. Watson L, Armon M. "Thrombolysis for acute deep vein thrombosis". Cochrane Database Systematic Review. 2004.
40. Weiss, Weiss. Doppler ultrasound findings in reticular veins of the thigh subdermic lateral venous system and implications for sclerotherapy. Journal of Dermatology Surgical Oncology. 1993;19(10):947-51.
41. Wikipedia database. http://en.wikipedia.org/wiki/Hypotension Accessed on 2nd August, 2010.

CHAPTER

9

Neurological Conditions

9.1: Examination of Neurological Disorders, Knowledge of Various Investigative Procedures Used in the Diagnosis of Various Neurological Disorders

Neurological disorders can be categorized according to the primary location affected, the primary type of dysfunction involved, or the primary type of cause. The broadest division is between central nervous system (CNS) disorders and peripheral nervous system (PNS) disorders.

CNS includes cerebral cortex, brainstem, midbrain, hypothalamus, spinal cord. (Fig. 9.1.1) The peripheral nervous system consists of the nerves arising from the motor nuclei or the sensory nuclei, the cytoplasmic extension, neurons in dorsal root ganglia, ventral horn of the spinal cord. These peripheral nerves may involve the sensory or the motor branches.

Neurological examination aims to assess the integrity of motor, sensory nerves, cranial nerves, higher mental functions (speech, hearing), body balance and equilibrium, coordination, mental status, behavior and the functioning of all these subsystems in efficient and coordinated manner. Neurological disorder affects the body's nervous system in form of structural, biomechanical, physiological functional alteration in the brain, spinal cord or the various nerves within the neurological network of body. This impairment may involve the muscle weakness, paralysis, poor endurance, poor coordination, motor or sensory loss, altered level of consciousness. The other factors responsible for causing the neurological disorders may include metabolic insult, hemorrhage, the ischemia, direct trauma.

The clinical examination is highly important to narrow down the possible factors responsible for the neurological impairment in the client, and the investigative procedures are further useful to identify those functions which are beyond the domain of the

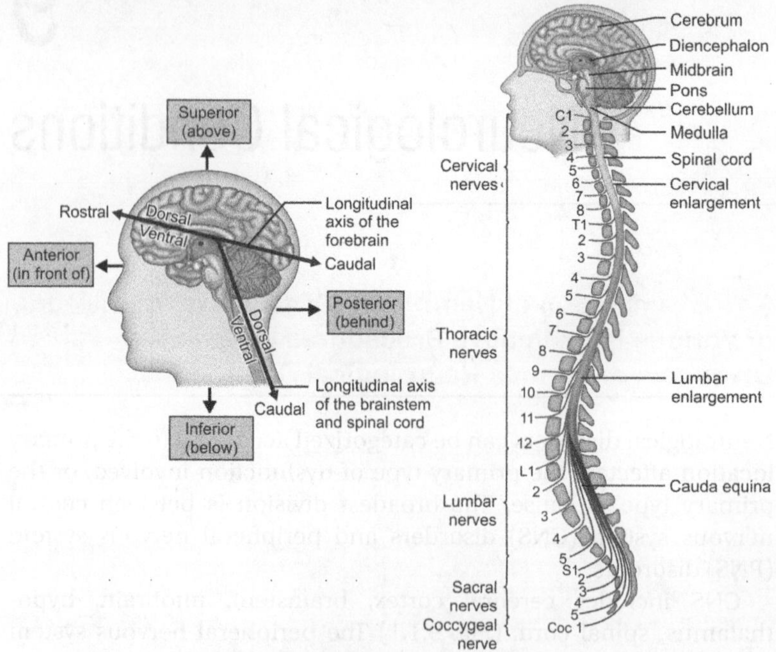

Fig. 9.1.1: The various components of central nervous system

clinical examination, and also these procedures could be useful for confirming the tentative diagnosis. The sample format for the neurological assessment of the client is described in (Table 9.1.1).

INVESTIGATIVE PROCEDURES USED IN THE DIAGNOSIS OF VARIOUS NEUROLOGICAL DISORDERS

Based on the findings of the neurological examination, client history, documentation of the signs and symptoms the specific investigative procedures can be used to confirm the tentative diagnosis. The vast options are available for being used as the investigative procedures. These options may include the X-ray, CT scan, MRI, nerve conduction studies (NCS), positron emission tomography (PET), electromyographic studies (EMG), the cerebrospinal fluid examination (CSF), nuclear magnetic imaging, etc.

X-rays are radiographs that are commonly used as cheap, fast, non-invasive and useful mean to check the gross integrity of the bony structures, and vertebral alignment. The low dose radiations are

TABLE 9.1.1 Format of neurological clinical assessment

Identification data	Name Age Gender Occupation Address and contact number Socioeconomic status Handedness Referral Informant
Chief complaint	
History and treatment	Second child from consanguineous or non-consanguineous marriage Age of mother at time of marriage
	Mother's history: • Pre-natal- duration of pregnancy; health during pregnancy; Ultrasonography; Labour pain • Natal- age of mother at time of delivery; type of delivery; delivery at home or in hospital • Post-natal- lactation; any post-delivery complication
	Child's history • Seizures • Delayed birth cry • APGAR score • Birth cry • Birth weight • Birth colour • Head and chest circumference during different phases of early life such as:- late neonate (7-28 days); infancy (1st year of life); early childhood (1-6 years); Late childhood (> 6 years) • Mile stone development
	Family history: Pedigree chart
	Psycho-social history: Behavior of child
Associated problems	• Hearing • Vision • Hearing • Speech • Feeding • Mental retardation • Fits • Developemental history • Repeated chest infections • Head banging • Attention deficit • Slow learning • Any abnormal posture adopted during sitting, walking, stair usage, etc.
On observation	Any type of problem: • Nutritional status • Aids and appliances

Contd...

Contd...

On EXAMINATION	
Higher functions	Speech and language • Articulation • Expression • Comprehension • Reading • Writing • Repetition/naming Auditory Vision Cognition and perception Cranial nerve examination
Reflex maturation	Primary innate Spinal level Brainstem reflexes Midbrain reflexes Cortical reflexes • Optical righting • Equilibrium—protective; fixation; righting
Developemental milestones	Gross motor Manipulation of objects General understanding Speech Vision—skills; acuity Sphincter control Projection skills Play Self-feeding skills
Motor system	General physical appearance Head and chest circumference Current height and weight Superficial reflexes such as abdominal reflex, cremastric reflex Skin Swelling Pain Tone • The tone must be evaluated in both agonist as well as antagonist muscle groups • The effect of change observed in the muscle tone while making changes in neck position, body position, speed of movement, fear, cold, stress must also be carefully examined and noted Voluntary control MMT (Manual muscle test) ROM (Range of motion) T/C/D (Tightness, contracture and deformity) DTRs (Deep tendon reflexes) Right/Left • Bicep jerk • Tricep jerk • Brachioradialis

Contd...

Contd...

	• Knee jerk • Ankle jerk Clonus • At wrist • At ankle • Patellar • Babinski's reflex
Sensory symptoms	Simple/protective • Touch • Pain • Temperature • Pressure Discriminatory • Proprioception • Kinesthesia • Localization • 2-point discrimination • Vibration • Paresthesia
Coordination	Equilibrium tests Non-equilibrium tests
Posture and gait	
Hand functions	Localizations Reach Circle drawing test Grasp • Hook grip—MP flexion and MP extension • Cylindrical grip—Thumb adduction and thumb abduction Disk Grasp and Release Grasp and throw Grasp and lift Grasp and place in a groove
Prehension	Tip to tip Tip to lateral Three jaw chuck Opponence Rotation Translation Shift

Contd...

Contd...

Bladder and Bowel control	• Control is completely or partially lost • The loss of control of these functions is consistently similar or transient • Whether loss of these function is associated with complete loss of sensation regarding leakage of urine or feces • Whether incontinence is of stress type, or true incontinence type or overflow incontinence
Oral—motor/communication	
Functional assessment	Quality of movement • Speed • Direction • Sequence • Rhythm • Range Dissociation • Eye-head • Head-trunk • Scapula-humeral • Shoulder-hand • Trunk-pelvis • Pelvic-femoral Eyes • Focus • Guide Patient's action • Active • Preparation to movement • During movement • End of movement Functional balance • Static/dynamic • Sitting • Kneeling balance • Standing balance • Walking balance Functional and non-functional ambulation *Activity of daily living (ADL)* • Feeding • Dressing: Upper portion, lower portion • Grooming: – Bathing – Combing – Brushing – Toileting • Locomotion – Wheelchair mobility – Walking mobility

Contd...

Contd...

	– Stair – Transfers—bed to chair; chair to bed; Transfers in bed; toilet mobility • Communication comprehension; expression • Social recognition
Home environment	• The attitude of family and family members towards the illness and limitations of the patient • Whether the environment of the family is supportive or cursing • Whether family has a supportive and optimistic attitude towards patients or it has pessimistic attitude
Work/school	
Play/leisure	
Mode of transport	
PT goals (physiotherapy goals)	Both short-term and long-term goals must be designed. Goal setting must be done comprehensively and must incorporate family members, working colleagues and other associated members so that patient gets facilitatory atmosphere at all spheres of life for rehabilitation
PT activities (treatment protocol)	
Home exercise program	

made to pass through the body and the imprint is taken on the X-ray sensitive photographic films. The integrity of bony structures, the alignment of bony structure with respect to each other, the regions of abnormal calcification and decalcifications can be located. The X-rays of skull, spine, chest are taken in routine for the neurological consideration.

The use of specific used contrast dyes can be used to enhance the clarity and prominence of the imprints.

The fluoroscopy involves the injection of the barium salt followed by the visualization of the real time dynamic imaging of the internal region of interest. The fluoroscopy involves the use of X-rays therefore the higher exposure of the radiation to the client.

Angiography procedure is invasive procedure to directly visualize the integrity, patency and continuity of the blood vessels including arteries and veins. The angiography is highly useful for detecting the degree of narrowing or obstruction of vessel; the detection of intraluminal tumor or obstruction; the internal aneurysm or dissection of the blood vessel. It involves the injection of a radio-opaque dye via

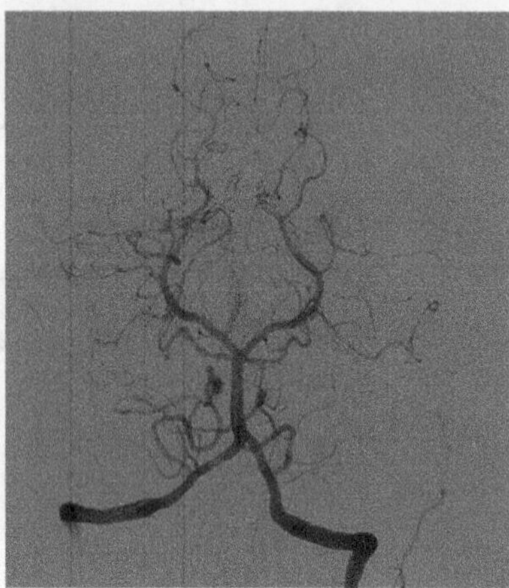

Fig. 9.1.2: The angiographic visualization of the vertebra-basilar artery

catheter into the major blood vessels of the region, followed by serial X-ray to identify the blood vessel architecture.

Cerebral angiography (Fig. 9.1.2) is the specific procedure for the visualization of the arterial, venous and blood vessels network in the brain. The catheter is passed via femoral artery and guided towards carotid artery. Via this catheter a radio-opaque agent is injected, and then the rapid series of radiographs is taken while the radio-opaque agent passes through vasculature.

Tissue biopsy involves the removal and examination of a small piece of tissue from the body. The tissue is examined in term of its histological, biochemical or the fibrous contents. The commonly used biopsy is used for the nerve, muscle, or the unexplained tissue lump (suspected tumor). Muscle and nerve biopsy are helpful to identify the neuromuscular disorder in cases where the pathology could otherwise not be confirmed by the other clinical or investigative procedures. The biopsy is relatively more invasive and uncomfortable procedures therefore it is reserved only in very few cases whenever needed. Moreover the biopsy alone is not sufficient to conclude a diagnosis, rather it has to be combined with the other clinical findings and features for the confirmation of diagnosis.

Brain scans are imaging techniques used to diagnose tumors, blood vessel malformations, or hemorrhage in the brain. These scans are used to study organ function or injury or disease to tissue or muscle. Types of brain scans include computed tomography, magnetic resonance imaging, and positron emission tomography (see descriptions, below).

Computed tomography, (Fig. 9.1.3) also known as a CT scan, is a noninvasive, painless process used to produce rapid (approximately 20 minutes scanning time), clear images of organs, bones, and tissues. This is relatively very fast procedures and can be helpful to assess the integrity of the bony structure or the location of hemorrhage or tumor or the space occupying lesion in the cavities within brain. The CT scan can be taken across any plane of the organ and therefore to locate the extent of lesion across any plane. This procedure is highly useful as first investigative mean in the unconscious patient due to the faster scanning in emergency state, the higher safety in case of presence of the metallic implants in the client body.

The clarity of the scan can be further enhanced by the injection of the contrast enhancing dye into the blood vessels supplying the region of interest. The contraindications of CT scan involve same as those of the X-ray radiation such as pregnancy, radio-sensitivity.

Cerebrospinal fluid analysis involves the laboratory analysis of the sample of the CSF fluid that has been removed in the small amount for the analysis purpose from the intra-thecal space. This analysis helps to understand removal of a small amount of the fluid that

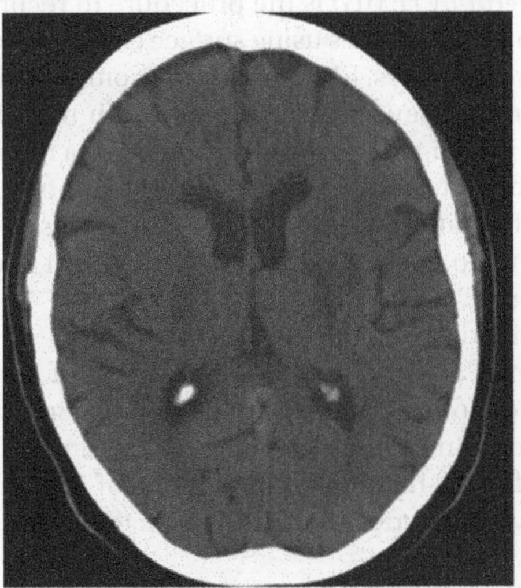

Fig. 9.1.3: The CT scan of skull showing the outline of skull bone and internal brain tissues

protects the brain and spinal cord. The fluid can show the presence of the blood, hemorrhage, infectious agent. For collection of the CSF, the lumbar puncture or the spinal tap procedure is done under the minor operation.

Discography is done in cases of the patients planned for the lumbar surgery and those who don't respond to the conservative treatments. The contrast dye is injected into the intervertebral discs. This is followed by the X-ray and CT scan imaging, to understand the regions of the damage of the disc.

Electroencephalography (EEG) is noninvasive procedure used to record and analyze the electrical activity of the brain through the skull. This can be helpful for the diagnosis of the seizures, head injuries, the activity of brain tissue under various tasks, inflammatory procedure affecting the brain and spinal cord. Also it is helpful for brain study in unconscious patients or to confirm the brain death. For EEG a series of noninvasive electrodes are attached to the patient's scalp using a conducting medium and a adhesive tape. The electrodes are connected to the EEG machine for recording the electrical activity of brain. The baseline electrical activity is recorded and then the activity of brain is recorded under variety of the external stimuli such as flash light, noise, voluntary activity, the reflex activities. The EEG recording is also important during sleep in cases of the seizures.

Electromyography (EMG) is the procedure to record and analyze the activity from the muscles using surface electrodes or the invasive intramuscular electrodes. EMG itself is not complete diagnostic tool, however its finding have to be combined with the clinical findings and the other investigative procedures to reach a definite diagnosis. The EMG study detects the normal and the abnormal activities of the muscle. The pattern of the electrical activities present variable forms and have to be studied carefully to detect the most logical pathological state.

- EMG examination is conducted in 4 stages:
  - Insertional activity (immediate record of activity at time when electrode is just inserted). During insertional activity (Kugelberg and Peterson, 1949) at the time of the insertion of needle the high frequency burst of –ve and +ve waves occurs which immediately stop when the needle movement is stopped.
  - At rest: When the muscle is not performing any activity and is at complete rest. Normally in state of the rest the muscle is almost

electrically silent and no spontaneous activity is present except low amplitude minute end plate potential recordable.
  - Upon minimal voluntary activity.
  - Upon maximal voluntary activity.

Presence of the spontaneous activity during resting state is always indicator of the abnormal pathological state of the muscle. These spontaneous activities in abnormal state are recorded irrespective of the voluntary activity of muscle. The common four types of spontaneous activities include the:

- Fibrillation
- Fasciculation
- Positive sharp waves
- Repetitive discharge.

During an EMG, very fine wire electrodes are inserted into a muscle (intramuscular electrodes) or are kept over the muscle belly (surface electrodes) to record the changes in electrical voltage that occur during movement and when the muscle is at rest or when muscle is functioning is the variable extent of contraction. The electrodes are attached through a series of wires to a recording instrument. This documentation of the electrical activity is also used extensively for assessing the muscle functions during the injury or the pathological state of the brain, spinal cord or peripheral nerve roots. Also it helps to determine the innervated or the denervation status of the muscles.

NERVE CONDUCTION STUDIES

The nerve conduction studies are used to determine the quality of the conduction through the peripheral nerves which are accessible through the superficial points in the course of the nerve. The peripheral nerves are electrically stimulated and the responses are recorded over the nerve or/muscle at some other points (proximal or distal). This can be done for sensory as well as motor nerves.

The important parameter which are evaluated or recorded in the NCS testing include:

- Latency between stimulation and the recording. It is the time in million-seconds from the stimulus artifact to the first negative deflection of CMAP (compound muscle action potential) (Gilchrist, 1993).
- The amplitude of the recorded wave or the CMAP. It represents the height of positive peak plus the depth of the negative peak.

The amplitude is important as it represents the number of nerve fibers.

- The velocity of the conduction across specific portions of the nerve.
- The data from NCS may be correlated with the clinical findings. The data and their records may be compared over period of time of weeks or months to determine whether the pathology is progressive or regressive in nature.

Data compared to normal data and interpretation is provided. The sensory conduction velocity is about 50 m/s (Gitter and Stolov, 1995). The latency represents the measurement of conduction in the fastest conducting motor fibers. The timing included in the latency are neuromuscular transmission time and the residual latency (the time between time along muscle membrane (Mishra and Kalita, 1999). The most common NCS are performed for the median nerve (Fig. 9.1.4) and radial nerve (Fig. 9.1.5).

- When the nerve is stimulated, a stimulus artifact appears followed by a latency period (gap b/w artifact and onset of recording potential).
- Action potential (evoked potential) makes M-wave which represents summated activity of all motor units in the muscle that responds to stimulation of nerve.

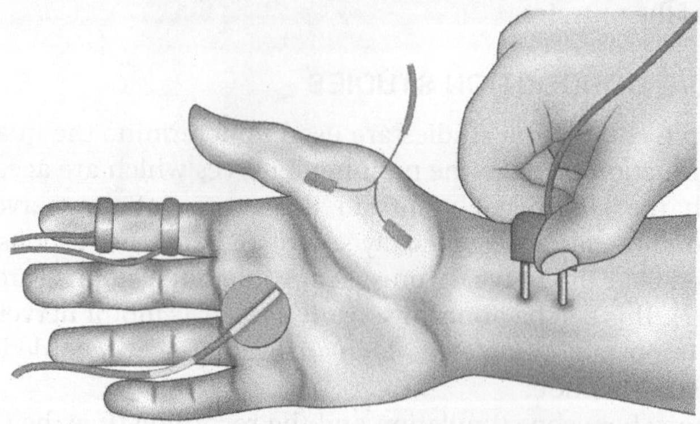

Fig. 9.1.4: NCV for median nerve

Recording electrode over abductor pollicis brevis

Ring electrode over PIP (proximal interphalangeal joint) and DIP (distal interphalangeal joint) of 2nd digit for SNCV (sensory nerve conduction velocity)

Ground electrode between recording and stimulating electrode

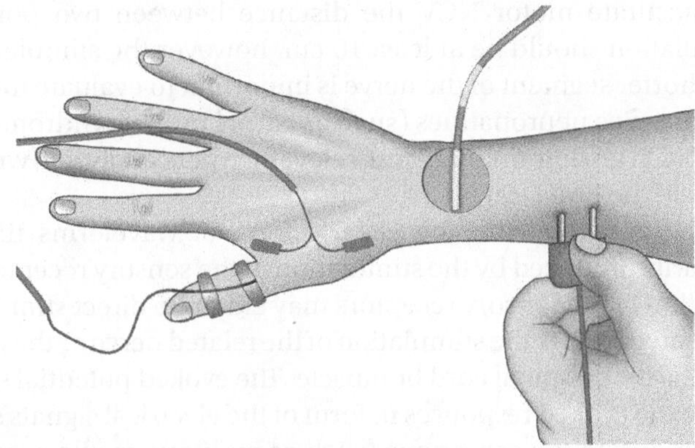

Fig. 9.1.5: NCV for radial nerve
Recording electrode over extensor indicis (1st MC—metacarpal dorsum)
Ring electrode over base and IP (interphalangeal joint) of thumb
Ground electrode between recording and stimulating electrode

- Nerve can be stimulated at proximal point (S1) or distal point(S2). As distance b/w recording and stimulating electrode increases, the latency duration also increases.
- CV is determined by dividing the accurate distance b/w two stimulation sites by the differences in latencies.

PRINCIPLES OF NCV TESTING (MISHRA AND KALITA, 1999)

- Motor or mixed nerve is stimulated at least at two points along its course.
- The pulse of stimulation can be adjusted to record a compound muscle action potential.
- The supra-maximal stimulation is advisable keeping the cathode close to active recording electrode.
- Ground electrode is placed between stimulation and recording electrode.
- During stimulation, the biphasic action potential with a initial negative phase is recorded.
- The conduction velocity is calculated by dividing the distance between two stimulation points in mm, which is divided by the difference of latency between both stimulating points:

$$\text{Conduction velocity} = \frac{\text{Distance between proximal and distal stimulation points (mm)}}{\text{Proximal latency (in msec) - distal latency (in msec)}}$$

- For accurate motor NCV the distance between two points of stimulation should be at least 10 cm, however the stimulation at the shorter segment of the nerve is important to evaluate the focal compressive neuropathies (such as carpal tunnel syndrome).

The NCV testing findings are relevant when analyzed with the findings of the EMG test.

Evoked potentials are the electric form of waveforms that are temporarily produced by the stimulation of the sensory receptor. The stimulation of the sensory receptors may either be direct stimulation of the related region, the stimulation of the related nerve or the related area of the brain, spinal cord or muscle. The evoked potential studies measure the evoked responses in form of the electrical signals sent to the brain during the sensations (such as auditory, tactile or visual). These potentials are measure to assess the variety of the neurological problems related to sensory involvement, brain organic pathology, multiple sclerosis. These are also useful for testing the sensations of the vision and hearing in the blind and deaf children; and also useful to confirm the brain death. These studies are helpful for the study of the waveform generated in the PNS as well as CNS, while the NCV testing measures the response in the PNS only.

BAERs (brainstem auditory evoked response) assesses the electric potential waveforms of the sound stimuli. These are useful to assess the hearing loss of the high-frequencies sounds; diagnose impairment of the vestibule-cochlear acoustic nerve and/or auditory pathways in the brainstem (Sohmer and Feinmesser, 1967). This includes the auditory input via one ear while the other ear is masked, and the response evoked potentials are recorded by electrodes placed over the scalp. The same procedure is tested with the second ear after blocking the first ear. The result findings are compared.

Visual evoked potentials is used to assess the loss of vision or the optic nerve damage (such as in multiple sclerosis patients). The patient sits close to a screen and is asked to focus on the center of a shifting checkerboard pattern.

Somatosensory evoked potentials evaluates the response from stimuli to the peripheral nerves to locate the pathology in the nerve, proprioceptors, spinal cords, etc.

Magnetic resonance imaging (MRI) uses high frequency computer-generated radio waves and a powerful magnetic field for generating the detailed images of body structures including tissues, organs, bones and nerves. This technique is highly useful for generating the images with different contrasting abilities. Therefore, it is useful for the detection of the infection, hemorrhage, inflammation, traumatic sequelae, vascular margins, blood vessels integrity. Besides this, the MRI imaging is also helpful for reproducing the images of spine, vertebral discs, the ligaments, the spinal cord or the various nerve roots. It is also a highly useful procedure to diagnose the disorders such as multiple sclerosis, demyelination, brain injury, brain ischemia, etc. This technique is highly sensitive to differentiate between the areas of hemorrhage and the ischemia. The image of the body part can be taken across any plane and any axis.

The machine generates a strong magnetic field and therefore not recommended in the patients with metallic implants, dental implants, the surgical fixation of the spinal fractures or pace makers.

The equipment consists of very large cylindrical magnet and a long hollow tube. The patient lies on a table in specific position. The principle of the MRI rests on the fact that body has rich amount of protons, when some external magnetic field is applied using the MRI machine apparatus, these protons get temporarily influenced and realigned along the direction of the magnetic field. After that the radiowaves of variable strengths are made to pass through the body tissues to detect the behavior of the magnetized ions. The orientation and the reorientation of water molecules (protons) create a kind of resonance which is processed by the computer to construct a two or three dimensional picture of the target tissue. The picture can be taken across any section at any angle and can differentiate between bone, soft tissues, fluid filled spaces, hemorrhage, tumors, inflammation and edema. The contrast between tissues and conditions may be further enhanced using the contrast dye.

Functional MRI (fMRI) is advanced version of the MRI to utilize the magnetic properties of the blood and to generate the real-time images of blood flow to specific region of the brain or organ. This can differentiate between the active or inactive regions; also documents the duration for which the portion of brain remains active upon the stimulation or the activity.

Sometimes, in clinical practice, it becomes important to choose between CT scan and MRI scans, to be prescribed for patients. During this time the basic differences between both scans (Table 9.1.2), their advantages, limitations, time consumption must be born in mind.

Myelography involves the injection of a water- or oil-based contrast dye into the spinal canal to enhance X-ray imaging of

TABLE 9.1.2 Differences between CT scan and MRI scan

CT scan	*MRI scan*
Uses X rays → high radiation exposure	Uses powerful magnetic field → no radiation exposure
Good for checking integrity of bony structure	Good for getting higher details of soft tissue (because soft tissues have more proton content and more magnetic field)
Cheaper than MRI	Expensive
Less time consuming (5 minutes) → first line of investigation in case of unconscious patient or head injury	More time consuming (30 minutes) → not used in emergency or for claustrophobic
Can be used safely over metallic implants and pacemakers → can be used in case of unconscious patient	Cant be used over metallic implants
Can take images only in one plane with one particular setting of machine	Can take images across many sections without realigning machine Advantages: • Uses non-ionizing radiation

the spine. Myelograms are used to diagnose spinal nerve injury, herniated discs, fractures, back or leg pain, and spinal tumors.

Positron emission tomography (PET) this procedure is generally performed after the MRI or CT scan has been performed. The purpose of this scanning is to develop the details of the area under pathology or concern. The low intensity radiotope isotope materials are inserted into the body blood vessels and made to pass through the brain tissues. The isotope emits the Gamma radiations which are collected by a special machine and the images are reconstructed to produce the two or three dimensional images. These can detect the organic pathology of brain, problems with tissue metabolism, blood flow, the presence of the tumors, etc.

A polysomnogram is a noninvasive used to measure the activity of brain or body during sleep to identify various sleep related pathologies such as sleep apnea, insomnia, the insomnabulism, and the brain activities during sleep. It is performed at specialized sleep centers where the electrodes are placed over the scalp to record the activity while the patients sleep at the center for the whole night.

Single photon emission computed tomography (SPECT), a nuclear imaging test functions similar to the PET (positron emission tomography) and produces a detailed three-dimensional image of blood flow and activity within the brain.

Neuro-ultrasound imaging, uses the ultrasound waves to generate the images related to the brain tissue perfusion, diagnosing the arterial narrowing, tumors or stroke; the problem related to the blood vessels in the brain system; the integrity of the ligaments or other soft tissues.

Repeated nerve stimulation technique (RNST) is the procedure to record the amplitude of the action potential upon the application of faradic current repeatedly at short intervals (Jolly, 1895). This technique is important to test the conduction ability across the neuromuscular junction (NMJ). In cases where the NMJ conduction is impaired, the RNST finds the progressively reduced amplitude of the recorded potential. This is a common finding in case of the myasthenia gravis.

The brief description of the findings of neurological tests in few common neurological states is described in (Table 9.1.3).

TABLE 9.1.3 The interpretation of clinical states as per various investigative procedures

Peripheral nerve pathology	• The presentation varies depending on the types of neuropathies in terms of relative onset of sensory and motor symptoms and NCS (nerve conduction study) changes. In initial stages, the NCS are helpful for assessment • Electrophysiological changes occur before the clinical manifestations • Sensory nerves get affected earlier than motor nerves thus sensory NCV test is most effective in early diagnosis, however motor deficits are more consistent with the pathology of supplied nerve • In the impairment persists for long time or axonal changes are significant than the EMG may be helpful to detect abnormality • EMG + NCS are valuable to decide the prognosis
Neuroprexia	• In neuroprexia, the nerve conduction is normal in proximal and distal portion of the blockage, however the conduction is impaired (though temporarily) across the blockage • Thus NCS shows increases latency across compressed area but normal NCV above and below that point • EMG remains normal in acute cases because Wallerian degeneration does not occur

Contd...

Contd...

Axonotmesis	• Neural surrounding sheath is intact but axonal damage has occurred • Wallerian degeneration occurs distal to lesion • +/- NCS abnormality with abnormal EMG findings occurs • NCS finding depends on types and numbers of axons affected • If larger axons intact → NCV is normal but amplitude of M-wave decreased (because less motor units are working now) • Abnormal EMG findings (positive sharp waves and fibrillation potential) after 2–3 week (findings may delay if axon injury point is close to the nerve cell body)
Neurotmesis	• Disrupted neural tube + total loss of axonal function • Total block of nerve conduction across cut point • NCS is absent because no evoke response can be elicited • Spontaneous potentials appear with the muscle at rest and even in absence of any voluntary attempt • Regeneration of axons may occur by collateral sprouting and it causes polyphasic potentials with voluntary attempt • Serial EMG may help to confirm regeneration or deterioration
MND	The degeneration of the anterior horn cells occurs **EMG** shows • Fibrillation potentials and positive sharp waves at rest • In advanced cases polyphasic motor unit potentials of increased amplitude and duration occurs due to re-innervation and collateral sprouting • Diminished motor performance coz less of motor neurons **NCV** • Motor NCV reduced, amplitude of motor attempt reduces • Sensory NCV remains normal
GBS	• MRI can show nerve root enhancement • CT scan helps to rule out other pathology • NCS – Studies show demyelination and establish the extent of injury – Sensory NCS abnormalities are less marked than motor NCS abnormality Changes on NCS should be present in at least 2 nerves in regions that are not typical for those associated with compressive mono-neuropathies (preferentially in anatomically distinct areas, such as an arm and a leg or a limb and the face)

NCS, nerve conduction studies; EMG, electromyography; NCV, nerve conduction velocity; +, present; –, absent

9.2: HEMIPLEGIA

Hemiplegia is the condition characterized by the abnormal functioning of the lateral half side of the body (either left of right) due to the rapid or acute onset focal neurological deficit resulting from the disease of the brain vasculature or its content.

Hemiplegia is the significant weakness or the complete paralysis of the lateral half of the body, (Fig. 9.2.1) while the hemiparesis refers to the weakness of the muscles of the lateral half of the body. The most common cause of the hemiplegia is the 'brain stroke' or commonly known as 'stroke' therefore the terms hemiplegia, stroke or brain stroke are used interchangeably though the stroke is a 'cause' and the hemiplegia is the 'consequence'.

Therefore, stroke is the acute onset of neurological impairment secondary to the abnormality of cerebral circulation, resulting in the signs and symptoms specific to the area affected.

Classification of the Stroke

The stroke can be classified (Table 9.2.1) on the basis of etiology, the changes in the presentation and the anatomical region involved. Following are the subdivisions of these broad classifications:

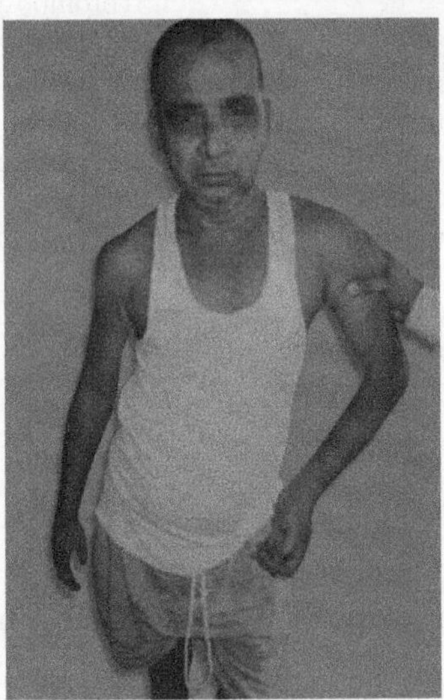

Fig. 9.2.1: The attitude of the joints in a typical hemiplegic patient (*For color version, see Plate 9*)

TABLE 9.2.1 The classification of hemiplegia

The basis of classification		*Type*
Etiology	Hemorrhagic (15% of all cases of stroke)	Rupture of the blood vessels of the brain Rupture of the cerebral vasculature aneurysm The dissecting aneurysm of the cerebral vasculature The bleeding disorders The intracerebral hemorrhage due to the trauma The hemorrhage can occur either: • Intracerebral hemorrhage (10%) when the bleeding occurs within gray matter of the brain • The subarachnoid hemorrhage (5%) when bleed occurs in subarachnoid region
	Ischemic (85% of all cases of stroke)	It can be due to the obstruction of the brain blood vasculature patency. It can further be classified in to two types: 1. Thrombosis (60%) 2. Embolism (25%)
Region of the brain involved	• Anterior cerebral artery (ACA) involvement • Posterior cerebral artery (PCA) involvement • Middle cerebral artery (MCA) involvement—most common artery involved in stroke • Pontine artery involvement • Lacunar stroke • Basilar artery involvement • Medullary syndrome • Brainstem syndrome	

Causes of Stroke

Vasculopathy: The blood vessels responsible for carrying the blood to important regions of the brain are affected or have impairment.

Coagulopathy: When the higher viscosity of blood slows down the blood flow across the blood vessels leading the higher risk of blood stagnation and the abnormal clotting in the blood vessels. The reduced capacity of the blood clotting (sickle cell anemia, the excessive dosage of blood thinners, the vitamin K deficiency, and lack of clotting factors in brain) may put the brain structure at the higher risk of developing the internal hemorrhage.

Aneurysm: Aneurysm is the abnormal dilation of the blood vessels, due to various possible etiologies. These aneurysms have delicate vessels walls and the higher risk of undergoing rupture when the pressure of the blood flowing through them increases. Therefore, the rupture of the aneurysm is important cause of the stroke.

Trauma: The trauma to the skull or the brain portion also affects the blood supply to the parts of the brain leading to their malfunctioning

Comorbid conditions: The other associated medical pathological states such as diabetes mellitus, the history of recent surgeries such as cardiac surgeries/brain or skull region surgery, the increased bed confinement due to fracture or the surgery, massive infections in the body, cardiac insufficiency are the other reasons of increasing the risk of developing stroke.

The unstable hypertension for prolonged period will also increase the risk of arterial rupture due to the higher pressure in vascular channel.

Differential Diagnosis of the Stroke

Following are the conditions that have to be ruled out for the diagnosis of the stroke:

- TIA—transient ischemic attack
- Severe migraine
- Partial seizures
- Metabolic pathologies—hypoglycemia, dys-electrolytemia, hyponatremia
- Convulsions and local vascular spasm
- Hysterial paralysis
- Subdural hematoma.

Assessment of the Stroke Patient

General Physical Assessment

- Integumentary system
- Lymph node enlargement

- Examination of the head, ear, nose, eyes, breast, skull region
- Abdominal color, sweating, temperature and warmth.

Neurological Examination

- Mental status examination
  - Level of consciousness (alert, lethargic, unresponding, Glasgow Coma scale rating, stupor, coma)
  - Attention—respond to the commands
  - Orientation—about the time, place and person
  - Language testing—fluency, content, comprehension, repetition, reading and writing ability
  - Memory—short-term memory, long-term memory
  - Cognitive functions—RLA (Ranchos Los Amigos) score
- Cranial nerve testing
  - *Facial nerve*: Sensory and motor examination. Bell's palsy has to be ruled out to the lower motor function evaluation of the facial nerve.
- Musculoskeletal system
  - Muscle tone (Modified Ashworth Scale)
  - Grade 0 = normal muscle tone; no increase in tone
  - Grade 1= slight increase in tone manifested as a catch and release or the minimum resistance at the end of range of motion, when the affected part is moved passively
  - Grade 1+ = slight increase in muscle tone, manifested as catch followed by minimal resistance throughout the range of motion when the affected part is moved passively
  - Grade 2= more marked increase in muscle tone, through most of ROM but the affected part can be moved
  - Grade 3= considerable increase in muscle tone, and the passive movement is difficult but possible
  - Grade 4= affected part is rigid in flexion or extension, and the movement is difficult to be carried out.
- Deep tendon reflexes (DTRs)
  - The standard method of documenting
  - 0 = no response; always abnormal
  - 1+ = a slight but definitely present response; may or may not be normal
  - 2+ = a brisk response; normal
  - 3+ = a very brisk response; may or may not be normal
  - 4+ = a tap elicits a repeating reflex (clonus); always abnormal

The normal or the abnormal labeling of the DTR rests upon the associated features such as muscle tone, muscle weakness, the neurological history, disease of the neurological weakness, etc.

- *Manual muscle testing*: According to the Oxford grading criteria:
  - The muscle strength testing is very important to be evaluated as the weaker muscle actions are always prone to cause the compensatory mechanisms that lead to the faulty movement pattern and the higher risks of developing the abnormal synergy patterns. In case of the hemiplegic patients, it is very important to differentiate between the actual muscle strength and the spastic or the hypertonic muscles.
  - The strength testing must be performed bilaterally and the normal side must be tested first, so as to have the knowledge of the actual muscle ability and to know what is normal. After the normal limb testing the abnormal limb testing must be done.
  - The strength performance of the muscles is documented on the standard scale using the Oxford grading scale (Daniel and Worthingham, 1995) as follows:
  - Grade 0= no muscle contraction can be appreciated either visually or by palpation.
  - Grade I= the minimal muscle contraction appreciable as a visual or palpable flicker over the tendon or the muscle belly, however the no movement of the bony lever occurs.
  - Grade II= when the muscle strength allows the bony lever to move through the complete range of motion in the gravity eliminated situation.
  - Grade III= when the muscle strength allows the bony lever to move through the complete range of motion against the force of gravity, without the additional resistance added.
  - Grade IV= when the muscle strength allows the bony lever to move through the complete range of motion against the force of gravity, with minimal additional resistance added.
  - Grade V= when the muscle strength allows the bony lever to move through the complete range of motion against the force of gravity, with maximal additional resistance added.
- ROM—range of motion assessment
- *Motor control assessment*: The ability of the client to perform physical functional task is analyzed in terms of the quality of movement.

- Sensory examination
  - Superficial sensations—light touch, pin prick, thermal sensations
  - Deep sensations- joint position or proprioception sense, kinesthesia, pressure, deep pain, vibration sense
  - Combined cortical functions
    a. Graphesthesia
    b. Streognosis
    c. Double simultaneous sensations
    d. Barognosis
- Coordination assessment
  - Non-equilibrium tests
    a. Finger to nose
    b. Finger to therapist finger
    c. Alternate nose to therapist finger touch
    d. Finger opposition
    e. Alternate pronation and supination
  - Equilibrium tests- balance assessment.
    a. OLST (one limb stand test)
    b. Rhomberg test
    c. Tendom walk test
- Gait assessment: During gait assessment the period of weight-bearing on each limb and the proportion of weight born on each limb must be assessed. The hemiplegic patients have tendency of having unequal bearing of weight between two limbs (Fig. 9.2.2).
- Bowel and bladder function assessment.
- Hand function assessment: The functional assessment of hand is very important aspect of hemiplegic patient rehabilitation. Various types of grips that must be evaluated for hand function assessment include the cylindrical grasp, spherical grasp, pinch grip, power grip, chuk grip, and the grip strength (Fig. 9.2.11).
- Environmental assessment.
- ADL assessment using standard scales for both basic activity of daily living (BADL) and instrumental activities of daily living (IADL).

PHYSIOTHERAPY MANAGEMENT OF THE HEMIPLEGIA

Principle of Treatment of Hemiplegia or Stroke during Flaccid Stage

- During this stage, the prevention of the further disability is the prime aim followed by with the aim of enhancing the recovery from the suffered impairment.

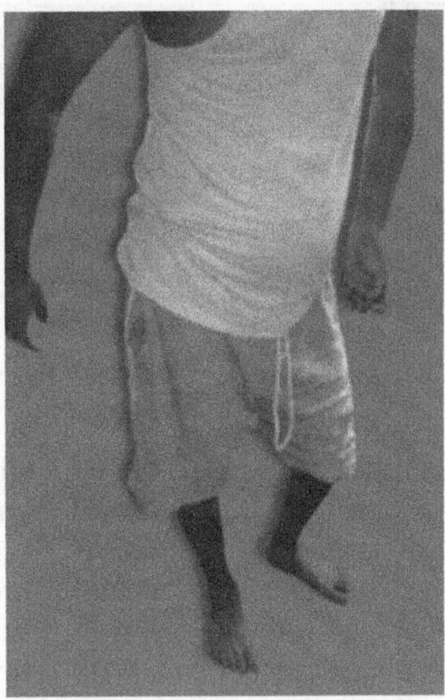

Fig. 9.2.2: The unequal weight-bearing between both the legs in hemiplegic patients

- The joint contractures and muscle shortening/contractures are prevented with the help of the full range of motion (ROM) exercises regularly.
- The prevention of the joint dislocation of the weakened joints such as shoulder joint is done with the help of the sling or support and the proper precautions or positioning and the adequate supports to the vulnerable joints with pillow, sandbag or the braces. However, whenever possible the splinting must be avoided as these impose the higher risk of forming pressure sores over the weakened muscles.
- Positioning of the limb is very important to prevent the development of the muscle impairment.
- The anti-synergy positions (Fig. 9.2.3) are implemented to prevent the development of the synergy abnormal movement patterns. For this purpose, the limb and the associated joints are placed in the position opposite to the abnormal synergy positions. The common synergy pattern of the upper extremity (Fig. 9.2.1) involves the flexion, adduction and the internal rotation of the shoulder. Therefore to prevent the development

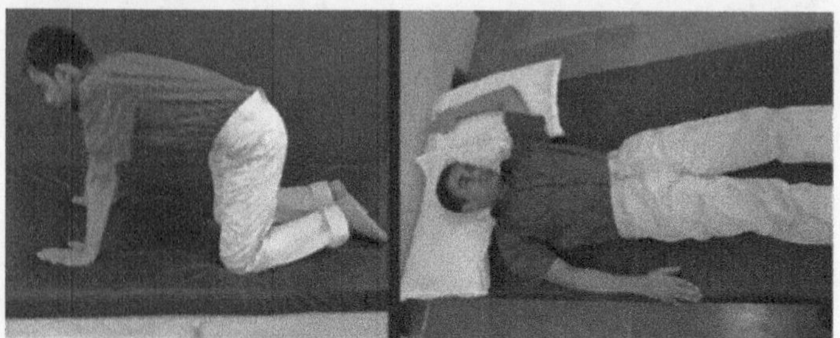

Fig. 9.2.3: Anti-synergy positions for hemiplegics

of this abnormal synergy pattern the upper limb is to be placed in the position of the shoulder extension, abduction and the external rotation fashion.

- The prevention of the sensory dissociation and the re-education of the sensory perception is also very important. For this, the
  a. Sensory feedback are feedback to the client.
  b. During passive limb movement, the client is asked to focus on the movement that is being carried out passively, and the client himself/herself attempts to carry out the movement along with the therapist assistance.
  c. If the patient remains lazy or inattentive or does not give attention to the movements being implemented by therapist, the benefits of the therapeutic interventions would remain sub-optimal.
  d. The increased sensory inputs may be given using Rood's facilitation techniques such as quick icing, brushing, gentle stroking, gentle tapping.
  e. Exposure of different textures and shapes; the exposure of hard and soft surfaces may be helpful.

- The earlier interventions during flaccid stage helps to prevent or at least minimize the degree of spasticity that is expected to occur as the recovery from flaccid state starts.
  - The gentle and the controlled weight bearing of the affected limb (Fig. 9.2.4) is permitted as this increases the joint proprioceptive inputs and also helps to prevent the development of the spasticity. However, the proper support or assistance or supervision is to be given to client to avoid unwanted fall or undue joint loading beyond the desired extent.

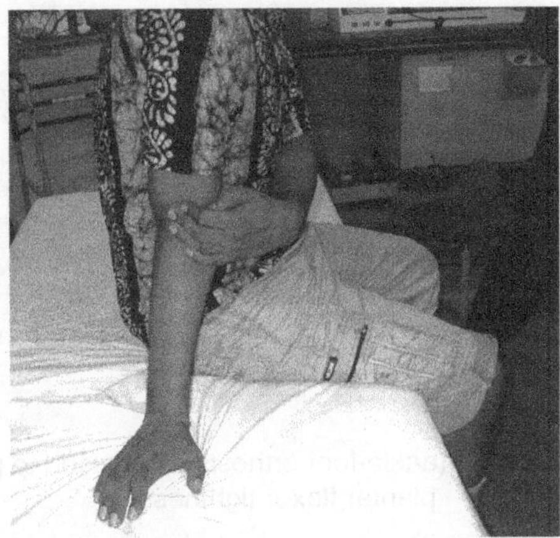

Fig. 9.2.4: The controlled early weight-bearing of the upper extremity joints

a. The shoulder joint is highly vulnerable to undergo inferior dislocation, therefore this joint must be paid special attention.
b. For preventing the development of the plantar flexor muscle contracture or tightness the AFO (ankle-foot orthosis) splint can be recommended (Fig. 9.2.5).

- The restoration of the functional independence is an additional highly vital aim of the hemiplegia management.
  - Right from the flaccid stage, the client has to be mentally prepared for becoming the functional independence.
  - For enhancing the movement response by the patient, the mat exercises (Fig. 9.2.6) are implemented to train the client for carrying out various bed immobility tasks such as initiating the turning from supine or prone position; the mobility exercises to assume sitting position from the side-lying or supine position, etc.
  - The common mat activities include turning from supine to side-lying to prone and vice versa; prone to prone on elbow; bridging activities; prone on elbow to prone on hand; prone on hand to quadripud; quadripud to kneeling; kneeling to half kneeling; half kneeling to standing with support; standing with support to the standing without support.

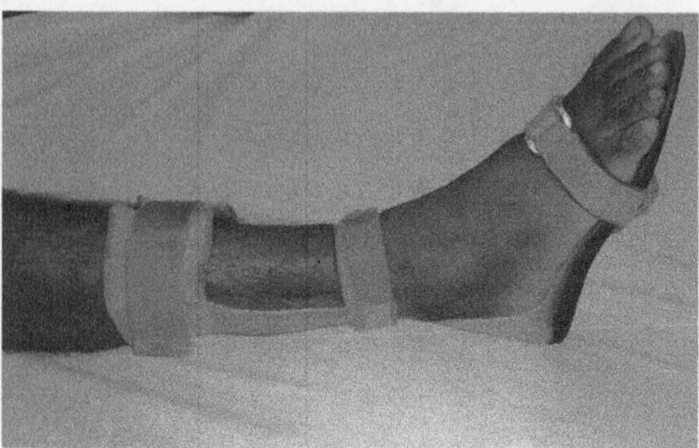

Fig. 9.2.5: AFO (ankle-foot orthosis) is advised to prevent plantar flexor tightness

- The various activities performed in the prone lying or quadripud positions include commando walking with elbow, commando walking to sides or forward or backward or in multiple directions (Fig. 9.2.6).
- The mat exercises may require the assistance or the support to carry out the movement, and as the performance of the client improves, the assistance may be diminished. When the active performance improves, the number of repetitions or the amount of resistance imposed on muscles can be increased. For example, when the client is able to perform the bridging satisfactory with both feet resting on couch in crrok-lying, the progression can be made by asking the client to cross one knee over another and take the weight only on one feet resting on floor (Fig. 9.2.6).

- The prevention of the sensory impairment aims to:
  - Prevent the development of 'hemineglect': The hemiplegics have the tendency of developing the negligence of the affected lateral half of the body and this is an important issue which has to be dealt at earliest so as to enhance the functional symmetry of the two halves of the body.
  - To avoid the development of the hemineglect the modifications are required in the home environment and the way of dealing with the client. The television, the table or almirah having utility items, the door of the room, etc. must be kept on the affected side of the body so that the client does not forget the affected

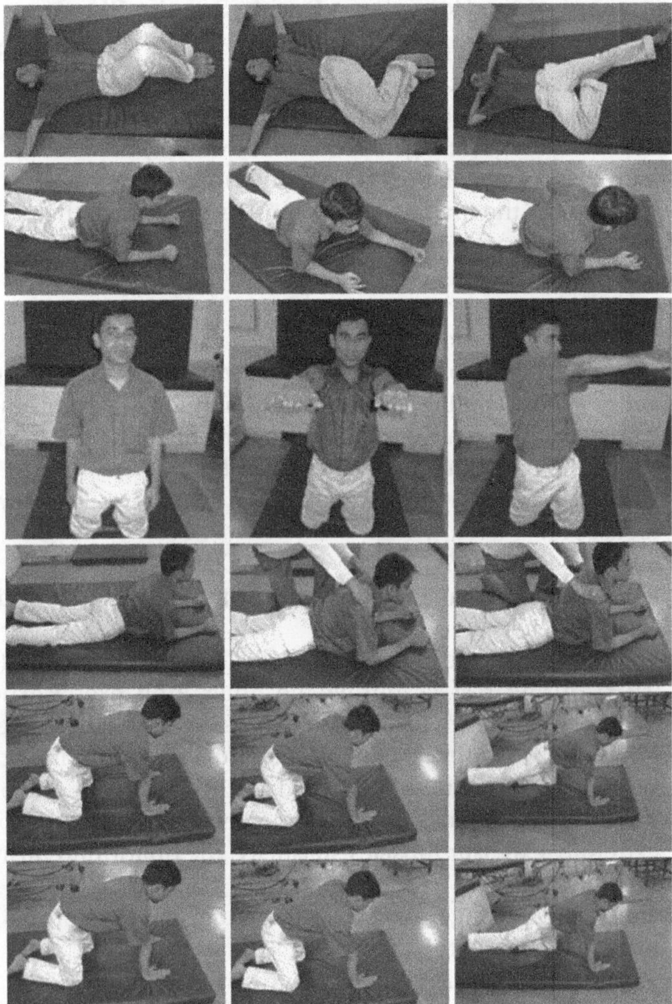

Fig. 9.2.6: Mat activities for the hemiplegic patients

part. The guests visiting the patients, the bed pan, the meal, the water, and the medicines all must be given from the affected half of the body to avoid the forgetting of this affected half.

- To minimize the sensory dissociation
- To prevent the development and the maturation of the synergy abnormal movement patterns.

Management of the Hemiplegia During Spastic Stage

The common problems encountered in stroke patients include the following (Aruine, et al. 2000):

- Deficits in motor control that involve
- Abnormal synergistic organization of movements
- Impaired force regulation (either due to muscle weakness or overactivity or the inability of the muscles to control the pattern of the muscle functioning
- Muscle weakness
- Sensory deficits, and
- Loss of range of motion.

Patients with stroke present with the asymmetry in the static (Fig. 9.2.2) and dynamic standing postures and during functional movements (Pai, et al. 1994). This is a risk factor for causing the impairment of the balance and the gait disorders (Wall and Turnbull, 1986).

The physiotherapy management of hemiplegics during spastic stage focuses to:

- Reduce the spasticity.
  - Early weight bearing for prolonged time is helpful to reduce the spasticity.
  - The position of the client in the reflex inhibiting posture (Fig. 9.2.3) during rest or during the other limb exercise helps to deal with the progression of the spasticity. These "reflex inhibiting postures" positions the joints and muscles in the position opposite to that adopted by the spastic muscle or by muscle synergy. For preventing the development of the lower extremity extensor muscles spasticity, the quadripud position is highly useful.
  - The gentle rocking, rhythmic, alternating, and the non-painful passive movements help to reduce the spasticity.
  - The prolonged and gradually progressive stretching (Fig. 9.2.7) of the spastic muscles at all the crossed joints, to the full extent helps to reduce the spasticity.
  - The cryotherapy for the prolonged time (over 20 minutes) helps to slow down the nerve conduction velocity and helps to cope with the spasticity.
  - The occurrence of clonus may be undesirable as this reduces the tendency of the client to bear weight on the affected extremity. Upon weight bearing as the muscles are stretched the ankle clonus leads to the unstable base for the weight

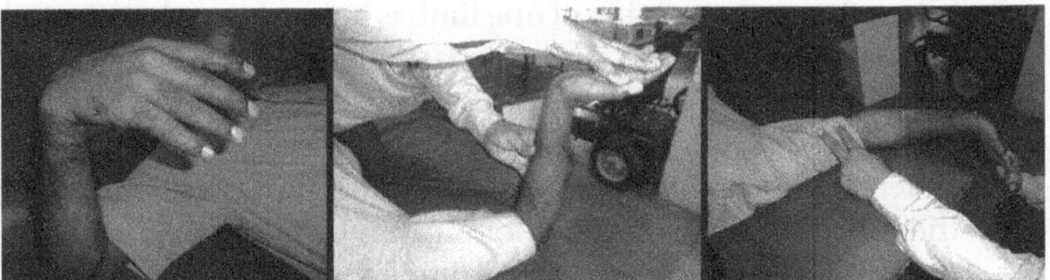

Fig. 9.2.7: Stretching exercises for the spastic wrist flexor

bearing and reduces the balance. To deal with the clonus the low grade sustained stretching of the spastic muscle helps.
- The isometric and isometric contractions of the spastic muscles; and the isotonic contraction of the antagonist muscle group (group opposite to the spastic muscles) is helpful.
- The relaxation exercises, the reduction of the pain, fear and anxiety helps the client to calm down and the better dealing with the spasticity. The isotonic contractions of antagonist muscles are advisable after the relaxation exercises to reduce the range of spasticity in the motion arc.

• Re-educate the muscles.
  - As the muscle spasticity is controlled and decreased, the further breaking of the abnormal movement pattern is possible by appropriate interventions. The interventions focus to enhance the use of the affected extremity in a controlled and desirable fashion. The active efforts of the normal tone muscles help to improve the correct movement learning by the affected brain.
  - The early stage movements must be as simple as possible and this movement recruits the single joint at a time. As the condition improves and the motor control improves, the multi-joint movements and progressively more complex movements may be advised.
  - The proximal joints provide the stable base; therefore the early movement focuses to improve the proximal joint control followed by the training of the distal joints.
  - For the training of multiple muscle groups and joints simultaneously in functional manner, the proprioceptive neuromuscular facilitation (PNF) patterns may be used (Fig. 9.2.8).
  - Those muscles are trained earlier which are important for the functional task and those which provide the stable base for the movement of the adjacent muscle groups.

- When the active training of one limb is being done, the affected limb has to be kept in the 'spasticity-inhibiting' or 'tone-inhibiting' or the anti-synergy position.

- To improve the strength of the weakened muscle.
  - When the flaccid state is over, the tone starts returning and therefore the muscle strengthening may be initiated to improve the strength of the weaker group of muscles. During this training, it is important to avoid the increase in the tone of the already spastic muscles. During spasticity in the hemiplegia, the weakness may be present in the spastic as well as the antagonist group of muscles. The sensory stimulation may be needed to facilitate the muscle activity after reduced state of the spasticity. The higher stimulation may be required for the muscles antagonist to the spastic muscles.
  - During strengthening those groups have to be paid special attention which have tendency to remain weak even during the development of the spastic movement patterns. Thus the strengthening of the hip extensors, hip adductors, knee flexors, ankle dorsi-flexors, elbow extensors, wrist extensors, finger abductors and extensors, etc. is important.
- To reduce the gait asymmetry and to improve the weight-bearing on the affected limbs.

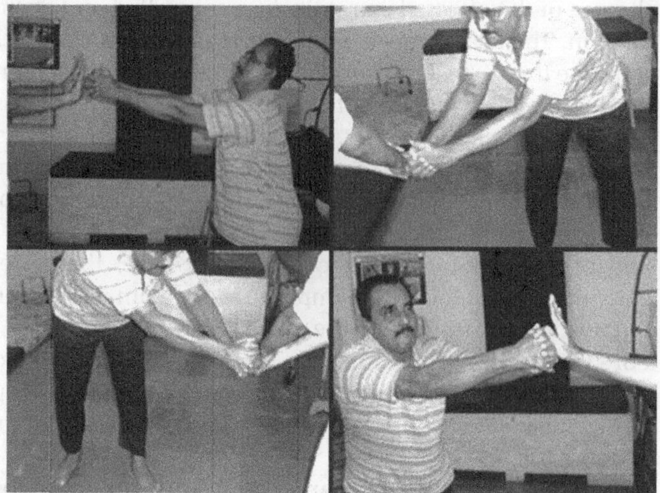

Fig. 9.2.8: PNF exercises for upper extremity and trunk control

- The equal bearing of the body weight on normal as well as the affected limb is important for facilitating the gait symmetry. Improvement of the gait quality is an important goal for the rehabilitation of the stroke patient (Wang, 1994).
- For improving the weight bearing on the affected extremity, the variety of the goal directed movements (Sax, et al. 1993) may be taught. These include the standing leg flexion, lateral trunk flexion, gait initiation (two steps forward), a hip shift maneuver, and lateral leg raising with a step (lateral step up), forward step ups (Aruin, et al. 2000; Sax, et al. 1993).
- Sit to standing activities; the isometric hip abduction activity with the standing position; verbal feedback and encouragement to initiate the goal directed movements, leading with the affected extremity are other useful methods to enhance gait and postural symmetry (Aruin, et al. 2000).
- These activities need to be supervised accurately to avoid the compensatory or trick movements, and the client must be encouraged to perform these drills as number of time as possible.
- Other common techniques used for improving the gait asymmetry, in physical therapy treatment including visual, tactile, or verbal cues or postural feedback devices to improve weight loading on the paretic limb (Sackley, et al. 1988; Shumway-cook, et al. 1988).

• To improve coordination and balance.
  - The hemiplegic patients present a variety of the imbalance related impairments and the higher fall risks secondary to the higher tone, high tendency of the rigid body segments, the diminished ability of the postural muscles to prevent the fall of body. Therefore, the balance training is an important intervention needed for improving the functional performance of the hemiplegic patients.
  - The coordination among different muscle groups, is important to be re-established for optimizing the motor performance.
  - The balance training aims to improve the body's ability to deal with the external or internal generated perturbations and disturbances which tend to outbalance the body.
  - The balance training exposes the patient to a large variety of the static or dynamic positions, which tend to shift the body's COG (center of gravity) in numerous directions, and, therefore,

imposes the variable demands of the muscle activity needed in the body to maintain the equilibrium and balance.
- The progression in the balance training can be made as follows:
  a. From lying position to the sitting and standing positions
  b. From sitting positions to the standing position
  c. From bilateral foot supported standing to the single foot supported standing
  d. From single joint tasks to the tasks involving multiple joints simultaneousy
  e. From active movement to the activities involving the movement of bony levers against external resistance of the weight cuff or dumble
  f. From the straight walking activities to the retro-walking, side walking, tandem walking, side walking involving the foot placement after foot crossover
  g. Step up activity to the front and then to the side step up.

- To re-educate the functional activities.
  - The muscle activity has to be facilitated or trained with appropriate progressions to improve the functional outcome.
- To enhance the ADL (activity of daily living) performance
  - The tasks mimicking the ADL activities must be incorporated in the daily practice regime. Some common activities include those activities, which are important to perform various daily routine tasks such as feeding, writing (Fig. 9.2.9) dressing, bathing, self hygiene, water drinking, the approach towards and grabbing the object by opening and closing hand and digits.
  - The residual irreversible impairments may be managed to certain extent by the training in a way which would utilize the remaining strength to gain better functional outcome.
  - For example, the patient with diminished ability of finger extensors but normal wrist flexors, may be trained to learn to open his/her hand/fingers to reach towards the object and then do wrist extension to bring about the finger/hand closing (due to the passive insufficieny or the tenodesis effect) to grab the object and pick it up.
  - The ADL training may be done initially in the laboratory or clinical setting, but this can not be considered useful or satisfactory until it has been incorporated in the situations (occupational set up, social scenario) where the client would actually use them practically.

- To maximize the independence.
  - The physiotherapy interventions aim to regain the highest possible level of independence in the hemiplegic patient, and to bring the patient back to the normal pre-stroke lifestyle and occupational rehabilitation.
  - The use of walking aids such as cane (Fig. 9.2.10), to increase the safety during walking, increasing base of support, and to assist the weight transfer. This also helps to curb the higher risk of the hemiplegic patients to fall towards the normal side or the backward direction.

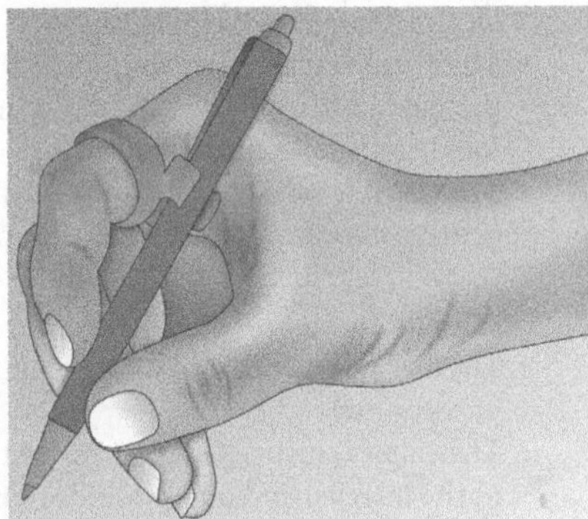

Fig. 9.2.9: Improving the writing ability in hemiplegics by giving writing aid

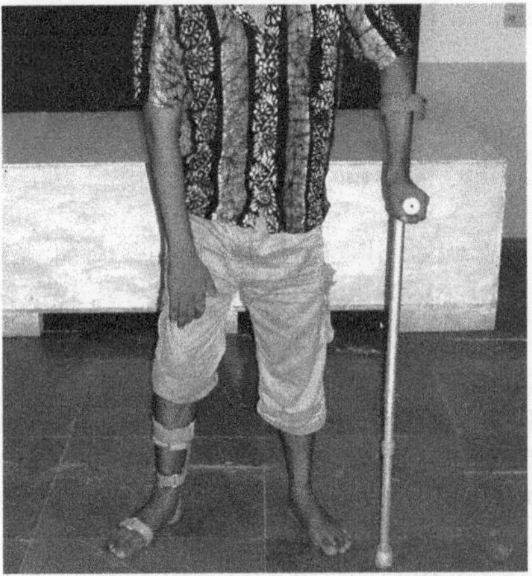

Fig. 9.2.10: Use of cane for improving gait

TABLE 9.2.2 The application of the PNF technique for improving the pelvis control (Wang, 1994)

PNF Technique	*Protocol*
Rhythmic initiation	• The client is asked to stay relax, and the pelvis is moved through available range of motion in the anterior elevation and to return the pelvis through posterior depression pattern (passive movement phase) • Then client is instructed to help the therapist to carry out the movement by adding the active efforts upon the command "now help me to move the limb" (active assisted movement phase) • The client is then asked to oppose the movement of the therapist by offering the resistance to the movement (resistance movement phase) • The client is asked to carry out the movement actively into the anterior elevation pattern, and the position is returned back passively to the starting position
Slow reversal	• The body part is moved to the lengthened position of the muscle • The client is instructed to perform the contraction of the internal and oblique abdominis muscles to elevate the pelvis with maximal effort against resistance added by the therapist • The therapist gradually switches the manual contact point to the posterior depression pattern • The client is asked to contract the quadratus lumborum, ilicostalis lumborum muscle to lower the pelvis against maximal resistance
Agonist reversal	• The pelvis is taken into the anterior elevated position; using the manual contact and verbal cues the client performs concentric contraction of the target muscles • The client is asked to offer resistance to the movement upon the command of the "make it hard for me to move the limb"

– The cane must be given only when the client has regained the gross independent ambulation, however needs a little support to boost the confidence and independence. The cane must not be given to client when he/she cant stand or walk satisfactory, as use of cane in these patients would increase the dependency

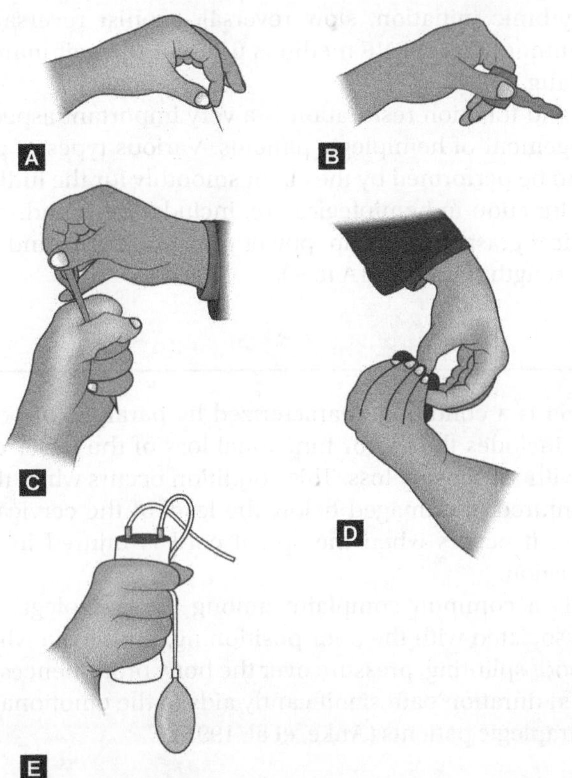

Figs 9.2.11A to E: The various types of grips which have to be evaluated: (A) Pinch grip; (B) Key grip; (C) Power grip; (D) Chuck grip; (E) Testing grip strength for hand function

on the walking aid. For the same reasons the quadruped or tripod canes are not recommended, and only the single leg cane is commonly used (Davies, 2000).

- Use of the PNF techniques (Table 9.2.2).
  - PNF (proprioceptive neuromuscular facilitation) techniques (Fig.9.2.8) are commonly used for the gait management and upper extremity control in the hemiplegic patients (Sullivan, et al. 1982). These PNF techniques aim to improve the control of the pelvis, the "key point of the control" to optimize the gait pattern (Sullivan, et al. 1982; Wang, 1994).

- Rhythmic initiation, slow reversal, agonist reversal are the commonly used PNF methods used for the gait management (Wang, 1994)

- The hand function restoration is a very important aspect for the management of hemiplegic patients. Various types of grips that have to be performed by the client smoothly for the independent hand function in hemiplegics are, include the cylindrical grasp, spherical grasp, pinch grip, power grip, chuk grip, and the good grip strength (Figs 9.2.11A to E).

9.3: PARAPLEGIA

Paraplegia is a condition characterized by paralysis of both lower limbs. It includes the motor functional loss of the lower extremity with or without sensory loss. This condition occurs when the spinal cord is injured or damaged below the level of the cervical region. Therefore, it occurs when the spinal cord is injured in thoracic, lumbar region.

Pain is a common complaint among the paraplegic patients, and is associated with the poor positioning, prolonged wheel chair sitting, poor splinting, pressure over the bony prominences, etc. The prolonged duration pain significantly aids to the emotional distress of the paraplegic patients (Anke, et al. 1995).

CAUSES OF PARAPLEGIA

The causes of the paraplegia include following: - the paraplegia may have its cause in the spinal cord or/and cerebrum itself. Broadly, the causes of paraplegia can be classified into 5 ts—trauma, tumor, tuberculosis, thrombosis and transverse myelitis.

- The extra growth which compromises the spinal cord such as epidural abscess, spinal tumors
- Transverses myelitis
- Traumatic spinal cord injury—during accedents, falls from heights, during mountain cycling, during diving, ballistic injuries during war
- The obstruction in the blood supply of the spinal cord by emboli, blood vessels injury or arteriosclerosis and in arteriovenous malformation (AVM), spinal hemangioma, ruptured aneurysm
- Developemental disorders such as spina bifida, meningomylocele

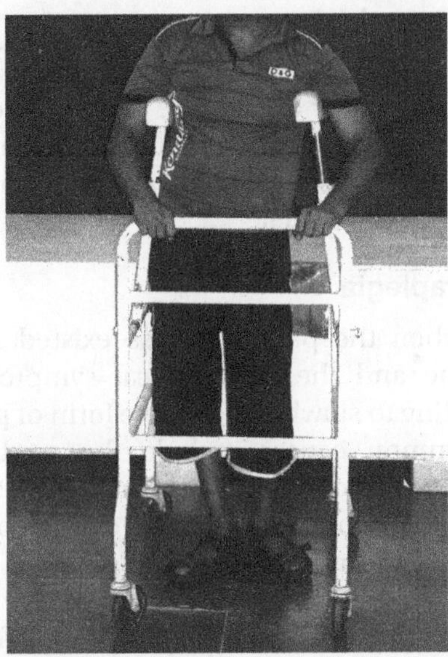

Fig. 9.3.1: Typical paraplegia patient, using the brace for supporting the injured site, using knee-ankle-foot orthoses (KAFO) for ambulation, using walker as walking aid

- Infective conditions such as spinal infection, transverse myelitis
- Compression of the spinal cord by tumors or the tuberculous spine (Pott's paraplegia)
- Non-compressive or systemic disease such as motor neuron disease (MND), multiple sclerosis (MS), syringomyelia, hereditary spastic paraplegia, Friedrich's ataxia
- Severe form of prolapsed intervertebral disc (PIVD)
- The tumors which cause paraplegia include myeloma, lymphomatous, chordoma, ependymoma, glioma.

CLASSIFICATIONS OF PARAPLEGIA

Depending on the etiology and the rapidity of progression, the paraplegia may be classified as sudden onset or slow onset. According to the clinical findings, the paraplegia may be spastic or flaccid. The spastic and flaccid paraplegia may again have their origin as sudden onset or slow onset. On the basis of presence or absence of the bladder or/and bowel control, the paraplegia can be classified as incomplete or complete paraplegia.

Sudden Onset Paraplegia

- This paraplegia occurs suddenly and during the early acute phases of the pathology or trauma. The pathology may include trauma, tubercular spine and inflammatory edema.
- During the sudden onset paraplegia, the prognosis is good for recovery of the neural deficit.

Slow Onset Paraplegia

- This occurs when the pathology has existed in the spine for prolonged time and the neurological symptoms have arisen gradually, leading to slowly progressive form of paraplegia.
- The most common causes include the gradually increasing pressure on the spinal cord such as during progressive mechanical compression of the cord, tuberculous debris compromising the cord, the spinal deformity (scoliosis, or gibbus).
- Due to the slowly progressive nature of the paraplegia, the symptoms have manifested gradually and the prognosis is relatively poor while compared to the sudden onset paraplegia because of the fact that the chronic nature of the disease might have lead to the irreversible damage to the cord structure.

Spastic Paraplegia

This is the form of paraplegia in which there occurs the spastic manifestation in the affected lower extremities.

Flaccid Paraplegia

- The shock or acute stage of the spinal cord injury, acute anterior poliomyelitis, acute infective polyneuropathy.
- During this stage, there is the complete loss of tone, the bowel and bladder control is impaired, and the deep tendon reflexes related to knee jerk and ankle jerk are lost.

PHYSIOTHERAPY MANAGEMENT OF PARAPLEGIA

The degree of lesion, the functioning of the residual musculature and the location of the lesion affects the prognosis of the functional independence. In as high location lesion in the cervical region the upper as well as lower extremity involvement occurs, which leads to the significant impairment and the extensive loss of functioning of the upper extremity, lower extremity and the trunk.

In the thoracic lesion the paralysis of the lower extremity predominates including hips, knee and feet. In case of the lower lumbar region involvement the loss of muscle functioning is not that much predominant, and the only the feet or knee or the intrinsic feet muscles may be involved.

The motor as well the sensory loss occurs in the spinal cord injury. The sensory loss may include the loss of sensation to the touch, proprioception, heat and cold. The loss of the autoregulation ability of the blood vessels also occurs which impairs the autoregulation to maintain the blood vessels tone important for the blood returns and the blood flow to and from extremity and vital organs. The loss of ability to maintain the adequate vascular perfusion to the important organs including brain, while assuming the erect standing posture. This leads to the frequent complaints of the orthostatic hypotension (Cariga, et al. 2002).

Loss of the skin tone and the sensations puts it at higher risk of developing the pressure sores and ulcers. The patients cared with the proper positioning; turning, sore preventing strategies are at lower risk of developing pressure sores, while compared to those who are devoid of such interventions (Aung and El Masry, 1997). To avoid these pressure sores, the bony prominences must be well padded, the prolonged pressure on any surface must be avoided. During wheelchair usage, the special emphasis must be given to prevent the pressure sores over the sacral, ishial, heel region and popliteal region. To avoid the continuous pressure over the ishial region the pressure must be dispersed using the air filled ring with empty space in the center.

The loss of muscle tone puts the joints in abnormal positions which over period of time lead to the development of the contractures and deformity at joint. In some cases the contracture potential may be reduced using the surgical approaches (Eltorai and Montroy, 1990) such as tenotomy (tendon cut), tendon elongation, joint capsulotomy, cutting the nerve supply to the large muscle group. The physical therapy interventions during postoperative management depends on the type of surgery performed.

After the period of the flaccidity is over the spasticity comes into picture which makes the movements stiff and difficult to occur. Also the abnormal positioning of joints under influence of the spasticity makes them prone to develop contractures. Number of conservative therapy based interventions are applicable to minimize the extent of spasticity development, and to avoid the associated complication.

In certain cases when the physical therapeutic interventions alone can not bring about significant reduction in spasticity or the rehabilitation approaches get inefficient due to excessive spascitity, the medicine interventions such as oral baclofen (Azouvi, et al. 1996) or injectable intrathecal baclofen or baclofen pump or intrathecal morphine (Soni, et al. 2003) are used to reduce the spasticity.

Osteoporosis is present to definite degree in the bones below the level of the lesion in all paraplegics (Frey-Rindova, et al. 2000) and this could be linked with the immobility, lesser muscle activity, the muscle atrophy below the level of lesion. Unlike other causes of osteoporosis (such as menopause, ageing) where the vertebral collapse occurs commonly; the osteoporosis linked to the spinal cord injury occurs more commonly in the hip joint and femoral region, without having reduced bone mass density of the vertebral region (Szollar, et al. 1997). The isometric exercises, the early weight bearing, the functional electrical stimulation can be helpful for prevention of the muscle atrophy and the associated bone density loss.

The acute phase management also consists of the deep breathing exercise, frequent turning, the passive position of the body segments, the passive range of motion exercises of the major joints of the body. The physiotherapeutic care deals with the:

- Prevention of the joint contractures and deformity
- The prevention of skin ulcers and pressure sores
- To minimize the deformity and disability
- Bowel and bladder care
- The orthotic prescription to maintain the functional status and enhance the mobility status
- The transfer training for the improvement of mobility including the wheelchair transfers and the transfers in bed.

The mat activities and transfer activity training aims to develop good physical condition and to improve the ability to perform daily skill activity with adequate independence. These trained activities must resemble the daily routine tasks so as to have maximum carry over effects. These activities are also important to develop strength, balance, coordination, endurance, and to gain the activation of the dormant muscles.

- Changing position
- Rolling from supine to side or prone position and vice versa

- Coming to sitting position from the supine position
- Mobility training in bed
- Balancing activity in sitting, standing, long sitting and short sitting
- The balance and strength training in static conditions
- The balance and strength training in dynamic condition
- Coordination activity in- sitting, standing in parallel bar, on stable surface and then on unstable surface, the coordination training in static and dynamic conditions.

The self active and active assisted movements of the body segments are important to prevent the development of contractures.

The training specific and similar to the activities used in the daily routine tasks.

The common examples of the mat exercise programs include following activities:

- Rolling from supine to prone and vice versa
- The prone push ups
- Sit ups
- The leg raises, the leg rolling and heel slides
- The pelvic shifting and pelvic turning
- Sitting push ups
- Trunk twisting and raising activities
- The pelvic hiking activity of the quadratus lumborum muscle
- The Frenkel exercise program
- The forward and backward reaching activities
- The commando walking in prone position in forward, backward and lateral directions
- Cat and camel exercises
- The trunk rolling and mobility exercises
- *The progression in following positions*: The supine to prone lying, prone lying on hand, quadripud position, the kneeling, the half kneeling, plantigrade positioning against table support, the erect standing with supports of walker, standing with axillary crutches, the standing with elbow crutches.

The wheelchair training is an important aspect of the training of the paraplegics to improve the functional independence. For the wheelchair use by the paraplegic patients, the shoulder girdle has to be very strong as this is the joint which would be the key weight bearing joint during ambulation (Bagley, et al. 1987), therefore this girdle has to be trained with special emphasis.

In order to document the shoulder functioning among wheel chair users, the Shoulder Pain Index is an important tool which measures the shoulder pain during daily task activities such as transfers, self care tasks (Curtis, et al. 1995).

9.4: TABES DORSALIS

Tabes dorsalis is a complex group of neurological symptoms and signs caused by syphilis. The main lesions are in the posterior columns of the spinal cord, and the symptoms are therefore primarily sensory. But there are also lesions affecting the autonomic nervous system, whose effects are on the viscera, the pupils of the eyes, and the limbs.

Tabes dorsalis is a slowly progressive degenerative disease involving the posterior columns (i.e. demyelination) and posterior roots (i.e. inflammatory change with fibrosis) of the spinal cord. Tabes dorsalis is a rare condition because this is the last stage consequence of syphilis which, in turn, is very rare now.

Degeneration of posterior column of spinal cord occurs in tabes dorsalis.

About 90% death in tabes occurs due to pneumonia because respiratory involvement during paralytic stage is common.

Weakness and bedridden patient occurs in paralytic stage.

Each stage of tabes grows very slowly over period of 10 years therefore it is very chronic stage disease.

Tabes dorsalis is progressive degeneration of:

- Posterior nerve roots
- Dorsalis root ganglia
- Fasciculus gracilis
- Fasciculus cuneatus

CAUSES

It is late result of syphilis.

SEX

Males are affected more than females.

PATHOLOGY

Due to the posterior column degeneration the sensory system of the affected region and dermatome supplied, gets impaired.

■ STAGES

The typically three progressive stages occur and each stage lasts for about 10 years:

- Pre-ataxic stage
- Ataxic stage
- Paralytic stage

Pre-ataxic Stage

Symptoms are confined to eye and sensory system.

Sensory symptoms include:

- Slight pain which may increase to sharp shooting pain
- Girdle sensation around chest
- Paresthesia or numbness of foot.

Eye symptoms include:

- Loss of pupillary reflex
- Diplopia
- Ptosis
- Squint
- Pupillary constriction
- Argyll Robertson pupil.

Ataxic Stage

Most important stage in terms of the progression of disease with respect to physical symptoms can be controlled to certain extent in this stage.

It is also important as intervention at this stage will help to build up patient's confidence therefore the response to therapy is good.

Symptoms Due to Loss of Posterior Column

- Loss of conscious muscle and joint sensation therefore the impaired sensation of joint position
- The imbalance occurs and fall become common
- Rhomberg sign positive
- The balance impairment is most prominent with eyes closed
- Sensory changes are very marked at this stage
- Hypotonia starts setting in and if not care has been taken than may progress to atonia
- Paresthesia and loss of reflexes in the affected area.

Motor Changes

Hypotonia which may progress to atonia.

Trophic Changes

- Dry skin
- Impairement of sweat glands
- Pale skin
- Perforating ulcers infections are very common
- Charcot joint may develop as painless joint
- Abnormal mobility.

Visceral Crisis

- Renal system is badly affected therefore bladder is involved and urinary tract infection occurs
- Gastric system may be involved
- Respiratory infections.

Paralytic Stage

The patient is unable to walk and becomes bedridden.

Bladder trouble increases therefore renal system conditions start getting worse, recurrent urinary tract infections therefore the chronic renal failure.

Respiratory system involvement increases, pneumonia occurs classically in tabes dorsalis in later stages.

PHYSIOTHERAPY MANAGEMENT

Physiotherapy interventions are mainly needed in ataxic stage and treatment is by Frenkel's exercises, maintenance of ROM, strengthening exercises and the prevention of pneumonia.

The assessment has to be done with detailed sensory assessment.

The management helps to maintain muscles flexibility and sensations.

Main management includes the Frenkel's exercises during ataxic stage.

Progression of Frenkel's exercises can be made:

- From ling to sitting and to static standing to dynamic standing
- Fast to slow speed
- Simple and single step movement to complex multi-step movement

- Preparing patient for paralytic stage in the ataxic stage itself
- The bed transfers activity and bed mobility is taught in the ataxic stage itself
- During ataxic stage also taught the respiratory exercises and respiratory care
- Prevention of bed sores.

Tabes dorsalis is not a reversible condition therefore the paralysis of this is permanent and irreversible.

Patients with tabes dorsalis often lose peripheral feedback from the legs; however they yet can still walk (Bannister, 1979). Though the movement pattern in these patients could be irregular in the absence of the sensory feedback, the sequences of movement could be trained using the central mechanisms of motor control which regulate the higher command for movement that central mechanisms may play a pivotal role in motor control. Advocates of programming theory suggest that motor programs are key central mechanisms that provide the commands for movement (Morris, et al. 1994).

Management of the tabes dorsalis also considers the dealing with the neuropathic joint. Tabes dorsalis has been the most common cause of neuropathic arthropathy (Troyer and Levin, 2009). In contrast to diabetes, this post-syphilis condition has been shown to preferentially affect the knee over the foot and ankle (Langford and Gilliland, 2008). Clinical presentation of a neuropathic knee typically demonstrates an excellent ROM with a significant amount of crepitus, ligamentous laxity, a large effusion, and increased calor. Occasionally, there will be associated erythema surrounding the knee, making it difficult to rule out a clinical diagnosis of infection (Troyer and Levin, 2009; Long and Scuderi, 2008).

9.5: SPINA BIFIDA

Spina bifida is a developmental birth defect involving the incomplete closure of embryonic neural tube resulting in an incompletely formed spinal cord. It usually occurs at the end of first month of pregnancy when two sides of embryo's spine fail to join together leaving an open area. The defect is most common in lumbar and sacral area.

The vertebrae overlying the spinal cord don't completely fuse and remain open → the underlying portion of the spinal cord may protrude through the unfused/unclosed portion of the vertebral column → there may or may not be a fluid sac surrounding the exposed spinal cord.

The caudal end of the neural tube or the primitive spinal cord fails to close before the 28th day of the gestation. It can be typically detected before the birth and could be treated to certain extent at that time. The location and degree of severity may result in varying degrees of paralysis, impaired skin sensation, and impaired bowel and/or bladder control, scoliosis.

CLASSIFICATION

Spina bifida malformations fall into following categories:

- Spina bifida occulta
- Spina bifida manifesta (myelomeningocele and meningocele).

Spina bifida occulta 9.5.1A is a milder form, as cord is unaffected and child has no health problems due to it. Only X-ray shows defect in fusion of laminar arch. No neurological symptoms but may have abnormal bladder control, urine retention, enuresis. Band of fibrous tissue between bone and skin so dimple in skin over vertebrae.

Spina bifida manifesta further involves two subtypes called as meningocele and myelomeningocele.

1. *Meningocele 9.5.1B:* Membranes (called as meninges) responsible for covering and protecting the brain and spinal cord, are pushed through hole in vertebrae and form a sac. No nerve is pushed through the defect so cord is normal. The sac is covered with skin. Though patient has no neurological problem yet to prevent any damage to sac due to friction in later life, the surgical correction may be required.
2. *Myelomeningocele (MMC) 9.5.1C*: This is the most severe form of spina bifida as the spinal cord or/and cauda equina is also pushed along with the meninges via the defect. The posterior arch of the vertebra is not formed. Child has paralysis with the extent depends on the level/region of the opening in the spine. Higher is the opening, the more severe and extensive will be the paralysis.

MAJOR DISABILITIES IN SPINA BIFIDA

- Paralysis of the trunk (none in spinal bifida occulta; moderate in meningocele and maximum in myelomeningocele).
- Paralysis of the lower limbs (none in spinal bifida occulta; moderate in meningocele and maximum in myelomeningocele). In case of myelomeningocele, there is usually a flaccid paralysis.

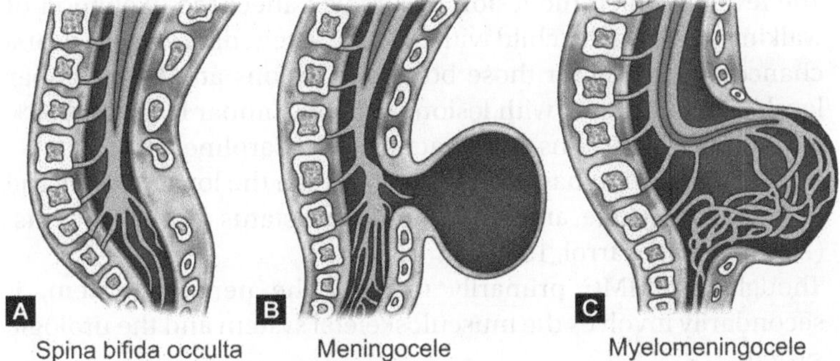

Figs 9.5.1A to C: Types of spina bifida

- Bony deformities: Trunk scoliosis and kyphosis and lordosis; hip joint dislocation or subluxation; foot—club foot, flat feet, rocker bottom foot are found in myelomeningocele whereas no bony deformity occurs in meningocele and spina bifida occulta.
- Loss of sensation: Complete loss of tactile, temperature and pain sensation occurs in the area below the level of defect in spinal cord. This puts the patient at higher risk of developing the pressure sore, burns, frictional injuries, and the cuts by sharp objects.
- Bladder paralysis: In case of myelomeningocele, there is always a loss of bladder control and the usually the voluntary control of micturition and defecation is always lost. There is bladder incontinence or may be the slow constant dribbling of the urine or the stagnation of the urine leading to the urine infection.
- The 80% of children with myelomeningocele usually also suffer from the hydrocephalous, i.e. accumulation of the fluid around and inside brain → may also suffer from learning problems and mental retardation.

Others

- Learning deficit, mental retardation, scoliosis (Brockelhurst, 1976), obesity, bowel and bladder problems, hydrocephalous, sensory/motor loss below the level of the affected region, osteoporosis due to loss of voluntary activity, neuropathic joints.
- For children born with MMC, walking onset is delayed by an average of 2 years compared with that in their peers with typical development (TD).

- The level at which the lesion occurs will affect the likelihood of walking ability of the child with MMC. Current data suggest a 20% chance of walking for those born with lesions at a high lumbar level, 80% for infants with lesions at a low lumbar level, and 90% for infants with lesions at the sacral level. (Caroline, et al. 2009).
- A good correlation has been found between the lower level of the myelomeningocele and the ambulatory status of the patients. (Desouza and Carrol, 1976).
- Though the MMC primarily involves the nervous system, it secondarily involves the musculoskeletal system and the urologic system.

INCIDENCE OF SPINA BIFIDA

- Spina bifida is one of the most common birth defect
- The incidence of this condition in India is about 8 per 1000 birth (Cherian, et al. 2005).

CAUSES OF SPINA BIFIDA

Exact cause of spina bifida is unknown however virus and unidentified harmful agents are found responsible especially during the initial 30 days of pregnancy.

MANAGEMENT

Spina bifida is preventable condition in majority of cases and the prenatal screening of mother along with the genetic counseling, amniocentesis examination, genetic mapping and detailed ultrasonographic study of the fetus may be helpful to identify any abnormal pathology which could have put the fetus at risk of developing spina bifida. Also these are helpful in identifying the disease in its early stage.

Medical and Surgical Management

- There is no definite treatment available for spina bifida. The surgical and medical aspect believes in preventing the damage to the nervous tissue and to prevent the infection of neural tissue. Also it focuses to minimize the progression of the pathology and associated disability.

- The management of the spina bifida is a multidisciplinary approach which utilizes the expertise of the urologist, neurologist, neurosurgeon, orthopedecian, physiotherapist, prosthetist, etc.
- In order to prevent the further damage to the nervous tissues, it is important in few cases to do surgical interventions for closing the opening defect. During this the nerve roots are pushed back to their normal places and a secured covering of the meninges and superficial layers is established.
- The nature of the intervention needed, varies according to the level of the spinal cord affected and the degree of the defect. Since the spina bifida is a congenital problem therefore the possibility of some other associated congenital deformity or abnormality always exists, and this needs appropriate consultation and intervention
- The bladder control may be impaired in majority of cases, and to manage this issue the intermittent catheterization may be needed along with other medical interventions to prevent urinary tract infection. Also the urologist opinion is important to rule out the other possible pathology of the kidney or urinary tract.
- Surgical interventions may also require placing the shunt to prevent the development and prevention of the hydrocephalous.

Aims of Physiotherapeutic Management

- To prevent the development of deformity
- To correct deformity wherever necessary
- Maintain ROM
- Maintain or increase the muscle tone
- Strengthening of weak muscles
- Orthotic devices to improve the ambulation and functional status
- Facilitation of motor development.

Physiotherapeutic Management

- Therapeutic management of the spina bifida lies on the management of the presenting disability, neuromotor deficit or associated complication. The preventive aspect to avoid the development of the possible complication or/and their progression is also important.
- Bracing is used to improve the ambulatory status and to reduce the high energy cost (Duffy, et al. 1996).

- Patients having a high level of lesion on the spinal cord may lead to the extensive paralysis of the muscles, and large number of muscles is affected therefore may need wheelchair, crutches or braces for ambulation.
- Management of the ambulatory deficits.
  - The assessment of the ambulatory deficits attempts to identify the affected musculatures, the degree of functioning of the antigravity muscles, the need of the orthotic interventions, and the degree of support that is needed to maximize the ambulatory ability.
  - Initially when muscles are weak then the appropriate interventions of orthosis may be needed to support the body while ambulating, however the degree of support may be reduced as the condition of the muscles improves.
  - The prognosis and the possibility of ambulation also lies on the segment of spinal cord which is affected in spina bifida.
  - Child with higher level of lesion usually learns the motor skills slower than the local located level of lesion (Sousa, et al. 1983).
  - The child having good hip abductors and extensors along with poor to fair plantar flexors develop most rapidly while compared to those groups where knee or hip musculatures are involved (Sousa, et al. 1983).
- The management of the anesthetic skin.
  - The diminished sensation in the skin may lead to the higher risk of developing frictional injury, burns and abrasions which go unnoticed due to absence of pain. This leads to increased risk of the progression of the lesions and also the risk of developing ulceration.
  - The proper education of the family members is important so as to regularly inspect the skin for development of any skin roughening or breaching or ulceration.
- The management of the scoliosis development and deformity.
  - The scoliosis development in the patient with spina bifida is not common however the scoliosis may develop in cases where the location of lesion is at higher segments of the vertebral column.
  - The scoliosis may develop due to the weak/paralyzed muscles as well as the bony abnormality (such as hemivertebra or vertebral body malformation).

- The flexible and less severe curves may be dealt with the bracing and appropriate positioning, exercises however the rigid curve compromising the spinal cord may require the surgical corrections.
- The management of the pressure sore.
  - In case of the anesthetic skin, the pressure sore developing risky areas must be given proper attention including the sacrum, scapula, ileac crest, malleolus.
  - Once the pressure sore has developed, the proper care must be taken to prevent the development of the infection in these sores.
  - In cases of the non-healing ulcers, the surgical interventions are vital and the physiotherapeutic interventions are performed according to the nature and the extent of the surgery.
- Functional training and vocational training.
  - With advancing age, the adulthood spina bifida patient may require the vocational training and the work related functional training so as to enhance the vocational abilities and the performance.

9.6: CEREBRAL PALSY

INTRODUCTION

Cerebral palsy is the group of disorders resulting in muscular in-coordination and loss of muscle control caused by damage to the motor area of the brain during fetal life, birth and infancy. Cerebral palsy (CP) is a heterogeneous group of permanent, non-progressive motor disorders of movement and posture caused by chronic brain injuries that originate in the prenatal, perinatal, or postnatal period (Kothari, et al. 2010). The variety of causative factors affect the motor regulating area (motor cortex) of the brain leading to the loss or impairment of the muscles presented or regulated by this particular region.

It is a incomplete form of brain paralysis.

The whole brain is not damaged only parts of it, mainly parts that control movement, are affected. The normal developmental milestones (Table 9.6.1) are not achieved by the child during developmental period of life.

Once damaged, the part of brain does not recover, nor do they progressively worsen more.

TABLE 9.6.1 Normal timeline of developing the milestones

Activity	*Appropriate age*
Able to control the neck independently and does not abruptly drops the neck	6–8 weeks
Motor co-ordination of eyes and head, is able to follow the moving object with the turning of neck	16 weeks
Able to respond to noise, by turning the own's head Smile at a mirror image	20 weeks
Transferring objects from one hand to the other Respond to a name	28 weeks
Postural control of the head from lying prone	6–8 weeks
Reaching activity to grab objects while lying prone Recognize mother's face	16 weeks
Postural control of the head while body is pulled up	8 weeks
Relationship of body with hands	8 weeks
Feet to mouth	20 weeks
Rolling over by him or herself	20 weeks
Sitting independently	20–28 weeks
Crawling by him or herself Reach out persistently for toys Respond to words	24–28 weeks 32 weeks 40 weeks
Control the body in standing with maximum support	6 months
Walk by him or herself	12–15 months

In the child with cerebral palsy the musculoskeletal changes occur as secondary complications to the motor problem.

Cerebral palsy is non-progressive and results indefinite motor abnormality. It may occur due to single or multiple lesion of brain.

CAUSES

Causes of cerebral palsy may occur before birth, during birth, or after birth. This is the most common cause of the physical disability in the childhood (Morris, 2007). The most important risk factors for CP are low birthweight, intrauterine infections and multiple gestation (Odding, et al. 2006). Prematurely born babies are at higher risk of developing the CP.

Causes before birth include:
- Problem such as diabetes
- Infection of the mother while she is pregnant
- Difference between the blood of the mother and child (Rh incompatability)
- Lack of oxygen in fetal brain
- Premature birth
- Metabolic disorders in mother
- Abnormal fetal position.

Causes during birth constitutes the maximum incidence of CP (Hagberg, et al. 2001) and may include:
- Lack of oxygen
- Birth injuries
- Prematurity
- Forcep delivery.

Causes after birth include:
- Very high fever
- Acute jaundice
- Brain infection
- Head injuries
- Lack of oxygen
- Poisoning
- Bleeding or blood clot in brain
- Brain tumor.

CLASSIFICATION

According to the area of brain affected the CP can be of following types:
- Spastic type: The most common form of the spasticity, makes upto 65% of all cases of the spasticity (Odding, et al. 2006).
  - Affected part is the motor cortex of brain
  - There is hypertonia in muscles which increase the spasticity and hinder movement
  - In these children voluntary movement may be possible. Jerky, slow or uncontrolled movement may also occur
  - The stretch reflex is exaggerated
  - The muscle first appear normal but in time secondary changes takes place such as wasting, contracture
  - The scissor gait is often most marked symptoms

- External factor can increase or decrease the tone depending on the stimulus and which part of the body affected
- The persistence of the abnormal neonatal reflexes beyond their normal timeline of integration. These abnormal reflexes can involve the TLR(tonic labyrinthine reflex), ATNR (asymmetric tonic neck reflex), STNR (symmetric tonic neck reflex),

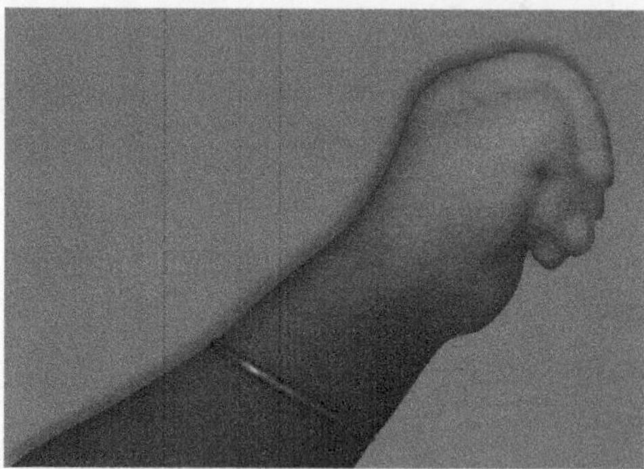

Fig. 9.6.1: The attitude of the cortical thumb in early age of the CP child

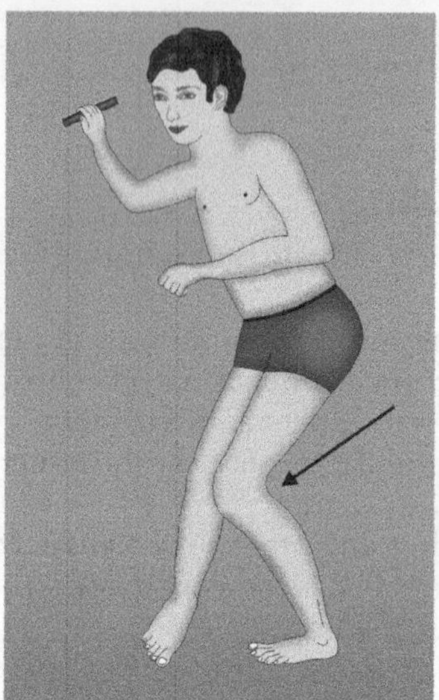

Fig. 9.6.2: The scissoring gait in spastic CP child

Parachute reflex, Gallant's reflex, the cortical thumb the flexed attitude of thumb (Fig. 9.6.1)
- Scissoring (Fig. 9.6.2) is the state when due to the excessive adductor muscle spasticity, the knees are pressed together or when at the time of ambulation the ankle and feet cross excessively medially crossing the midline
- The excessive stiffness in the hand (Fig. 9.6.1) and knee may force them to adopt the attitude of the finger and knee flexion. Sometime the excessive tone in the trunk extensor muscles may be seen while lying supine.

- Athetoid type
  - Athetosis is due to injury of basal ganglia of brain
  - Involuntary movements are the most striking symptoms—strange, slow twisting movement of the hands and arm or other parts. The patient may assume very strange positions if excited
  - Reflexes are normal and the muscles are able to contract but the movement produced is abnormal and slow. This is due to rigidity of muscles (not spasticity)
  - The muscle of speech and mastication may be involved
  - Athetoid movement cease during sleep but choreiform activity continues
  - In-coordination and slow acquisition of the motor skills occurs.
- Ataxic type
  - Cerebellum of the brain is affected
  - Ataxia is less common and is mild type which tends to improve
  - Balance and equilibrium being disturbed
  - Hypotonia
  - Nystagmus and dysarthria
  - The child typically assumes the broad based gait with high steps
  - The poor balance and frequent falls are easily noticed when child stands or walks without support.
- Mixed type
  - These may be two area of the brain affected example, spastic athtoid, ataxic athetoid
  - Incidence of the CP varies on the basis of etiological factors however reported incidence are (Hagberg, et al. 2001)
  - Spastic hemiplegic make 33%
  - Spastic diplegic make 44%
  - Spastic tetraplegic subtypes accounted for 6%

- Dyskinetic CP for 12%
- Simple ataxia for 4%.

According to the body parts affected (Kuban, et al. 2008):

- Hemiplegia affects the upper and lower extremities on one side of the body only
- Paraplegia—affects the both lower limbs
- Diplegia—affects the both lower limbs and some affect in the upper limb also.
- Quadriplegia—affect of both upper and lower limb.

CLINICAL FEATURES AND ASSOCIATED CONDITIONS

- At birth a baby with cerebral palsy is often limp and floppy or may even seen normal.
- *Slow development*: Compared to other children in the society, the child is slow to hold up his head to sit or to move around.
- *Feeding problem*: The babies may have difficulties with sucking, swallowing and chewing.
- *Communication difficulties*: The baby may not respond as normal baby. This may be due to floppiness, stiffness or lack of arm gesture or control of face or limb muscles
- A large proportion has some kind of cognitive impairment; the prevalence varies with the type of CP and especially increases when epilepsy is present (odding, et al. 2006).
- *Intelligence*: They appear mentally slow, but we have to remember that many of these are not mentally deficient but mentally backward because they are deprived of normal perception or/ and response, opportunities of accruing information specially if their speech be affected.
- *Speech defects*: Movement disorders can affect speech giving dysarthria or speech may be affected by deafness or mental retardation. Chewing and swallowing may be problem in some of the severely handicapped children.
- *Vision and hearing*: This can vary from normal to severe visual handicap or blindness. Low visual acquity occurs in 75% kids with CP (Odding, et al. 2006). If the damage has affected the auditory center or pathways the child may have impaired hearing or even may be deaf. Up to 80% have at least some impairment of speech (Odding, et al. 2006).

- *Fits*: Epilepsy related convulsions occur in 20–40% cases of cerebral palsy and it is most common among the hemi- and tetraplegics (Odding, et al. 2006).
- *Deformities*: As result of abnormal movement or lack of movement. May be due to adaptation of wrong posture.
- Stunted growth or overweight is also common.

OTHER IMPORTANT POINTS

- Sense of touch, pain, hear, cold and body position are not lost because cerebral palsy affects only motor component and not the sensory.
- It is not contagious and it does not spread from one person to other.
- Severity varies from child to child because of extent of the lesion in brain.
- Children of cerebral palsy person are not at risk of developing CP.

RADIOLOGICAL ASSESSMENT

Although no radiological investigation is necessary to diagnose the CP yet the MRI (magnetic resonance imaging) may reveal the site of the lesion, which has strong correlation with the clinical findings. Brain MRI scans may reveal the white-matter lesion including periventricular leukomalacia (PVL) (the most common finding) or basal ganglia lesions (12.8%), cortical/subcortical lesions (9.4%), malformations (9.1%), focal infarcts (7.4%), and miscellaneous lesions (7.1%). Only 11.7% of CP children had normal MRI findings (Martin, et al. 2006).

PREDICTION OF THE FUNCTIONAL ABILITY OF THE CP CHILD IN FUTURE

- CP course during life is highly variable and it is yet to be established that whether the future possibilities of the functional ability of kid can be predicted, from the presentation in his/her early childhood.
- CP though itself is non-progressive yet the presentation may vary depending on the muscle fatigue, pain, associated comorbid conditions (Jansen, et al. 2004) and the deformity, contractures.
- Around >50% of children with CP are able to achieve the independent walking without any walking aid by 8- to 17-year

age however of the remaining, around 25% remain unable to walk (Koman, et al. 2004).

- Walking ability varies strongly with CP type. Unilateral and ataxic CP types have the best while dyskinetic and bilateral CP types the least walking ability (Kuban, et al. 2008).
- The dystonic and dyskinetic form of CP are usually identified later in age. The presence of spasticity may mask the feature of dystonia (Kuban, et al. 2008) and the features may be missed out very easily because dystonia occurs intermittently.

THE PHYSIOTHERAPY ASSESSMENT OF CP

- The assessment starts with careful documentation of the pre-birth, during birth and post-birth history.
- The pre-birth history must carefully document the history of infection, drug abuse, convulsion to mother. It must also document any previous history of the miscarriage before this child birth.
- The birth history must document whether there was any delay in the birth cry, or the any reported symptom or sign of birth asphyxia. The weight of baby at the time of birth must also be documented.
- The early development history must keep a meticulous look or documentation of the normal milestone achievement. This includes the details about the social smile, speech development, motor development, the pattern of movement, the timing of achieving the supported sitting, independent sitting, neck control, crawling, standing with support, standing without support, walking, etc.
- In small kids, the integration or persistence of various neonatal reflexes is highly important. The persistence of the neonatal reflexes beyond the age of their normal integration reveals the risk of delayed achievement of milestones. Also the presence of the abnormal reflexes and their severity indicates the possible interference in the functional ability.
- During examination the therapist must document the walking ability, i.e the primary way of walking at 5 years of age graded as unaided walking,walking with aids, or unable to walk.
- The assessment of the muscle tone as per modified Ashworth scale which is a reliable tone Assessment Scale relating to response to

passive movement at various joints, except the ankle (Gregson et al, 1999).

- Assessment of the tightness, contracture or deformity of the joints.
- The ability to execute the functional tasks—hand gripping, hand release.
- The grasp ability—pinch grip, spherical grip, cylindrical grip.
- The walking ability, ability to use the walking aid.
- The presence of other associated pathological states, such as autism, low IQ, cardiac pathology, etc.
- The balancing ability in the sitting, lying and standing position.

MUSCULOSKELETAL LIMITATIONS IN A CEREBRAL PALSY PATIENT

Pattern of Involvement

A group of muscles acting together is called as pattern. The pattern may be presented in form of extensor pattern or the flexor pattern.

- Restriction in range of motion (ROM).
  - When musculoskeletal changes takes place in the body, it can be either in form of tightness, contracture, and deformity (Fig. 9.6.3).

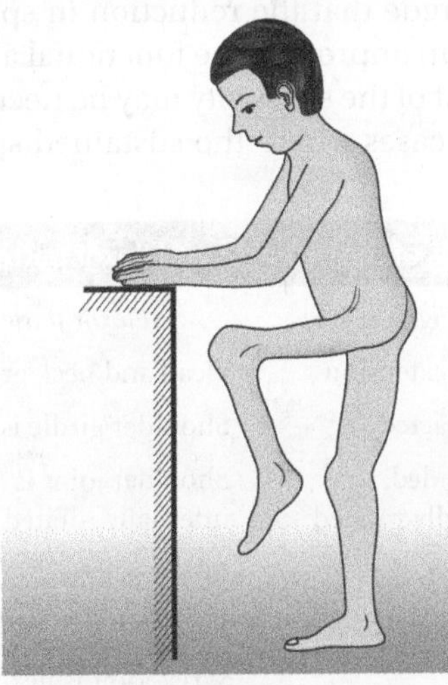

Fig. 9.6.3: The hip flexor, knee flexor and ankle plantar—flexor contractures in CP

- Tightness s when restriction in range of motion is reversible.
- Contracture is when restriction in range of motion is irreversible.
- Deformity when the limitation in muscles forced the abnormal positioning of the controlling joint.

- Musculoskeletal deformities. These occur according to the affected part.
  - Diplegia: Kyphosis, lordosis, subluxation/dislocation of one or both hips. Equinovalgus deformities of feet are common.
  - In quadriplegia: Scoliosis or kyphoscoliosis, flexor deformities of hip/knees, subluxation or dislocation of hip joint.

MEDICAL MANAGEMENT OF CEREBRAL PALSY

- The medical management of the spasticity believes that the existence of spasticity may interfere, mask or impede the existing voluntary motor function. In order to manage the spasticity the most common theapy include the baclofen therapy, whose effect is well established in case of spastic CP however the effect on the dystonic CP is yet to be explored (Butler and Campbell, 2000).
- In contrast to this, few others (Sahrmann and Norton, 1977) believe that the spasticity in fact may provide the necessary stiffness which is needed for the ambulation and functional tasks, therefore they argue that the reduction in spasticity may in fact impair rather than improving the functional ability.
- The management of the spasticity may be necessary with the help of medicines in cases where the sustained spasticity may place

TABLE 9.6.2 Features of the extensor and flexor pattern of spasticity

Extensor pattern (Fig. 9.6.4.A)	*Flexor pattern (Fig. 9.6.4.B)*
Head and neck are in extension	Head and neck are in flexion
Shoulder girdle is retracted	Shoulder girdle is protracted
Shoulder joint is extended, abducted, and externally rotated	Shoulder joint is flexed, adducted and internally rotated
Elbow joint is extended	Elbow is flexed
Radioulnar joint is supinated	Radioulnar joint is pronated
Wrist is extended	Wrist joint is flexed
Thumb is abducted and finger fisted	Thumb is adducted and fingers extended

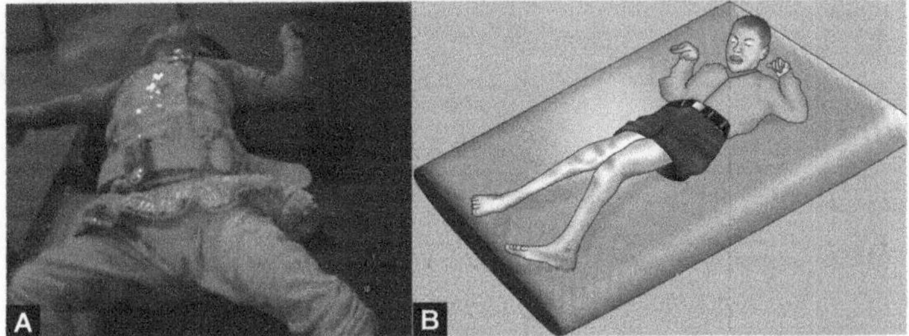

Figs 9.6.4A and B: Patterns of spasticity: (A) Extensor pattern, (B) Flexor pattern

the child at higher risk of developing contractures. The studies have revealed that the use of baclofen for reduction of spasticity reduces the need of the orthopedic surgical interventions (Gerstzen, et al. 1998).

MANAGEMENT OF CEREBRAL PALSY

- General instruction to parents about the care of child physically, supportively and psychologically.
- Helping the child to achieve better position so as to maximize the comfort, minimize the progression of abnormal reflexes, abnormal positioning of the joints and neck.
- Good nutrition of the mother.
- Avoiding the premature conceiving. Girl should get pregnant only when she is over 18, is medically and nutritionally fit, and free from the infections.
- The genetic counseling may help to avoid the risk arisen due to the blood group incompatibility.
- Pregnant lady must avoid the unnecessary medicines and alcohol during pregnancy.
- Vaccination is important for mother during pregnancy to avoid the infections such as rubella, mumps and measles.

MANAGEMENT OF SPASTIC CEREBRAL PALSY

- The rehabilitation and health needs of adults with cerebral palsy need to be addressed. The CP client may not be able to succeed without proper physiotherapy interventions (Barry, 1996).

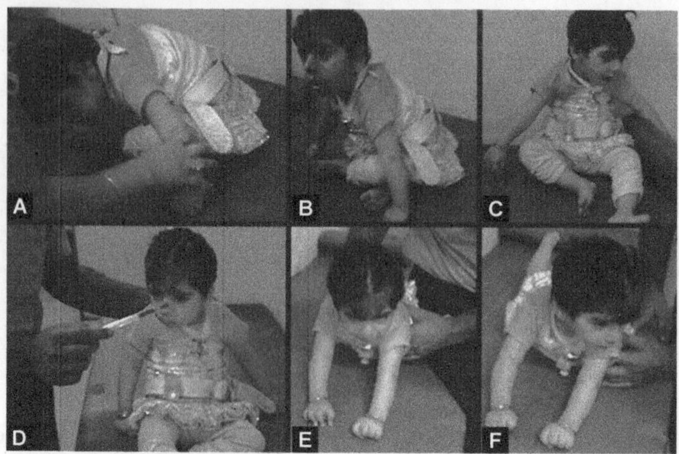

Figs 9.6.5A to F: Activities to improve neck and trunk control: (A) Supported sitting in cross legged position on floor; (B) The assistance to assume straight position of trunk; (C) The supported sitting against the wall support; (D) Use of toys to draw attention of child and help in developing active neck control; (E) From the prone position the child is brought to prone-on-hand position and the tickling stimulation is given to posterior aspect of neck to guide the child to actively extend neck; (F) From the previous position the weight is shifted towards right or left forearm so as to allow the deviation in the trunk and develop the trunk control

- In spastic child, the parents must be taught the positioning and regular range of motion with stretching to avoid the development of contracture which could have developed due to disproportionate pull and secondary shortening of the spastic muscle.
- The training is important to help the child to progress through subsequent stages of the milestone development. For example, if the child is not able to control the neck or trunk, the exercises or sports activities must incorporate the skills that will help to develop neck or trunk control (Figs 9.6.5A to F).
- Must be taught to care for the child who has already developed the contracture.
- The properly fabricated splints, callipers or braces are used to maintain the proper positioning of the joints and avoid the contracture formation.
- Passive movement helps to regain ROM and reduce the spasticity.

- Movements must be rhythmically and slowly. No joint should be neglected while doing the passive movement for prevention of contracture formation.
- Active exercises—simple active movement of the weak antagonists or the spastic muscles.
- Games can have important places during the spastic stage both for the educational purpose and for the recreational purpose. The child must be kept in position so as to maximize his/her functional performance. The activities during the games must also be designed so as to maximize the voluntary movements in controlled manner. Examplé—during the ball passing game the child can be made to sit on stool or riding horse or bolster so as to provide the trunk stability and adductor lengthening during upper extremity activity.
- In order to improve the walking performance the use of toy tricycle, various type of crutches, walking in parallel bars, etc. may be used.
- The hydrotherapy may be useful for providing the assisted movement and balance training during the initial stages to assist the movement. In later phase, the resistance may be imposed to augment the strengthening of muscles.
- Strategies to reduce the spasticity may include:
  - Smooth slow gentle passive range of motion exercises
  - Gentle rocking rhythmic movement
  - The slow sustained but comfortable stretching of the spastic muscle
  - The music therapy to synchronize the voluntary activity of child with that of the music beat
  - Prolonged cryotherapy also reduces spasticity. This is due to the fact that cold decreases metabolic activity, slows nerve conduction, produces analgesia, lessens muscle tone, and inhibits spasticity. For this purpose the icing must be used for about 20 minutes every time before the stretching exercise session (Basford, 2007)
  - The spasticity increases in response to the stress, pain and fear therefore the adequate support, reduction of fear and the pain due to any cause, must be minimized to reduce the spasticity.
- The music therapy is also helpful to regulate the features of the cerebral palsy to certain extent. It helps the child to alleviate his/

her anxiety; help them to express themselves in this way. Athetoid child respond more effectively to the music therapy.

- The Phelps method of treatment: Phelps used 15 special techniques or modalities or combined them according to the type of patient to be treated. These techniques included:
  - Massage
  - Passive movement
  - Assisted active movement
  - Free active movement
  - Resisted movement
  - Conditioned movement
  - Automatic or confused movement
  - Rest, relaxation
  - Movement from relaxed position
  - Reach and grasp skills.

  For example, if a hemiplegic child can't do the dorsiflexion of ankle, he is asked to do hip and knee flexion, then he will be able to do ankle dorsiflexion.
- Bobath method of management.
  - Madam Bobath considers that dominance of the postural reflex system upsets the rhythm of both voluntary and involuntary movement. This is the main cause of the disorders in the patients. Bobath concept is commonly known as NDT (neurodevelopment technique) and aims to improve the motor and functional deficits in the children and adolescents with cerebral palsy (Weindling, et al. 2007; Bobath and Bobath, 1984). NDT aims to influence muscle tone and improve postural alignment by specific handling techniques and attempts to facilitate improved active participation and practice of relevant skills (Knox and Evans, 2002).
  - Bobath and Bobath (1984) the main cause of the motor problems of cerebral palsy is the central nervous system (CNS) dysfunction which interferes with the development of normal postural control against gravity and impedes normal motor development (Butler and Darrah, 2001). Therefore, the goal of NDT is to establish the normal motor development and function and/or the prevention of contractures and deformities. The NDT approach focused on sensorimotor components of muscle tone, reflexes and abnormal movement

patterns, postural control, sensation, perception and memory (Butler and Darrah, 2001). Handling techniques control various sensory stimuli and therefore is important to inhibit spasticity, abnormal reflexes, and abnormal movement patterns and also to improve the motor and functional deficits of children and adolescents with cerebral palsy (Butler C and Darrah, 2001).

- PNF techniques (proprioceptive neuromuscular facilitation technique).
  - PNF techniques were firstly developed by Dr Kabal, physiotherapist Margaret Knott (1966) and Drrothy Voss (Levine, et al. 1955) for the management of the cerebral palsy kids for the first time. It makes use of functional pattern of movement rather than individual muscles or groups. These patterns all include rotator and diagonal components. This is the most valuable for muscle weakness.
  - Beside this during PNF application the resistance is applied to various target muscle groups to enhance their strength. However, it must be born in mind that the amount of resistance applied to muscles must be "maximal" as per the client's ability and not the "heavy resistance" as the application of the "heavy resistance" will lead to the development of the abnormal muscle tone in the muscles and would further aggravate the motor performance.
  - Besides this, it is useful to implement the "dynamic system approach" for the management of the cases of neuro-developmental delay, as it is believed to bring more rapid and beneficial changes in developmental delay. This approach involves the simultaneous stimulation of multiple systems such as physical therapy, cognitive, motivational and sensory inputs. Children receive multiple input and greater demand is placed upon them and show greater improvement in a shorter period of time (Cook and Horak, 1986).
- Rood techniques.
  - Miss Rood makes use of different types of stimulation both cutaneous such as stroking and deep such as muscle stretching in order to activate or inhibit motor activities. The techniques for facilitation include quick icing, quick brushing, tapping, hacking, rapid movements. The inhibitory means include the prolonged icing, prolonged weight bearing, painful stimuli.

9.7: GUILLAIN-BARRE SYNDROME

Guillain-Barre syndrome (GBS) is an autoimmune disorder where the immune system of the body starts working against the own nervous system leading the inflammation of the nerve and its impairment leading to the extensive peripheral neuropathy (Shy, 2007).

■ CAUSES

The exact cause of the GBS is yet to be confirmed,

It is believed that some triggering factors lead to the overactivation of the autoimmune mechanisms within body and this in turn leads to the damage or the impairment of the multiple nerves in the body.

The most common believe is that after the triggering infections, the antibodies are synthesized in body against the invading organism, and in cases of the autoimmunity or GBS these antibodies fail to differentiate between foreign particles and the body's own cells. This causes the attack of these antibodies on the nerve and their sheath.

The patients of the GBS report the history of the fever or some other infections (gastrointestinal or the pulmonary or the upper respiratory tract infections) 3–4 weeks prior to the onset of the features of the GBS.

GBS may be more common as the comorbid condition among those who had a history of the infections or the other pathological conditions little time back, such as recurrent pulmonary infections, the AIDS, bacterial infections, the hypersensitivity disorder such as systemic lupus erythematosus (SLE) etc. The most common infective agents believe to provoke the GBS are *Campylobacter jejuni* (Yuki, 2008) and the influenza virus (Tardy, et al. 2009).

■ FEATURES

The presentation of the GBS varies according to the type of nerve affected and the severity of the nerve involvement. Usually, the features of the GBS appear very quickly, and the symptoms may progress within hours to several weeks. The fever is absent during the sudden onset weakness however patient might be having history of having fever 3 or 4 weeks back.

The autoimmune mechanism start producing the antibodies against the myelin sheath of the nerves to result in the demyelination, causing the impaired conduction of the impulses across these nerves, and therefore the variable degree of impaired functioning of the concerned nerves. Depending upon the degree of involvement, the nerve functioning may be either partially or the completely impaired.

The impairment of the nerve functioning can be presented in the form of the tingling, altered sensations, the muscle weakness, the extreme muscle paresis or the paralysis.

The involvement of the GBS is usually ascending in nature, and the lower extremity muscles are involved first and later on the upper extremity muscles. The distal group muscles are involved earlier than the proximal group of muscles.

The bilateral involvement, both sides of the body are involved.

The paralysis is ascending type in nature.

The initial features may be in form of tingling, pain, altered sensation, the difficulty inbreathing, weakness in the affected muscles.

The significant involvement of the nerve may present the loss of reflexes in the concerned nerve root, the autonomic presentation such as (impaired blood pressure control, the impaired blood flow regulations across muscles, postural hypotension, the repeated syncope), the weakness of the related muscles, the numbness, sensations.

The nerves supplying the respiratory muscles (such as diaphragm and the intercostals muscles) may also get damaged, leading to the impaired respiratory capacity of the patient. The partial or complete respiratory failure may occur leading the emergency requirement of the ventilator support.

The muscle or the muscle groups may be affected leading to the in-coordinated movement.

The neuralgia along the affected nerve or the muscle pain/muscle cramps in the muscles innervated by these impaired nerves.

INVESTIGATION OF THE GBS

The sudden onset weakness or the nerve impairment related features with the history of the infections few weak prior, may hint towards the possibility of the GBS.

The other causes of the possible neuropathy, multiple neuritis complex, the toxic neuropathy, etc. have to be ruled out.

The sudden onset motor or sensory presentation might be confused with the stroke. The CT scan and MRI scanning helps to rule out the stroke.

The sensory examination reveals the altered sensations in the multiple dermatomes or the peripheral nerve regions.

The motor examination reveals the progressive weakness, the ascending type paresis and the bilateral involvement. The tendon reflexes are found to be diminished or absent according to the affected nerves.

The autonomic nervous system testing reveals the impaired control of the blood pressure, the heart rate, respiratory rate, the auto-regulation, the dry/clumsy or scaly skin.

The blood oxygen analysis or the arterial blood gases (ABG) analysis may indicate the constituents of the blood gases, the amount of oxygen in the blood, etc.

The cerebrospinal fluid (CSF) analysis helps to rule out the infections such as meningitis, encephalitis, etc.

The electromyography (EMG) testing rule out the other pathological conditions (such as myopathy), which could mimic the multiple muscles weakness or paralysis.

Pulmonary function testing (PFT) indicates the degree of the functioning of the pulmonary systems.

TREATMENT

In the absence of the confirmed etiopathogenesis, there is no definite medical cure for the GBS, however its associated complications and the symptoms may be dealt with.

The medical and the physiotherapy interventions also are useful for speeding up the recovery process.

The symptomatic management are important till the time some spontaneous recovery occurs, and the acute phase of the disease is suppressed.

The acute phase medical management of the GBS include:

- The mechanical ventilation for the respiratory support. In majority of cses of the GBS the period of the ventilator support is not very prolonged, therefore rarely the tracheostomy is needed.
- The immune-suppressants help to suppress down the autoimmune mechanisms of the body, and prevent the damage to the myelin sheath of the nerves.

- The removal of the autoantibodies already formed in body, can be speed up with the process of plasmapheresis (Huges, 2003; Meythaler, 2003) or by the injection of intravenous immunoglobulins (Huges, 2009).
- To reduce the inflammation the anti-inflammatory medicines are prescribed.
- To deal with pain the analgesics are not much effective therefore the narcotics may be needed.

The appropriate electrolyte management is important as the bed-ridden patients are more prone to suffer dyselectrolytemia, which in turn further worsens the neurological status of the patients and the nerves.

The fluid management is important to maintain the adequate perfusion pressure in the vascular channels and for regulating the blood flow in the vital organs of the body.

Physiotherapy Management of the GBS

During Acute Phase

- The respiratory management:
  - To maintain the healthy status of the respiratory airways
  - To prevent the accumulation of secretions and the development of the pneumonia or lung collapse
  - To maintain the oxygen saturation pressure in the body
  - In case of ventilated patients, the physiotherapy interventions are important to prevent the formation of the excessive secretions secondary to airway irritation
  - To maintain the air spaces for gaseous exchange to occur
  - To facilitate the expulsion of the accumulated secretions if the secretions have already formed.
- The management of the mechanically ventilated patient, and to help the multidisciplinary team during the weaning off the patients from mechanical ventilation.
- In the conscious and cooperative patients, the deep breathing exercises (DBE), ACBT (active cycle of breathing technique), coughing and huffing maneuvers help to dislodge the secretions and to promote their expulsion by directing them towards main bronchus and pharyngeal region.
- In the unconscious patients, the above-mentioned active interventions are not much useful, therefore other means

have to be used such as postural drainage, manual techniques (percussion, vibration, shaking techniques), steam inhalation, the nebulization are important to dislodge or loosen up the secretions. In order to remove the secretions from the airways, the mechanical suctioning is useful.

The management of the paralytic limb(s).

The prevention of the decubitus ulcer.

Prevention of the muscle contracture and the joint deformity is important.

The splints or the supports may be provided to prevent the overstretching of the muscles under the influence of the gravity and the external forces.

The Recovery Phase Management

Once the patient has been weaned off from the ventilator, the physiotherapist is helpful to improve the cardiopulmonary fitness of the client.

- The management of the residual paralysis or impairment
- Functional enhancement
- The orthotic interventions to support the weak joints
- The assistive devices to improve the independence and the quality of life (QOL)
- The functional electric stimulation
- The balancing exercises.

PNF exercise (proprioceptive neuromuscular facilitation) are helpful to improve the sensory inputs via proprioceptors and to increase the functional demands from the muscles.

During any kind of exercise or exertion based management during recovery phase, it must be kept in mind that the recovering patient has tendency of undergoing early and prolonged fatigue, therefore the adequate rest interval is important between the bouts of exercise to allow the complete recovery from the fatigue imposed by the exercises.

Gait training—to deal with the residual impairments such as foot drop, high stepping gait.

Recovery

Most of the cases of GBS recover spontaneously within weeks to years. Grossly the GBS is non-fatal and the death directly related to disease itself. Therefore, the prognosis of the GBS is considered to be good. However, in long-term the complications and the residual impairments may be present such as joint deformity, the permanent paralysis of some muscles, the pressure ulcers, the lung parenchyma damage.

9.8: PARKINSONISM

Parkinson disease (PD) is a chronic progressive neurodegenerative disease of nervous system characterized by rigidity, impaired gait, akinesia, bradykinesia, tremors, diminished expression and postural instability (Baatile, et al. 2000).

EPIDEMIOLOGY

Parkinson's disease (PD) occurs in about 1% of population older than 55 years of age and becomes increasingly common with advancing age reaching proportion of 2.6% of the population by age of 85 years.

Mean age of onset is 58–62 years.

Majority of cases have their onset between 50 to 79 year of age.

10 % cases develop young onset PD which is defined by appearance of initial symptoms before the age of 40 years.

Sex incidence—male:female = 3:2

Familial incidence is 5%.

ETIOLOGY

- The term Parkinsonism is used to refer to group of disorders that produce abnormality of basal ganglia functioning.
- Parkinson's disease or primary Parkinsonism is the most common cause affecting approximately 78% of the patients.
- Secondary Parkinsonism result from the number of different causes including inherited and acquired neurodegenerative disorders.
- Parkinson's disease
  - Also called as primary parkinsonism.
  - Two distinct clinical subgroups have been identified:
    a. The first group consists of individuals whose dominant symptoms include the postural instability and gait disturbances (PIGD)

b. The other group includes the individual with tremors as main features they demonstrate few problems with bradykinesia or postural instability

- Post-infectious parkinsonism
  - Also called as secondary parkinsonism.
  - The influenza epidemics or encephalitis lethargic that occurred from 1917 to 1926 affected large number of individuals.
  - The onset of parkinsonism symptoms typically occurred after many years giving rise to the theory that the slow virus was infecting the brain.
  - There has been no recent recurrence of this influenza and the incidence of this type is decreasing in frequency.
- Toxic parkinsonism [secondary parkinsonism]
  - A form of secondary parkinsonism which occurs in individuals exposed to the certain industrial pollutants and chemicals.
  - The manganese is most common and represents serious occupational hazard to many miners.
  - Other causative chemicals include the carbon-disulphide (CS_2), carbon mono-oxide (CO), cyanic (CN-), methanol (CH_3OH).
  - Severe and lasting classic parkinsonism has been inadvertently produces in individuals who injected a synthetic heroin containing the chemical MPTP.
- Pharmacological parkinsonism
  - A variety of drug can produce extrapyramidal dysfunction that mimics the sign of PD.
  - These drugs are thought to interfere with the dopaminergic mechanism either presynaptically or post synaptically. They include following:
    a. Neuroleptics chloropromazine—haloperidol (haldol), thioridzine, thiothizen
    b. Antidepressants—amitriptyline, amoxapine, trazodone
    c. Antihypertensive drugs—methyldopa, reserpine

High doses of these medications are particularly problematic in elderly and severity of effect noted may be related to subclinical PD. Withdrawal of these agents usually reverses the symptoms within a few week although in some cases effect will be long lasting.

- Metabolic causes
  - Parkinsonism can be caused by rare condition by metabolic conditions including disorders of calcium metabolism that result in basal ganglion calcification.

- The common conditions associated with parkinsonism include hypothyroidism, hyperparathyroidism, hypoparathyroidism, and Wilson's diseases.
- Akinetic/rigid syndrome with parkinsons features:
  - This is also called as parkinson plus syndrome.
  - A group of neurodegenerative diseases can affect the substantia nigra and produce parkinsonism symptoms along with other neurological signs.
  - These diseases include striatonigral degeneration, progressive supranuclear palsy, and cortical basal ganglionic degeneration.
  - Parkinsonism symptoms can be exhibited in atherosclerosis and Alzheimer disease. Early phases of these diseases may present with rigidity and bradykinesia, therefore the differential diagnosis from PD may be difficult.
  - Parkinson plus syndrome typically do not show measureable improvement from the administration of antiparkinson medication such as (L- dopa) therapy.

PATHOPHYSIOLOGY

- Basal ganglion is a collection of interconnected gray matter nuclear masses deep within the brain. It is now considered to be composed of the caudate nucleus, putamen, globus pallidus, subthalamic nucleus, substantia nigra.
- Basal ganglia play an important role in the production of voluntary movement and control of postural adjustments associated with voluntary movements.
- Cerebral cortex and thalamus send input of caudate and putamen to initiate the activity.
- Widespread cortical area involved in sending the signal to basal ganglia including the sensory and motor association area.
- The striatum also receives the input from substantia nigra and pedunculopontice tegmental nucleus of midbrain. Output is channeled primarily through the globus pallidus and substantia nigra via thalamocortical projection to prefrontal and premotor cortex area.
- Within the basal ganglia information is integrated and modulated from the cerebral cortex and thalamus through multiple parallel circuits.

Damage to the basal ganglia results in the motor disturbances that can be:

- Hyperkinetic disturbances characterized by excessive or abnormal movements such as chorea, dyskinesia, dystonia.
- Hypokinetic disturbances are characterized by slowness or lack of movement such as akinesia or bradykinesia.
- The substanstia nigra pass compacta (SNPC) works to facilitate movement through both direct and indirect pathways of motor loops.
- Parkinson disease is associated with degeneration of dopaminergic neuron that produce dopamine. They have their all bodies in SNPC and send their axons to striatum.
- A degeneration of 80% of neurons is estimated to occur before signs of disease become clinically evident. Niagral cells loss is more prevalent in the ventral cell group and loss of melanin containing neurons produces characteristic changes in depigmentation. There are deficiency of other neurotransmitter as well including serotonin and nor-epinephrine; however the effects of this depletion are less well understood.
- As the disease progresses and neurons degenerate they develop characteristic cytoplasmic inclusion body called as Lewy's body.
- Other site of predilection include dorsal motor nucleus of vagus, hypothalamus, cerebral cortex, autonomic ganglia.
- Loss of dopaminergic neuron influence leads to a reduction in spontaneous movement. Thus the patient wants to move but cannot move. Tremors and rigidity are viewed as released phenomenon representative of loss of inhibitory influences within basal ganglia.
- Significant changes may also occur in the dopamine receptos resulting in decreased binding sites for dopamine in basal ganglia.
- This may explains the loss of clinical effectiveness of L-dopa (a dopamine substitution treatment) during the later stages of Parkinson.

Neuropharmacology

Some drugs can induce the features of extrapyramidal syndrome affecting the movement disorders.

Neurotransmitters

- Neurotransmitter substances are synthesized and stored pre-synaptically when release by appropriate stimulus they cross the synaptic gap, and get combined with specific receptors of post-synaptic cell. Neurotransmitters that modulate the effect of neurotransmitter in the basal ganglia are substance P, encephalin and somatostatin.

- Acetylcholine is synthesized by small strial cells, where its quantity is maximum. It has excitatory effect on the basal ganglia.
- Dopamine is made by cells of substantia nigra and has inhibitory effect on the basal ganglia.
- The amount of the excitatory neurotransmitter (acetylcholine) and the inhibitory neurotransmitter (dopamine) are in balance. The dopamine excess leads to the movement disorder called as chorea. The dopamine depletion results in the movement disorder called as parkinsonism.
- Beside this the GABA (gamma aminobutyric acid) is synthesized from glutamate in the striatum and globus pallidus and has the inhibitory action and deficiency is associated with Hutington's Chorea.

CLINICAL FEATURES OF THE PARKINSONISM

Rigidity

It is the resistance to passive motion that is not velocity dependent.

It is the clinical hallmark feature of PD.

The complaint of the patient includes the heaviness and stiffness in the limbs.

It affects the agonist as well as antagonist group of muscles therefore it affects the movement in both the directions.

Rigidity is present regardless of task amplitude or speed of the movement.

Two types of rigidity are common:

1. *Cogwheel rigidity*: It is a jerky catch-like resistance to passive movement as muscles alternately tense and relax.
2. *Lead-pipe rigidity*: It is a constant uniform resistance to passive movement with no fluctuation.

The rigidity is typically unequal in distribution. It affects proximal muscles first especially shoulder and neck. It progresses to involve the muscle of face and extremity. It may affect the left or right side eventually spreading to involve the whole body.

As the disease progresses, rigidity become more severe. Rigidity decreases the ability of patient to move easily. For example bed mobility or loss of reciprocal arm swing during gait is often related to degree of truncal rigidity.

Active movement, mental concentration, emotional tension may all increase the amount of rigidity present.

Prolonged rigidity results in decreased available range of motion thus may put the high risk of developing contracture and postural deformity. Rigidity also has a direct impact on increasing the resting energy expenditure and fatigue levels.

Reflexes

Spinal stretch reflexes are normal.

Long latency reflexes are enhanced.

Akinesia and Bradykinesia

Akinesia is the difficult in initialing movement. The moments of freezing may occur and are characterized by sudden break or block in movement.

Akinesia is due to deficit in the preparatory phase of movement control and can be directly influenced by degree of rigidity as well as stage of disease and fluctuation in drug action.

Bradykinesia refers to slowness and difficulty in maintaining movement. Movements are typically reduced in speed, range and amplitude termed hypokinesia. Rigidity and depression also influence bradykinesia.

Micrographia

It is abnormally small hand writing that is difficult to be read.

Patient has difficulty in performing simultaneous and sequential tasks. Patient freezes up when carrying out another motor task while walking. The patient shoe and hesitant or unable to switch from one movement to another during a transfer sequence.

Freezing episode may also be triggered by confrontation of competing stimuli. Example—the patient slows or stops walking when exposed to a narrowed space or obstacle. To compensate for impaired control individual with PD may resort to slower visually guided movement to ensure movement accuracy.

Motor learning may also be impaired particularly for sequential task and procedural learning.

Torque production is decreased at all speeds resulting in functional difficulties and muscles weakness.

It is thought to be caused by insufficient neural activation of muscles.

EMG studies reveal that motor unit recruitment is delayed. A common perception among patient is an increased sense of effort associated with movement that is manifested by difficulty in activating and sustaining responses.

Tremors

Tremor is the initial symptoms in 50% of the PD patients.

It is an involuntary oscillation of body part occurring at slow frequency 4–7 cycles per seconds.

Parkinson's tremors are described as resting tremors, because it is typically present at rest and disappears with voluntary movement. This is usually manifested as pin rolling tremors of the hand although resting tremors may also be seen in the feet, lips, tongue or jaw. Some individual demonstrate postural tremors when muscles are used to maintain a position against gravity relieving factor.

Tremors tends to be less severe when patient is relaxed and unoccupied, it is diminished by voluntary effort and disappears completely during sleep.

Aggravating factors include emotional stress and fatigue.

In early stages tremor is usually unilateral, quite mild and occurs only for short periods whereas in later stages tremor can be severe interfering with daily function. Fluctuation in frequency and intensity are common.

Postural Instability

Patients with PD demonstrate abnormalities of posture (Fig. 9.8.1) and balance.

As the base of support narrows (tandem stance or single limb stance or as attention demands vary (divided attention situation), the postural instability increases.

Patient experiences increasing difficulty during dynamic destabilizing activities such as self initiated movement such as functional reach, walking, turning.

Frequent falls and fall injury are the result of progressive loss of balance reaction with about 1/3rd of the patient experiencing falls and 13% fall more than once a week. Most of the falls in PD occur during the dynamic mobility tasks such as getting up from chair or during freezing of gait (Bloem, et al. 2001; Keus et, al. 2007), therefore the fall risk assessment must consider the evaluation of mobility during these situations and the interventions programs must be tailored to meet these circumstances (Keus, et al. 2007).

Patient tends to respond to instability with abnormal pattern of co-activation resulting in rigid body and as inability to utilize normal postural synergies to recover balance regulating feed forward anticipatory adjustment of postural muscles during voluntary movement.

Postural reaction becomes easily impaired as the disease progresses.

Contributing factors include—rigidity, decreased muscle torque production, loss of available ROM particularly of trunk motions and weakness.

Extensor muscle of trunk demonstrates weakness than flexor muscles contributing to adoption of a flexed, stooped posture with increased flexion of neck, trunk, hip and knees (Fig. 9.8.1).

This results in a significant change in the center of alignment position, positioning the individual at the forward limits of stability.

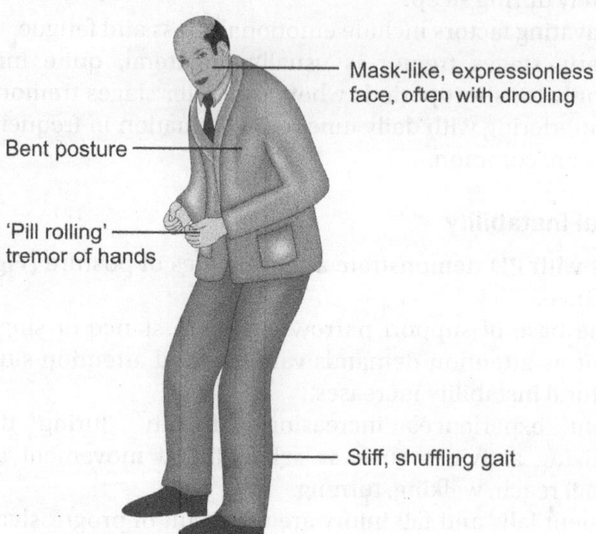

Fig. 9.8.1: The features of the parkinson patient

Patients with PD also demonstrate an inability to adapt movement strategies to changing sensory condition.

Visuo-spatial impairment is correlated with lower score in mobility. Some patients are unable to perceive the upright or vertical position, which may indicate as abnormality in processing of vestibular, visual or proprioceptive information contributing to balance.

Poverty of Movement

Overall decrease in the total number and excursion of movement.

As the task complexity increases the movement difficulty increases.

This provides evidence of central deficit in motor planning in patients with PD.

Rotation movements are reduced, resulting in uniplanar movement.

Automatic or unconscious movements are impaired or lost. Example—loss of reciprocal arm swing during gait.

Loss of automatic movement leads to increased cortical demand on the patient, who is required to think about movement to execute it successfully. There is constant combat with effect of bradykinesia, rigidity and movement impoverishment. It further leads to loss of motivation and mental fatigue.

Fatigue

Difficulty in sustaining activity.

Patient Experiences increasing weakness and lethargy as the day progresses.

Repetitive motor acts may start out strong but decreased in strength as the activity progresses.

First few words spoken may be loud an strong but diminish rapidly as speech progresses.

Performance decreases dramatically with great physical effort or mental stress.

Rest or sleep may restore mobility.

When L-Dopa therapy is initiated, the patient may notice a dramatic improvement initially and the less fatigue is felt.

In long standing diseases and drug therapy, the fatigue typically reappears.

Masked Face

Infrequent blinking and lack of expression.

Smiling may be possible on command or with volitional effort.

Musculoskeletal Changes

Most of the PD patients are elderly therefore the musculoskeletal changes are almost always associated.

Generalized musculoskeletal deconditioning occurs.

Muscle weakness, loss of flexibility, lack of movement in any body segment leads to the risk of contracture development of both contractile and non-contractile tissues.

The common problems of the spine may include kyphosis and scoliosis.

Reduced activity and poor diet may lead to secondary osteoporosis.

Lack of automatic movement and poor balance reactions lead to frequent falls and fracture of osteoporotic bones. Furthermore, the fracture healing may be delayed.

Gait Disturbances

Gait pattern of the patient with PD is characterized by impoverished movement and decreased velocity.

Hip, knee, ankle motions are reduced. There is generalized lack of extension at all three joints.

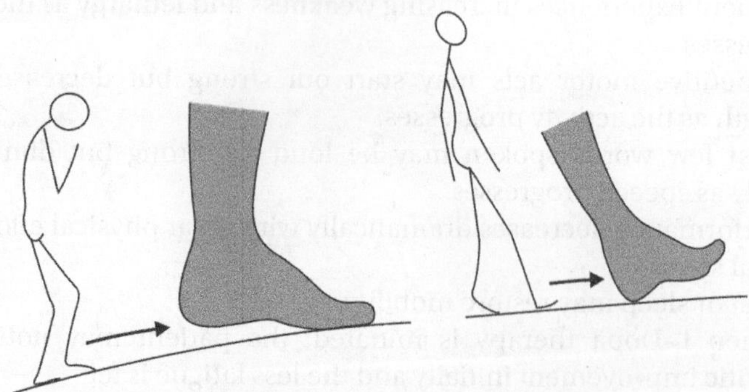

Fig. 9.8.2: The weight is born on toes instead of heel in case of parkinson patients

Trunk and pelvic motions are also diminished resulting in decreased stride length and decreased reciprocal arm swing.

Patients characteristically walk with small shuffling steps.

There is loss of normal heel toe progression (Fig. 9.8.2). Stance phase double support is lengthened, the more weight is born on the toes instead of heels. Period of single limb support is shortened. Asymmetries of gait are common.

Abnormal stooped posturing can contribute to development of a festinating gait.

Characterized by progressive increased in the speed with a shortening of stride.

Patient takes multiple short steps to catch up with his or her center of mass and avoids falling and may eventually break into a run or trot.

Propulsive gait has a forward accelerating quality whereas the less common retropulsive gait has a backward accelerating one.

Swallowing and Communication Dysfunction

Dysphagia is impaired swallowing is estimated in 50–95% of patients. Dysphagia leads to chocking or aspiration pneumonia and impaired nutrition with significant weight loss.

Nutritional inadequacy leads to fatigue and exhaustion.

Dysphagia is due to reduced mobility, rigidity and restricted range of motion.

Individuals with PD have problem in all four phases of swallowing oral preparatory, oral, pharyngeal and esophageal.

Patient demonstrates abnormal tongue control, problems with chewing and bolus formation; delayed swallowing response; peristalsis.

Patients also typically experience excessive drooling (sialorrhea) as a result of increased salivatory production and decreased spontaneous swallowing.

Impaired Speech

The speech is impaired in 50–73% of patients.

Hypokinetic dysarthria is characterized by decreased voice volume, monotone or monopitch speech, imprecise or distorted articulation, uncontrolled speech rate.

Difficulty in initiating and maintaining speech.

Cognitive and Behavioral Dysfunction

Dementia occurs in 1/3rd of the patients with PD.

Deficits include loss of executive function, reasoning, abstract thinking, judgment, memory impairment.

Bradyphrenia is disorders of intellectual function. It is characterized by slowing of thought process, lack of concentration and attention, problems with selective attention, problems with shifting attention, learning deficits especially with procedural learning, increased practice time may be required for learning, perceptual deficits.

Basal ganglia and frontal lobe appear to play an important role in integration of sensory information.

Deficits have been reported in vertical perception, topographic orientation, body scheme, spatial relation.

Depression occur in 25–40% patients.

Depression suggest endogenous cause that may be related to underlying changes in serotoninergic system.

Symptoms of major depression are apathy, passivity, loss of ambition and enthusiasm, changes in appetite, changes of sleep, dependency, suicidal thought may be present. Patient may demonstrate a dysthymic disorders characterized by variability in dysphoric mood, atypical depression, intermittent episodes of severe anxiety.

Behavioral changes may occur due to sensory deprivation.

Drug related psychosis can occur including hallucination and delusion due to L-dopa toxicity.

Autonomic Dysfunction

Common problems include excessive perspiration, greasy skin, and increased salivation, thermoregulatory abnormalities (uncomfortable sensation of heat or cold).

Bladder Dysfunction

Increased urinary frequency, urgency, nocturia.

Low appetite, decreased motility of GIT (gastrointestinal tract), constipation.

Cardiopulmonary Dysfunction

Orthostatic hypotension, low resting blood pressure, arrhythmia due to leva dopa toxicity.

Pulmonary dysfunction impairment occurs in 84% patient.

Airway obstruction air trapping, most frequent problem lung insufflations.

Restrictive dysfunction occurs in 28% patients and it has been linked to decreased chest expansion.

Lower forced vital capacity, higher residual volume, higher airway resistance and lower forced expiratory volume.

In long standing disease the lower extremity may exhibit circulatory changes owing to venous pooling as a result of decreased mobility and prolonged sitting. Patient present with mild to moderate edema of the foot and ankle which usually subsides during sleep.

DIAGNOSIS

Early diagnosis of PD is difficult. Diagnosis is usually made on the basis of history and clinical examination, handwriting samples, speech analysis and physical examination.

A diagnosis of PD can be made if at least two of the four cardinal features are present.

PROGNOSIS

Factors (Baatile, et al. 2000) that affect the progression of PD are age at onset, duration of the disease, onset of tremors, dementia and gait disturbances.

PHYSIOTHERAPY MANAGEMENT

Examination

It includes the examination of:

- Rigidity
- Bradykinesia
- Balance
- Gait impairment
- Posture

Rigidity primarily affects the muscles of respiration, trunk and extremities.

Balance assessment includes

- Assessment with eyes open
- Assessment with eyes closed
- Tandem walking

- Standing on a unstable surface
- Gait velocity

Dynamic balance testing involves functional reach test while maintaining the body balance on a single extremity.

Gait assessment involves:

- Assessing the ability of client to alter speed
- Time necessary to complete transitional movement
- Sit to stand ability
- Standing to sitting ability

Handwriting ability—it must be periodically sampled
Active and passive range of motion
General muscle strength
Chest expansion
Evaluation should include performance of sequential task.
The alternate movement patterns and spontaneous movement must be given special emphasis during assessment.

GENERAL GOALS OF TREATMENT

- Increasing the range of motion (ROM) of trunk and extremities
- Increasing the range of movement in both extremities and trunk
- Improving chest expansion
- Improving the balance reaction
- Maintaining or restoring functional abilities

The major problems which cannot be dealt with medicine regime alone and definitely require the physical therapy interventions include:

- Mobility deficits
- Difficulty in transfer (Keus, et al. 2007)
- Difficulty in maintaining the posture, balance and equilibrium (Keus, et al. 2007)
- Difficulty in maintaining the independent ambulation
- Loss of independence (Garrett, et al. 2004; Keus, et al. 2007)
- Higher risk of falls
- Large period of inactivity—higher risk of osteoporosis, cardiovascular problems (Garrett, et al. 2004)
- Reduced quality of life (Schrag, et al. 2000)

Parkinson disease patients have significant difficulty in performing the simple tasks of daily living such as eating, dressing, bathing in safe and time effective manner. The need and concern of individual patients must be paid proper attention. In order to manage these simple tasks the simple (Lyon and William, 2003) strategies are useful:

- The work timing may be rescheduled according to the time when the effect of the medicines is maximum during the day time
- Regular exercises help to maintain the strength and flexibility necessary to do the daily work safely
- Adaptive equipments to aid the mobility, and perform work hygienically
- Strategies to enhance the mobility and transfers in chair, bed and space
- Workstation modifications may be needed to tackle the problems associated with the work and occupational activities
- Correct instruction and methods to perform daily work such as cooking, laundry
- When the patient is able to perform work safely in individual setting, the social group services may be utilized to enhance the mobility in the community
- Physical activity is important for the comprehensive management of PD. The studies have shown that participation in the regular moderate intensity exercises reduces the progression of PD (Sasco, et al. 1992)
- In early course of treatment, the home exercise program are helpful
- The regular sessions are needed for the reassessment, modification of goals, and to compare the progression and resolution of symptoms
- When the client can perform home exercise program individually with confidence and safely, the community resource centers can help to maintain the therapeutic regime, boost the patient's motivation and introduce the group therapy approach.

Regular exercise can help reduce changes in motor disability, muscle strength, ambulation and quality of life (Scandalis, et al. 2001). The exercises commonly used for the PD patients are stretching exercises of the ventral aspect of the body, strengthening exercises of the postural antigravity group of muscles, relaxation exercises. Exercise programs should be tailored according to individual ability and interest levels.

The recommendation is that after taking the medicines, the client must do one hour rest and then perform the exercise program. This is important to achieve the maximum benefit (Goetz, et al. 1993).

The relaxation activities may include deep breathing, guided imagery, massage therapy, music, or involvement in forms of creative expression (Lyon and William, 2003).

Studies have found that the ambulation ability of the PD patients can be improved by providing the cues during active gait training (Nieuwboer, et al. 2001). Cues are stimulus available within environment or produced by the patients, to facilitate the automatic or/and repetitive movements (Keus, et al. 2007). These cues are believed to compensate for the ill-supplied internal rhythm of basal ganglia; corrects the motor deficiency or facilitate the cerebellar visual-motor pathways (Keus, et al. 2007; Rubinstein, et al. 2002).

The types of cues that have been found to be effective for being used in PD patients are following four (Keus, et al. 2007):

- Auditory cues (Marchese, et al. 2000)—use of walkman with rhythmic music; Metronome or counting by patient/partner
- Stepping over the differently colored or bulged stripes on floor (Marchese, et al. 2000; Lewis et al. 2000)
- Focusing on a fixed object such as clock (Lewis et al. 2000)
- Tactile cues (Marchese, et al. 2000; Muller, et al. 1997)—tapping on hip or portion of limb
- Cognitive cues (Gauthier, et al. 1987; Morris, et al. 1996)—using a mental image of appropriate step length and position.

To improve the motor performance during transfer skills, the cognitive movement strategies are useful (Keus, et al. 2007). In cognitive movement strategy (Nieuwboer, et al. 2001) the complex movement task is broken down into series of component movements, which are to be executed in a fixed order. All components are relatively simpler, are to be practiced adequately with appropriate feedback, and are arranged in a sequentially progressively manner using conscious efforts. When the components become acceptably perfect, they can be arranged together to perform whole task at once.

PRESCRIPTION FOR ASSISTIVE DEVICES

Treatment procedure:

- Functional activities that incorporate complex motor activities
- Participating in gait and balance activities

- Strengthening of muscle groups in functional activities
- Movement through full range
- Relaxation of the rigid group of muscles.

To reduce rigidity
- Relaxation techniques
- Gentle slow rocking movement
- Rotation of extremities and trunk
- Yoga.

The progression of exercise must be from distal to proximal muscles.

Once the rigidity reduces via relaxation training, the movement therapy must be initiated.

To reduce tremors—the relaxation techniques

Start movement from distal joint to proximal joint. Bilateral symmetrical pattern first, followed by diagonal pattern.

To add trunk rotation, the PNF patterns and Rhythmic initiation may be used.

The neurodevelopment treatment (NDT) and mobilization techniques may be useful to increase scapular and pelvic mobility.

Rhythmic and auditory cues facilitate movement.

Both auditory and visual stimuli should be used in treatment of parkinson gait disorders.

Aerobic exercises to improve pulmonary function

Balloon dancing is a rhythmic therapy for patient with parkinson.

Gait Rehabilitation

It must include improving the:
- Walking in crowd
- Walking through doorways
- Walking on different surfaces
- Walking with altered stride lengths.

Balance

Balance exercises and equilibrium reactions to improve balance.

Rhythmical stabilization: To improve static balance.

The timing of resistance should be sufficient to allow the client to develop during first set of muscles before increasing resistance.

Dynamic balance exercises must include turning the body and turning the head.

For bedridden patient: Mat activities are important.

Group therapy and home program are also important for the treatment rehabilitation.

For PD patients, the balance training combined with visual or vestibular feedback, and the lower extremity strength training is important for improving the balance performance, while compared to the balance exercises alone (Hirsch, et al. 2003; Toole, et al. 2000).

9.9: DISSEMINATED SCLEROSIS (MULTIPLE SCLEROSIS)

Disseminated sclerosis (multiple sclerosis) is the autoimmune pathological state, which affects the myelin sheath around the axons of the CNS (brain and spinal cord), to cause the demyelination of these CNS structures. Therefore, the MS is considered to be a chronic inflammatory disease of CNS (Klefbeck and Nedjad, 2003). After the demyelination the scattered patches of the sclerosis or scarring appear in the brain or/and spinal cord.

The dissemination means the scattered, the "sclerosis" means scarring or patches, and the word "multi" signifies that many patches are present in the brain or/and spinal cord.

PROGRESSION AND FEATURES

- The onset of MS mostly occurs between age of 20 and 30 years
- The disease is a chronic and progressive in nature (Mc Alphine, 1972)
- The disease commonly starts during the third decade of life in adults and may affect either gender.

CAUSES

- The exact cause of the MS or disseminated sclerosis remains unexplored
- The most widely accepted mechanism involves the autoimmune reactions
- The genetic factor, environmental factors or the infection related factors are also believed to play important role.

RISK FACTORS

Following are the several risk factors which are believed to trigger the onset of the multiple sclerosis:

- Viral conditions such as cold, influenza
- The infections such as gastroenteritis, diarrhea
- Other autoimmune diseases
- The clients with the hypersensitive disorder such as SLE (systemic lupus erythromatosus), anaphylactic reactions, etc.

PATHOPHYSIOLOGY

The cause of the disseminated sclerosis or MS is believed to rest upon the autoimmune mechanisms. The autoimmune reactions impair the myelin sheath of the nerves, and impair the inter-neuron conduction and the ability of the body cells to communicate with each other effectively (Compston and Coles, 2002).

In case of MS the PNS (peripheral nervous system) is least affected however the CNS (the parts of brain or/and spinal cord) are primarily affected.

Due to the previous infections or other pathologies the body's blood-brain barrier remains excessively permeable to the large number of cells and substances. In MS due to the autoimmune defense mechanisms, T-lymphocyte cells (less rarely B-cells) cross the blood-brain barrier and reach up to the brain. These cells mistakenly identify body's own cells (including the myelin sheath of the nerves) as foreign body and start the inflammatory process. This produces inflammation, swelling and damage to the cells in the white matter of the cerebellum, brainstem, spinal cord, optic nerve, and the myelinated nerves of nervous system. The oligodendrocytes cells and myelin sheath are damaged leading to the impaired conduction of the signals between nerves. Due to repeated attacks or progressive attacks, the irreversible damage occurs.

CLINICAL FEATURES

- The any form of the neurological feature can appear in the disease.
- The functional disability is common and the prolonged disability can lead to the emotional and/or cognitive disability (Compston and Coles, 2002).
- The presentation of MS could involve in any form of the neurological feature, and may involve sensory or motor features either in isolation or in combination.

- The sensory presentation could involve changes in sensations, diminished or absent sensation, hypoesthesia or paresthesia. Loss of sensation to the touch, pain, pin prick, heat or cold.
- Motor presentation could involve the muscle weakness, spasm, difficulty in moving. The structure damage of the brain and its part may lead to the upper motor neuron lesion type (UMNL) appearance or the spasticity in different muscle groups.
- The features of in-coordination could include the ataxia, loss of balance (Kraft, et al. 1986), impaired performance during walking or daily routine tasks.
- The other commonly faced tasks include nystagmus, ataxia, dysarthria, dysphagia, optic neuritis, double vision (diplopia), and blindness. Most of the patients complain of the pain in the majority of the body joints and/or muscles. Patients with bulbar lesions may have both laryngeal and pharyngeal dysfunction, causing symptoms such as dysphonia, dysphagia, and aspiration (Troyer and Pride, 1985).
- Due to its chronic and almost continuously progressive nature, the majority of patients present with the cognitive or psychological distress which imposes severe restriction in the functional abilities and the compromised quality of life.

In advanced stage three typical symptoms which are seen include:

- *Nystagmus*: Oscillatory movement of eyeballs when the client watches sideways or operator's finger in the alternating right-left directions.
- *Intentional tremors*: At rest, there is no tremor but the tremors appear when the client attempts to perform some definite movement or task, and as the task progresses the intensity of tremors also progresses. This makes him difficult to perform the finger to nose movement or the toe to shin movement. The degree of tremor is asymmetrical on both sides of body.
- *Scanning of speech (staccato speech)*: Every syllable of every word is pronounced separately.

In almost all the patients the significant reduction in the physical activity occurs due to the fatigue (Ericson, et al. 1989). Fatigue is the major problem (Sharma, et al. 1995) encountered by the physical therapist while rehabilitating the MS patients and this fatigue is believed to be central in origin (Freal, et al. 1984).

TABLE 9.9.1 Various types of multiple sclerosis (MS)

Relapsing Remitting	80-90% of all cases of MS The type is characterized by the alternate period of remission (complete absence of the symptoms) and the relapses (when the features of MS are evident). The period of remission may vary from months to years This is the most common form of MS and makes up to 80-90% of all cases of MS After the period of relapse the symptoms may resolve in months or may take years In majority of cases, the early diagnosis is not possible as the client may recover from the relapse phase completely
Secondary progressive MS	65% of all cases of MS After the period of relapse, the client starts recovering, however before complete recovery, the next relapse phase occurs. Thus the client is never able to recover from the previous relapse phase and the symptoms gradually keep on progressing. The period of relapse is prolonged and the remission is smaller. This type of MS is also known as "galloping multiple sclerosis"
Primary Progressive MS	15% of all cases of MS The period of symptoms occurs continuously while the remission period is either absent or minimal, therefore the symptoms continue to progress without any period of the significant recovery (Reingold, 1996)
Progressive Relapsing MS	In these patients the symptoms continue to progress similar to the primary progressive form, but in addition to this progression the clients also suffer the superimposed additional attacks. This form of MS is uncommon, however possibly the cases could not be documented or could not been identified due to lack of reporting

TYPES

The MS may present in many forms and the features do vary significantly with the type of the MS (Table 9.9.1). The classification of the MS into various forms is according to the definitions of the NMSS (national multiple sclerosis society) criteria (Reingold, 1996). The four types are described in Table 9.91.

In majority of cases, the symptoms do recover to certain extent after the period of exacerbation is over. However, in advanced cases, the irreversible damage to the nervous system has occurred and it leads to the failure of the recovery from the symptoms.

TREATMENT

Assessment from physical therapy view includes the detail assessment of the presented complication and limitations.

The Up and Go test (TUG) is commonly used to evaluate functional mobility. This test measures, in seconds, the time taken by a person to stand up from a standard arm chair, walk a distance of 3m, turn,walk back to the chair, and sit down again (Podsiadlo and Richardson, 1991).

Modified Ashworth Scale is used to determine the level of spasticity on a five point ordinal scale for assigning the grade of spasticity according to the resistance encounterd during manual passive elongation of muscle (Bohannon and Smith, 1977).

Balance assessment is important and the postural sway, sway velocity can be measured by the AccuSwayPLUS force platform apparatus (DeBolt and McCubbin, 2004)

The three approaches are used in MS patients:

1. *Palliative treatment*: It aims to improve the performance of the affected part.
2. *Compensatory treatment*: When the impairment is irreversible, the compensatory treatment is used to train the unaffected or minimally affected parts of body, to support the functioning of the irreversibly impaired part
3. *Preventive treatment*: Aims to prevent the development of the complications and their severity.

Physical Therapy Management

In the clients of the spasticity, the physical therapy treatment aims to prevent the contracture; to regain the mobility; to regain muscle power.

Rehabilitation program are important for improving the functional independence and optimize the functional performance (DeBolt and McCubbin, 2004).

Lower extremity strength is most important predictor of the functional recovery of the adult MS patient (Skeleton, et al. 1994).

Resistance Training

During advancement of the MS, the ascending type of weakness is seen where the lower extremity are affected first and the upper extremity are involved later on (Smeltzer, et al. 1988).

Resistance training of weak muscles is helpful to improve the strength in MS adults. For this purpose, the progressive resistance exercises (Kasser and McCubbin, 1996) and aquatic therapy (Gehlsen, et al. 1984). Generally 4–8 weeks resistance exercise program are required to improve the endurance, to delay the fatigue (Swensson, et al. 1994) and improved strength.

The sample resistance exercise program for MS patients:

- *Chair raises*: The patient is asked to rise form arm-less chair, with arms crossed across chest × 10 repetitions
- *Forward lunges*: Patient is asked to step forward, bend opposite knee towards ground, and push back the lunged leg to starting position × 10 repetitions with right leg and then 10 repetitions with left leg
- *Step-ups*: Patient performs the step up on different height steps depending on their capacity
- *Press-up*: Exercise in prone lying position
- Lifting medicine ball from waist to head by shoulder flexion and extension
- Moving medicine ball while holding, and move in different directions
- In crook lying position carrying the medicine ball by both hands from shoulder to opposite hip
- In crook lying position carrying the medicine ball by both hands in different patterns (D-1 flexion, D2 flexion, D1 extension, D2 extension) of PNF (proprioceptive neuromuscular facilitation)
- Heel-toe raises—the client rises up on toes and heels alternatively
- Leg curls—with appropriate weight cuffs

During resistance training, it is important to keep the number of repetitions and the intensity of exercises low initially and giving adequate rest between sets, so as to minimize the fatigue and maximize the recovery. Later on, as the situation of the client improves, the rest period may be reduced, the intensity may be increased.

The exercises have double advantage of simultaneously strengthening of the girdle and trunk musculatures as well as improving the circulation.

Management of Fatigue

Fatigue is the major problem presented by the MS patients. To avoid the fatigue in MS patients multiple strategies have been employed.

These exercises help to improve the strength and endurance of the respiratory muscles, use of resistive breathing devices, and improvement of the aerobic capacity of the individual.

The study by the Klefbeck and Nedjad (2003) shown that the inspiratory threshold training by 3 sets, 10 loaded inspirations using IMT (inspiratory muscle training) device, on alternate days for 10-weeks period significantly improves the peak inspiratory and peak expiratory flow.

The general body aerobic activities such as swimming, skipping, running, jogging, stationary bicycle, rowing, general upper extremity ergometry, the girdle active exercises are useful.

Respiratory Management

During the progressive MS, the weakness of the respiratory muscles is inevitable leading to the higher risk of developing the respiratory complications and mortality conditions in MS patients (Sadovnick, et al. 1991).

Due to the ascending type weakness in MS, the expiratory muscles and abdominal muscles are affected first and later on the intercostals muscles and finally the inspiratory muscels are impaired (Smeltzer, et al. 1988; Klefbeck and Nedjad, 2003)

Therefore, in progressive MS the respiratory muscles training, the mobilization of pulmonary secretions and the preservation of respiratory status is important to maintain the respiratory muscle weakness and to improve the cough ability.

The effective cough training can be done by training for deep inspiration, deep elastic recoil, increased abdominal muscle pressure by increased abdominal contraction and the cough attempt against closed glottis (Hough, 1996).

Management of Spasticity

Spasticity is not the major problem in MS patients due to its less severity. The common areas presenting with the higher muscle tone include the legs and lower trunk. Spasticity is not severe and generally diminishes itself with the improved functional status.

Management of In-coordination

In-coordination is a major problem in MS and not been completely treated till date. However, its severity can be significantly reduced with the physical therapy interventions.

The simpler tasks which are lighter in nature are helpful to improve the coordination. However, the tasks including forceful muscle activity are not recommended as it would induce fatigue and would further deteriorate the in-coordination.

9.10: AMYOTROPIC LATERAL SCLEROSIS

ALS is the most common form of MND. Adult ALS is a neurodegenerative disorder characterized by loss of motor neurons in the cortex, brainstem, and spinal cord manifested by the upper motor neuron lesion (UMNL) and lower motor neuron lesion (LMNL) signs and symptoms. It results in bulbar, limb, respiratory muscles paralysis (Francis, et al. 1999).

There is a massive loss of anterior horn cells of the spinal cord and motor cranial nerve nuclei in the lower brainstem resulting in mixed LMNL and UMNL type features.

Demyelination and gliosis of the corticospinal and corticobulbar tracts caused by the degeneration of the cerebral cortex cells results in UNM symptoms termed as lateral sclerosis. The wasting of muscles is called as amyotrophy.

ETIOLOGY

Males are more affected than females.

The age of onset is around 50-70 years.

Exact etiology is unknown however certain theories are prevalent such as:

- Toxic theory—increase accumulation of lead and aluminium and the abnormalities in calcium and magnesium ions
- Deficiency of nerve growth factor
- Excess extracellular glutamate in the Central nervous system (CNS)
- Glutamate excitotoxicity (Francis, et al. 1999)
- Autoimmunity to calcium channels
- Cytoskeletal abnormalities
- Oxidative stress (Francis, et al. 1999)

CLASSIFICATION

Following are four distinct subtypes of ALS.

- Classical ALS

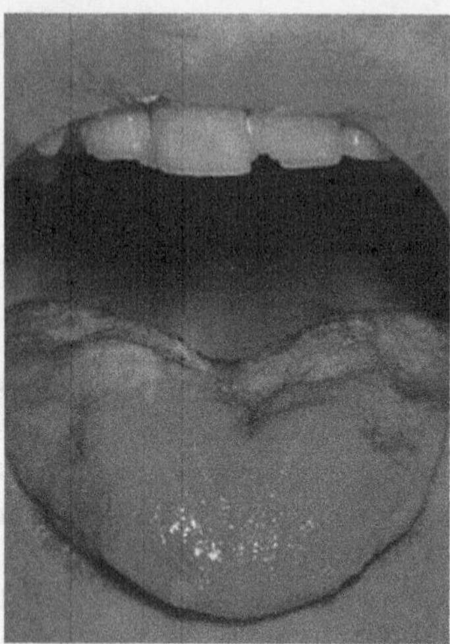

Fig. 9.10.1: Tongue muscle atrophy in ALS

- Makes about 90% cases of ALS. Characterized by mixed UMNL and LMNL features
- UMN features in classical ALS are hyperreflexia, clonus and spasticity
- LMN features include weakness, atrophy and fasciculation
- May affect trunk / limb and bulbar muscles
- Tongue muscle atrophy occurs (Fig 9.10.1)

- Progressive muscular atrophy (PMA)
  - The lower motor neurons signs and symptoms which affect limb and trunk musculature
  - Rarely affects the brainstem
- Progressive bulbar palsy
  - Affects motor neurons in the brainstem and presents with bulbar dysfunction only
  - UMNL and LMNL features of bulbar muscles only.

PHYSIOTHERAPY EVALUATION OF ALS

- To check the medical records to have an idea of the previous functional status and the rapidity of the disease progression
- To evaluate the ADL (activity of daily living) ability
- Respiratory status evaluation

- Psychological evaluation
- Assessment of pain, bulbar symptoms.

GOALS OF PHYSIOTHERAPY MANAGEMENT

- To maintain the muscle and strength till maximum possible time
- Prevention of associated deformities and problems
- To help in better deal with the impairments and disability imposed by the disease
- To preserve the respiratory status
- To maximize the nutrition status by helping them with the strategies to improve the food intake compliance.

TREATMENT OF MND

No definite treatment is available for treating MND.

The disease is progressive in nature, if the disease is non-progressive it is not probably the MND.

The damage that once has occurred in MND is irreversible and cannot be cured; however with help of proper used therapeutic and medical management the progression of symptoms may be delayed and the quality of life could be improved before the death (Francis, 2010).

The Riluzole is the only approved drug available for the treatment of ALS after the few studies showing few positive effect of this drug in ALS patients (Francis, et al. 1999). This is a glutamate antagonist and sodium channel blocker which improves the lifespan of MND patients by few months (Wikipedia, 2010).

Physical Therapy Management of MND

Due to the absence of the definite treatment available, the treatment believes to deal with the associated discomfort, problems. Until as definite treatment or cure is available for ALS, the multifaceted and multidisciplinary approach is needed as a best hope for improving the health and survival in this fatal illness (Francis, 2010).

The management of the MND or ALS has been suggested in accordance with the grading of the disease and the presented pathological features. These stagewise managements are described in Table 9.10.1.

Spasticity is a common problem in MND or ALS patients, and worsens the muscle dysfunction, compromises ADL activities and

TABLE 9.10.1 Management of MND/ALS in different stages

	Stage	*Clinical features*	*Management*
Independent phases	Stage I	Mild weakness Patient is ambulatory and independent in ADL	Encourage the activities to prevent disuse atrophy Start ROM exercises Strengthening exercises Psychological support
	Stage 2	Moderate selective weakness Slight decrease in ADL Patient is ambulatory	Stretching exercises to prevent contractures Strengthening exercises Orthotic supports Use of adaptive equipment to facilitate ADLs
	Stage 3	Severe weakness in ankle, wrist and hand Moderately decrease in independent ADL Easy fatigability with the long distance ambulation Slight increase in respiratory efforts	Continue the stage 2 progression Keep the patient physically fit and independent Deep breathing exercises, postural drainage is needed Wheelchair may be needed

Contd...

Contd...

Partially independent phases	Stage 4	Pain in shoulder Edema in hands Severe lower extremity weakness Patient able to perform ADL but quickly fatigues	Heat and massage Preventive anti-edema regimes AROM, resisted exercises or PROM exercises Encourage isometric contraction of all muscles Give arm sling Give wheelchair
	Stage 5	Severe impairment of lower extremity function Moderate to severe weakness of upper extremity Patient is wheel chair dependent Constant prolonged positioning in wheelchair causes sustained pressure on skin and ulceration	Courage family to learn proper transfers, positioning, turning The prevention of pressure sore strategies must be employed using pressure bed or water bed May need the respiratory unit at home to support breathing Modifications may be made at home to aid the patient's mobility and independence
Dependent phase	Stage 6	Patient's ambulatory status is lost Functional performance is totally dependent Patient unable to walk and becomes bedridden Respirator efforts is significantly increased	For breathing problems may need deep breathing exercises, postural drainage, anti-edema measures, positioning, stretching exercises, PROM

deteriorates the quality of life (Ashworth, et al. 2006). No conclusive study has been conducted till date to document the effect of spasticity management strategies for MND patients.

Approximately 80% of ALS patients report the difficulty with speech due to bulbar muscle involvement (Gubbay, et al. 1985; Caroscio, et al. 1987) and dysarthria. Nasal intonation of voice, changed oral movement rate (Yorkston, et al. 1993), harsh vocal quality, vocal cord malfunctioning, reduced vital capacity (Dworkin, 1979; Hillel, et al. 1989).

The other problems commonly reported by ALS patients include the swallowing difficulty; nasal reflux, poor food manipulation, mouth breathing, coughing or choking during meal (Robbins, 1987). Due to these factors, these patients tend to avoid the regular meal which compromises their nutrition and further aggravates the problem (Francis, et al. 1999). Loss of upper extremity function also compromises the self-feeding abilities, psychological fear of choking, interfered oral/food intake (Francis, et al. 1999; Kasarskis, et al. 1998; Slowie, et al. 1983). This poor nutrition status further aggravates the weakness of the respiratory muscles pulmonary system (Arora and Rochester, 1982).

The other common problem seen in these patients is the difficulty in eating or drinking due to failure to maintain the open oro-pharynx while putting food/drinking in mouth. This is due to the neck protraction and flexed position secondary to the poor strength of neck extensors. In these clients, it is important to maintain the chin-tuck position or erect neck position during eating. This can be achieved by using the straw which maintains the recommended chin-tuck position during consumption of semi liquid diet.

ALS is fatal neurodegenerative and without mechanical ventilation the death occurs due to respiratory failure within 2–5 years of onset of symptoms. Therefore, the mechanical ventilation becomes important to improve the survival and the quality of life among the MND patients having normal to moderately impaired bulbar symptoms, however in cases of the poor bulbar symptoms patients only the sleep apnea improves slightly while without affecting the survival (Raduvonic, et al. 2009).

In non-tracheostomized patients of severe respiratory muscle weakness but preserved bulbar muscles, the need of the mechanical ventilation could be delayed to significant limit by the respiratory training using *glossopharyngeal breathing*. This is a specialized form of breathing which involves taking the 6 to 9 gulps of bolus of air into lungs, to aid the deep breathing of the client. This specific form of breathing can be taught during early stages of ALS so that in the advanced stage when the respiratory weakness is prominent, the client can manage to maintain the appropriate ventilator status (Francis et al, 1999).

9.11: SYRINGOMYELIA

Syringomyelia is a disease characterized by the presence of longitudinally disposed cavities within the spinal cord (Williams, 1980). Syringomyelia originates in embryonic life as a result of the overdistention of the neural tube (Gardner, 1965).

The pathology lies in the possibly that during embryonic life in these cases the syrinx cavity is not cut off and is kept distended with the fourth ventricular fluid that enters it because the outlets of the fourth ventricle does not develop properly (Gardner, 1965).

In progressive cases the syrinx progressively expands and elongates along the length of the spinal cord. This causes the damage to the gray matter of the cord and leads to the weakness and sensory symptoms in the affected segments of the cord (Schurch, 1996). The most common feature involves the pain, weakness and stiffness in the trunk and extremities. The glove stocking type of sensation loss is common, especially in hands. The presentation of the symptoms varies according to the location and extent of the involvement of the spinal cord.

Causes

- Usually the symptoms are manifested slowly in nature, however sometime the weakened cord may develop the sudden onset features during the activities which increase the pressure within the spinal cord such as coughing, sneezing, weight lifting.
- The excessive accumulation of the cerebrospinal fluid (CSF) with in central canal of the spinal cord is called as hydromyelia. The excessive pressure with in central canal of the cord is responsible for the seepage of CSF into surrounding tissues. This causes formation of the cavity called as syrinx.
- The increase in the CSF pressure with in central canal of the spinal cord may occur in a variety of conditions such as: congenital

obstruction of the CSF drainage (Arnold-Chiari-malformation; the brainstem malformation; cerebellar tonsil herniation), or the excessive formation of the CSF fluid such as in case of the arachnoiditis.

- The post-traumatic syringomyelia is also a common cause of the syringomyelia (Schurch et al, 1996). The resolution of the hematoma in case of traumatic events also is a major factor leading the development of the post traumatic syringomyelia (Williams, 1980).

Pathology of Syringomyelia

The cerebrospinal fluid (CSF) is responsible for transporting nutrients and waste products, acts as shock absorber of the spinal cord and brain, and helps in providing the security to the brain and spinal cord. Sometime in few pathological states such as spina bifida, spinal tumor, Arnold-Chiari-malformation, scoliosis the excessive accumulation of the fluid in central canal of spinal canal is called as hydromyelia. This excessive pressure of the fluid caused the ependymal cells of the canal to break off and the seepage of fluid occurs within the surrounding white matter of the spinal cord. The seepage of fluid into the white matter of the cord forms a cavity called as syrinx. When the formation of the syrinx has occurred than this condition is known as syringomyelia. Once the syrinx cavity has formed, the CSF move towards this cavity due to the less pressure faced at this interface compared to the brain where the resistance encountered is high. This results in to the progressive enlargement of the cavity size, therefore in majority of cases the syringomyelia the size of the syrinx size and the severity of spinal cord damage is progressively increasing in nature.

Features

- Syringomyelia is characterized by the formation of cavities (known as cyst or syrinx) within the spinal cord along-with the dilation of the central canal of the cord. This is a rare condition and involves the scattered dissociated anesthesia and paralysis. The loss of sensations of pain and temperature occurs in these patients, however the sensation to touch or muscle proprioception is preserved in the same region.
- The major symptoms of this complication are pain, which may be localized centrally or which may radiate into the arm or trunk,

sensory impairment and increasing weakness. It appears to be more common in tetraplegic than in paraplegic patients (Rossier et al, 1985).

- The most common complaint in patients with syringomyelia is the pain which could be localized centrally or may radiate into arm or trunk. The sensory impairment and progressive weakness is also common. These complications are more common among tetraplegics while compared to the paraplegics (Rossier et al, 1985).
- The muscle atrophy and paralysis may be faced if motor cells of the spinal cord are affected. The weakness and atrophy starts distally first (in hands) and then it progresses proximally (towards forearm and arm). Usually the lower segment of the cord is affected first, and with progression of disease the upper segments of the spinal cord may involve. With further advancement of the disease the medulla and brain stem could get involved leading to the bulbar symptoms.
- In the advanced form when the significant part of the spinal cord is damaged, the posterior column involvement causes ataxia and the spastic paraplegia results from the involvement of the pyramidal tracts.
- The common complications of the syringomyelia include the scoliosis, burns, pressure sores, kyphoscoliosis.

Physiotherapeutic Management of Syringomyelia

- The aim of the physiotherapy interventions include to delay the muscle atrophy, to preserve the muscle functioning till best possible time; to maximize the functional ability of the client with in limits of available strength and irreversible impairments.
- The physiotherapy management deals with the complications associated with the impaired functioning of the spinal cord. These impairments could include the features of paraplegia, tetraplegia, the bowel-bladder involvement, the sensory loss or the motor weakness.
- In recent year the stem cell therapy has been found to be effective. During this treatment the embryonic spinal cord tissue of the embryo is implanted (Johnson, 2001) in to the patients with post traumatic syringomyelia, and the physical therapy interventions after that are useful for successive rehabilitation of the client.

- These patients are prone to develop burn and pressure sores, therefore the proper education is important to avoid these complications.
- The associated complications such as kyphoscoliosis and scoliosis are generally reported much before the established diagnosis of syringomyelia, therefore these are dealt inappropriate way using proper positioning, bracing, muscle strengthening, etc.
- The tight muscles may be maintained to their appropriate length, however the appropriate overstretching must be avoided as it would lead to irreversible muscle fibrosis.
- Once the ataxia sets in, the coordination exercises (Frenkel's exercises) are recommended similar to that recommended in the Tabes Dorsallis management.

9.12: MOTOR NEURON DISEASE

In the human body nervous system is sub-classified in to central nervous system (CNS), Peripheral nervous system (PNS) and Autonomic nervous system (ANS).

The CNS consists of spinal cord and brain. This is responsible for the determining, regulating and executing the basic as well as most vital and complex functions of body. The centers located in this are responsible for the regulating motor functioning, sensory perception, thirst, hunger, body temperature autoregulation, respiratory and circulatory control, social personality, intelligence, etc.

The spinal cord has additional functions of transmitting the impulses originated in brain to the PNS and the visceral organs. This is important for providing the pathways to the ascending tracts (which carry sensory information) and descending tracts (which bring the execution information from brain to the organs).

The neurons are responsible for conducting the current impulses in the nervous system network. The neurons can be considered as UMN (upper motor neurons) and LMN (lower motor neurons) (Table 9.12.1). The upper motor neurons conduct the impulses either in the brain itself or carry the impulse from brain up to the anterior horn cells of spinal cord. The anterior horn cells and its further conducting neurons constitute the LMN and carry the motor impulses from the spinal cord to the peripheral muscles. The anterior horn cells are under the higher control of cerebral cortex by

the corticospinal tracts. The bulbar nuclei are under higher control of brain by the corticobulbar fibers.

TABLE 9.12.1 Differences between UMNL (upper motor neuron lesion) and LMNL (lower motor neuron lesion)

UMNL	*LMNL*
These are the lesion of the neural pathways above the anterior horn cells or above the motor nuclei of the cranial nerves	These are the lesions of the neural pathways which travel from the anterior horn cells of spinal cord or from the bulbar nuclei of the brain
The supplied muscle appears hyper active, very stiff	The supply muscle appears flaccid, weak and paralyzed
The tone of muscle is variably increased compared to the normal muscle	The tone of muscle is either reduced or completely absent which compared to the normal muscle
The deep tendon reflexes of the affected nerve(s) are exaggerated and brisk	The deep tendon reflexes of the affected nerve(s) diminished or absent
When asked to contract the muscle, the contraction may be brisk, abrupt and hyperactive	When asked to contract muscle, either the muscle contraction is absent or it is weak/absent
Muscular atrophy is not prominent or unapparent	Muscular atrophy is prominent
The UMNL of the bulbar neurons leads to the features like difficulty in swallowing, spasticity in facial muscles, speech problems	
The nerve supply to the corresponding remains intact however the regulating body (anterior horn cell or bulbar nuclei) of this nerve has lost its higher neural regulation	The denervation of the corresponding muscles occurs which leads to the features such as muscle • Muscle paralysis • Fasciculation • Fibrillation • Flaccidity
Examples of the UMN include the lesion of the corticospinal tract and corticobulbar tract	Examples of the LMN lesion include the lesion of anterior horn cell and bulbar nuclei

Note: If corticospinal tract are impaired but the AHC and its peripheral nerves are intact the presentation will be of UMNL type lesion in the corresponding peripheral nerve and its supplied muscles. In contrast to this if corticospinal tracts are impaired and the AHC or/and its distal projected peripheral nerve is also affected the presentation will be of LMNL type in the corresponding peripheral nerve and its supplied muscles.

The CNS and PNS together control the activity of the skeletal muscles. The CNS and ANS together regulate the activity of the visceral organs and the smooth muscles.

The motor neurons are those neurons which are located in the CNS and project neurons out of CNS to directly or indirectly controlling the muscles. In CNS the two types of motor neurons are located namely bulbar neurons and peripheral neurons. The bulbar neurons are associated with the functioning of cranial nerve nuclei (also called as bulbar nuclei) which further regulate the vital functioning of the body such as deglutination, respiration, swallowing of food/ liquid in pharynx, vocal cord functioning. The peripheral neurons regulate the functioning of the peripheral muscles such as motor activity, locomotor activity, muscle tone, etc. most important bulbar nuclei (cranial nerve) nuclei are those which are associated with glossopharyngeal nerve (9th), vagus nerve (10th) and hypoglossal nerve (12th).

The lesion of the UMN and LMN are respectively known as UMNL (upper motor neuron lesions) and LMNL (lower motor neuron lesions). These lesions are characterized by different features and presentation (See Table 9.12.1).

Motor neuron disease (MND) refers to the group of pathological disorders where only the motor neurons are selective affected. The affected motor neurons may involve those controlling the peripheral muscles or those which control the bulbar muscles.

Pathology of MND

- The exact cause of the MND is not established.
- The familial link is not found as most of the MND patients lack the family history of MND.
- The genetic link is yet to be established and the researches are being done to explore the mutation related etiology of MND.
- Researches are yet being done to understand the pathological events behind the MND. Most of the researches are evaluating the effect of oxidative stress, autoimmunity to calcium channels, cytoskeletal abnormality, mutation of the gene coding for superoxide dismutase (Francis et al, 1999).

The impairment of the function of the corticospinal tract (the UMN lesion) impairment of the higher neural control of AHC (anterior horn cell) the ventral nerve roots undergo atrophy; the UMNL features in the corresponding muscles.

Classification

Depending on the location of the lesion the MND can be classified into following disorders:

- Amyotrophic lateral sclerosis (ALS) most common form of MND
- Progressive muscular atrophy (PMA)
- Primary lateral sclerosis (PLS) rare form of MND; makes about 4% of MND
- Bulbar palsy—This is further classified as progressive bulbar palsy and pseudobulbar palsy.

Types and Features of MND

ALS is most common form of MND and unless the type of MND is specified in a MND diagnosed patient, it is considered that ALS is the type with which patient is suffering. Depending on the type of the MND involved the sign and symptoms may be present. The mixed symptoms of UMNL and LMNL may occur (Table 9.12.2). Usually the symptoms associated with MND include the progressive increase in the features and ultimately majority of the cases become permanently handicapped or do not survive for long duration.

In ALS the corticonuclear fibers regulating the output conduction of the cortical nuclei in to the corticospinal tracts are affected. In early stage the AHC and its peripheral nerve is intact, therefore the UMNL symptoms occur in the muscle groups, however over period of time

TABLE 9.12.2 The following table presents the brief description of the MND types that have to be screened for

Type of MND	*UMNL like presentation*	*LMNL like presentation*
ALS	Yes	Yes
PMA	Yes	No
PLS	No	Yes
Progressive bulbar palsy	No	Yes
Pseudobulbar palsy	Yes	No

due to the neural deprivation the AHC and its related peripheral nerve degenerated, therefore later on the LMNL type features also are noticed. Therefore in ALS both UMNL and LMNL features are seen.

In PMA only the AHC or/and its distal peripheral nerves are affected, therefore it is a LMNL type MND. Therefore, the spasticity and UMNL features are absent. The presenting features include the fasciculation, fibrillation, atrophy, muscle flaccidity, loss of deep tendon reflexes. The EMG study of the affected muscle shows the death of the AHC in the most affected muscle as well as in some of the unaffected muscles.

In case of PLS (primary lateral sclerosis) the cortical nuclei responsible for the corticospinal tract conduction are degenerated. Thus, the proximal higher neural supply of the AHC is affected therefore it is a type of UMN lesion. The UMN symptoms in PLS leads to the problem in maintaining body balance, spasticity in hand/feet/legs, stiffness, excessive tone of the plantar flexors leading to dragging of foot.

In case of the pseudobulbar palsy the UMN and the cortical nuclei the corticobulbar fibers get affected leading to the UMN features in the bulbar muscles. The dysphagia, dysarthria, shrill cry may occur. Also the exaggerated jaw reflex, slow indistinct speech, normal to brisk gag reflex may occur. In such cases the emotional lability occurs, where the client fails to control the cry or emotions once provoked.

In case of progressive bulbar palsy, the bulbar nuclei (located in cerebral cortex, brainstem and pyramidal tracts) get degenerated. This leads to the LMN type presentation in the bulbar-innervated muscles. The excessive drooling may occur, the regurgitation of fluids may occur, the paralysis of the facial and pharyngeal muscles may occur leading to the failure of the respiration. This may lead to the speech problems due to facial muscles involvement, difficulty in protruding the tongue, difficulty in chewing/talking, weak movement of tongue and palate; the excessive drooling also occurs. The excessive drooling of saliva may be aspirated leading to pneumonia and death in about 3 years.

The common presentation in MND include the muscle weakness which is progressive, muscle fasciculation, muscle wasting, spasticity, muscles atrophy, brisk tendon reflexes, paralyzed muscles, foot drop, unilateral or bilateral wasting of hand, regurgitation of the fluid, slurring of speech. In MND any muscle group can be involved in peripheral and/or bulbar region.

Prognosis of the MND Subtypes

The Prognosis of PMA is litter better compared to ALS, due to the fact that only LMN of the peripheral nervous system (PNS) are affected. The higher centers (located in brain) remain intact therefore no loss of higher control loss. However due to the progressive nature later on it may involve the extensive area of the body including the vital muscles. Therefore, the survival rate in PMA patient is about 5 year (in 33% cases) to 10 year (in 12 % cases) after the onset of the disease (Wijesekera et al, 2009; Wikipedia, 2010).

Differential diagnosis of MND (Wikipedia, 2010; Francis, 1999):

- Multifocal neuropathy
- Kennedy's disease
- Hereditary spastic paraplegia
- Spinal muscular atrophy
- Monomelic amyotrophy
- Juvenile ALS
- Madras syndrome

Diagnosis of MND

The diagnosis of MND is clinical one and depends on the clinical neurological examination. No definite diagnostic criteria are available for the diagnosis of MND. The investigative procedures such as EMG, electrolyte testing, hormonal testing, NCV, genetic screening may be carried out to rule out the other diseases mimicking the presentation of MND.

The diagnosis still lies on the method of excluding the other similar pathologies. Because of its progressive nature the early diagnosis is highly warranted, however in absence of the definite criteria the diagnosis usually is established after the long time of establishment of the pathological processes.

Treatment of MND

The ALS is most common type of the MND. For the management of the MND see the chapter of ALS in this text.

9.13: PERIPHERAL NERVE, CRANIAL NERVE LESIONS, BELL'S PALSY AND FACIAL PALSY

The peripheral nerve injury means partial or total impairment of the nerve functioning as a result of some traumatic insult.

■ ANATOMY AND ORGANIZATION

The Peripheral nervous system (PNS) consists of the spinal nerves and the cranial nerves (except I and II cranial nerves).

Each peripheral nerve has sensory, motor and autonomic function. The sensory functioning is by the dorsal rami, while the motor function is executed by the ventral nerve roots.

Each nerve is surrounded and supported by the endoneurium, perineurium and epineurium.

Causes

The cause of this injury may be in form of:

- Overstretching, traction and avulsion
- Laceration
- Compression in the route of nerve (Lundberg, 1993) such as in carpal tunnel, Guyon tunnel, cubital tunnel
- Crush injury
- Mechanical trauma due to the adjacent joint dislocation
- Ischemia
- Shearing/frictional injuries—such as tardy ulnar nerve palsy
- Infections
- External compression—the pressure of prosthesis, orthosis, the Saturday nerve palsy, axillary nerve palsy
- Accidents
- Iatrogenic factors—such as traction to nerve during surgery, plaster casting.

Classification

Nerve injuries can be classified on the basis of the degree of pathological change in the nerve. The Grade I, II and III are the common grades of the classification of nerve injury which are more commonly known as neuropraxia, axonotmesis and the neurotmesis.

Suddon's classification of the nerve injury includes neuropraxia, neurotmesis and axonotmesis.

Neruroprexia (Grade I) is the mildest form of injury and the pathological changes occurring, are reversible in nature. There is temporary impairment of the nerve conduction due to the local pressure over the nerve, and there is no loss of nerve continuity.

Axonotmesis (Grade II) form of nerve injury is more severe injury. There is the impairment of the fibers of the axon fibers, without any pathological affection of the surrounding nerve sheath (connective tissue sheath of the nerve). Recovery may occur completely.

Neurotmesis (Grade III) is most severe form of nerve injury where the nerve axons as well as the surrounding connective tissue sheath of nerve are affected. The common events which lead to the neurotmesis include the burning, crushing, laceration, sharp object cuts, glass cut injuries. The functional loss of the nerve function is complete and almost irreversible if no surgical intervention is done to re-establish the integrity of the nerve fibers. Even with the surgical interventions the prognosis remains uneventful.

Features of Nerve Injury

The presenting features of the nerve injury depend on the type of nerve injury, type of nerve affected, the severity of involvement and the duration since when the causative factor is working.

The affected nerve may be of motor, sensory or mixed form. When the affected nerve is motor in nature then the injury leads to the loss of motor functions of the supplied muscles. If sensory nerve is damaged then the sensations of the supplied region get compromised. If a mixed nerve is injured, the mixed features are seen. The involvement of the autonomic nerves leads to loss of temperature regulation, blood pressure, the skin vascularity, the muscle tone of the blood vessels, and heart rate, etc.

The nerve recovery may or may not occur in case of the axonotmesis however in neurotmesis the nerve recovery does not occur without surgical intervention. The recovery of the nerve can be predicted to minor extent by the location of the injury on the route of the nerve. The injury site is more closer (pxominal) towards their origin from spinal cord, lesser are the chances of recovery.

ASSESSMENT OF THE PERIPHERAL NERVE INJURY

- History: The careful history has to be considered regarding the onset of symptoms, the progression or the deterioration, the changes in the presentation of the features since the time of injury, the extent of the weakness, the regions of the altered sensations, etc.

- Careful note is to be made about what is the most concerned complaint of the patient. Whether the complain is pain, tingling, altered sensation, weakness, or the extensive pain.
- General observation reveals the extent of external injury and suggests the regions which have to be screened out for the possible injury.
- The examination includes the sensitivity to the various sensations such as light touch, deep touch, cold, temperature, two-point discrimination, the pin prick, the proprioception. The presence of the Tinel's sign must be noted and also the location of the Tinel's sign must be accurately noted.
- The motor examination includes the testing of the muscles concerned with the injured nerve, the deep tendon reflex related to the supplied nerve.
- The functional examination has to be done.
- The electrodiagnostic findings must include the NCS (nerve conduction studies) to report the velocity and the amplitude of the tested nerve; EMG study to test the muscles supplied by the injured nerve; the H-wave or Reaction time, the evoked responses also have to be done for accurate assessment.
- The autonomic functions such as vasodilation, sudomotor function (sweating function), trophic changes (skin or hair changes) must also be noted carefully (Lundy-Ekman, 1993).

Treatment

Surgical Options for the Nerve Repair

In majority of the traumatic cases the wait has to be done to allow some spontaneous recovery up to the 3 months, if the electro-diagnostic findings do not get majorly deteriorated within this time period. However if the electrodiagnostic findings get drastically deteriorated, or reveal the complete transaction of the nerve, along with no apparent sign of nerve recovery, the surgical options have to be considered.

The direct repair to join the cut ends of nerves to re-establish the continuity, either with or without use of the nerve graft. It is a very delicate surgery and needs a good skill and experience to perform surgery.

Nerve grafting is used when the ends of nerve have retracted and some portion of the nerve has irreversible damaged leaving a gap between cut ends of nerves.

Nerve transfer can be used when the gap between cut ends is large or the nerve injury is located in excessive proximal location.

In case of nerve root avulsion the avulsed nerve cannot be reconnected with the proximal portion therefore the nerve transfer is the only option left.

In cases of the crushed injury where the exact extent of nerve damage cannot be identified with any other mean, the direct opening of the part to directly visualize the nerve and repair the concerned damage simultaneously can be done.

The surgical repair can either be done as primary repair or as the secondary repair. The *primary repair* involves the repair where the cut ends of the nerve are directly approximated and sutured. The secondary repair is done when the nerve injury is associated with other open injury or infection. The secondary repair involves the early management of the secondary infections and the open wounds while the nerve repair is done after some weeks or days.

Medical Therapy

Upon diagnosis of the nerve injury, it is very important to identify and remove the causative factor.

Meantime the supportive therapy starts with the:

- Minimizing the further trauma to nerve and the connective tissue structure
- The supporting the paralyzed portion of the extremity
- Avoiding the burns, cuts, frictional or other injuries which may occur due to the sensory or/and motor loss of the region
- To perform the electric stimulation of the supplied muscles.

The *medical treatment* focuses to cure the causative mechanism and the reduction of the associated inflammation or infections. The use of corticosteroid medicines or injections to reduce the swelling and edema; and the analgesics for the relief of neurogenic pain. The use of nerve growth factors and erythropoietin has been shown to have success in enhancing the speed of nerve recovery after nerve injury.

The initial orthopedic *treatment* focuses to deal with the orthopedic aspect of the injury including the stabilization of the dislocated joint or the fractures.

The *Physiotherapeutic management* starts immediately after the vital signs of patient are stable. The physiotherapy interventions include the:

- Early mobilization of the patient to minimize the complications associated with immobility.
- The maintenance of the passive range of motion to prevent the development of contractures, tightness and deformity, however the care has to be given to avoid the unnecessary stretch over the repaired portion of the nerve so that recovery can occur without hindrance.
- The strengthening of the remaining muscles or weak muscles to prevent the further loss of function and maintaining muscle strength in unaffected muscles.
- The use of the therapeutic currents has been studied extensively in case of nerve injuries to establish its therapeutic advantages.
- The completely denervated muscles may be stimulated by the use of large duration galvanic currents to deliver the large phase charge to stimulate muscle tissue. As the recovery of nerve occurs, the required phase charge reduces and the stimulation may be carried by relatively shorter duration of the current impulses.
- After the transfer or the nerve repair the muscles are generally weak, therefore the electrical stimulation may be required for improving the strength of the muscles and to make them re-perform the lost function.
- Beside re-educating the nerve function the low-frequency electrical stimulation can be used to speed up the recovery process of the nerve. When the majority of the nerve fibers have degenerated the galvanic current is needed to cause stimulation, but when the nerve fibers regenerate or escape injury the stimulation can be done with small phase charge faradic, surged faradic current and alternating current.
- Immediately post-operatively the bulky dressing is in place for around 2-3 weeks, therefore the work can be done only on the proximal and distal portion of the repair site while allowing the complete rest to the repaired site. Late on when the dressing is removed and the wound has healed the repaired site could also be subjected to the physiotherapy interventions.

- The sensory and motor re-education procedures may be used to augment the sensory and motor performance of the concerned regions of the repaired nerve. The sensory re-education may include the exposure to the variety of stimuli. These may include the tactile stimulation with the objects of different size, texture, and shape. The "contrast bath" may also help to improve the sensitivity of the region.
- For the neurogenic pain the long-term usage of the TENS (transcutaneous electric nerve stimulation) is advised which works by pain-gate theory to block the nociception (Gutman, 2001).
- Enhance the strength and the motor control of the affected extremity.
- Biofeedback to improve the control of the affected extremity.

The *orthotist management* aims to design the splints and slings or braces to support the affected extremity so as to minimize the adverse affect of gravity and other forces which could aggravate the condition of nerve injury. Splinting in the functional position is important to minimize the shortening or adhesion formation in the connective tissues including the ligaments, collateral ligaments. In case of radial nerve injury the cock-up splint may be used to maintain the position of the wrist and hand in case of wrist drop (Colditz et al, 1987). In shoulder dislocation cases the shoulder sling are important to prevent the downward directed forces on the underlying nerves.

CRANIAL NERVE

The spinal nerves were the nerves which had origin from the spinal cord while the cranial nerves are the nerves having origin directly from the brain including the cerebrum and brain stem.

The cranial nerves in human body are 12 pairs in number and are numbered in Roman numerals and each nerve has specific functions (Table 9.13.1). The assessment of the cranial testing is also specific (Table 9.13.2).

The sequence of the cranial nerves can be learned by following mnemonics indicating the first alphabet of the nerve's name:

On Our October Trip To Amarnath Found Very Great Views Across Hills

The first (Olfactory) and second (Optic) cranial nerves arise from the cerebrum while the remaining ten nerves (3rd to 12th nerve) originate from the brainstem.

TABLE 9.13.1 The cranial nerves and their functioning

Sequence of cranial nerve	*Name*	*Origin*	*Nature*	*Function*
I	Olfactory	Cerebrum	Sensory	Transmit sense of smell
II	Optic	Cerebrum	Sensory	Transmit sense of vision to brain Transmits the vision sensation to the brain Visual acuity is regulated by this nerve Regulates the ability to the see the peripheral vision Helps in the regulation of the direct (putting light in one eye causes constriction of same eye) and indirect pupillary reflex (putting light in one eye causes the constriction of the opposite eye too)
III	Oculomotor	Midbrain	Motor	Innervates muscles of eyes to regulate most of the eye movements with trochlear and abducens nerve Supplies sphincter papillae of eyes to control the accommodation reflex of eyes (as object moves towards eyes, the eyes converge and pupil constricts)
IV	Trochlear	Midbrain	Motor	Innervate the superior oblique muscle of eyes to depress, intort and extort eyeball Regulates accommodation reflex of eyes
V	Trigeminal	Pons	Both (sensory + motor)	Receives sensations from face Innervates the mastication muscle Regulates corneal reflex Regulates jaw reflex
VI	Abducens	Posterior margin of pons	Motor	Regulates accommodation reflex Innervates lateral rectus for abducting the eye

Contd...

Contd...

Sequence of cranial nerve	*Name*	*Origin*	*Nature*	*Function*
VII	Facial	Cerebellopon-tine angle	Both	Motor innervation to facial expression muscle and stapedius muscle of ear Taste form anterior 2/3rd of tongue Secretomotor to lacrimal and salivary gland
VIII	Vestibule-cochlear or stato-acoustic nerve	Cerebellopon-tine angle	Sensory	Transmit the sensation of hearing, balance and movement gravity Transmit sensations from semicircular canal Helps in maintaining the balance and equilibrium
IX	Glossopharyngeal	Medulla	Both	Regulates taste sensation from posterior 1/3rd of tongue Secretomotor to parotid gland Motor innervation to stylopharyngeus muscle
X	Vagus	Posterolateral sulcus of medulla	Both	Supplies laryngeal and pharyngeal muscles Regulates gag reflex Carries taste sensation from the pharyngeal wall Supplies palatoglossus muscle of tongue
XI	Accessory or cranial accessory or spinal accessory	Cranial and spinal root	Motor	Supplies muscles of shrugging the shoulder and neck movement
XII	Hypoglossal	Medulla	Motor	Regulates motor movement of tongue Regulates bolus formation of food Regulates speech articulation

TABLE 9.13.2 Assessment of different cranial nerves

Name	*Function*	*Test*
Olfactory	Smell	Test the each nostril separately with objects of different odors such as pungent smell, clove oil If unilateral loss is found rule out other causes of smell loss
Optic	Visual acuity	Visual acuity is checked by asking them to read the alphabets with progressively smaller size using Snellen chart
	Visual field Pupillary light reflex	Test the visual field with the perimetry and the fundoscopy putting light in one eye causes constriction of same eye (direct reflex) and putting light in one eye causes the constriction of the opposite eye too (indirect pupillary reflex)
Oculomotor	Pupillary reaction	Shine light in the eye and observe the constriction of same and opposite side eye
Trochlear	Eye movement	Check for presence of the abnormal features such as ptosis, eye position, nystagmus, accommodation Follow finger without moving the head to check the movement of the eyeballs
Trigeminal	Facial sensation	Check the touch sensations with a cotton wisp over the different branches of the trigeminal nerves
	Motor function	Check for the pain and temperature sensations too
	Jaw jerk	Ask the client to clench the teeth and palpate the temporalis region for the atrophy of temporalis and massector muscle Ask client to keep the jaw relaxed open, keep finger over the chin and tap it with reflex hammer. The jaw will reflexly close while tapped
	Corneal reflex	Touch the lateral aspect of cornea with a small cotton wisp, the blinking of the touched eyes show normal corneal sensation. The blinking action is motor activity executed by facial nerve therefore the facial nerve must be intact to check the corneal reflex too
Abducens	Motor function	Lateral eye movements especially towards abduction Check for presence of the abnormal features such as ptosis, eye position, nystagmus, accommodation of eyes

Contd...

Contd...

Name	*Function*	*Test*
Facial	Motor function	Check the strength of the facial muscles performing the action of smiling, frowning, wrinkle face, puff cheeks, whistle, closing eyes forcefully and against resistance of therapist While asked to close eye forcefully in the absence of motor activity the eyeball will roll upward and this phenomenon is called as Bells phenomenon. Platysma is checked by asking the client to draw down the angles of mouth while tightening the neck muscles
	Sensory	Taste sensation from the anterior 2/3rd of the tongue Put a litmus paper on the lateral corner of the eyelid, if this paper turns blue due to the secretion of eye it shows normal nerve functioning Ask the client for the presence of the Hyperacusis due to the paralysis of the stapedius muscle
	Secreto-motor	Ask the client about the complaint of the dry mouth, dry eyes (xerophthalmia)
Vestibule-cochlear	Hearing	Whisper the sound in front of each ear and check for the any difference observed in any of the ear Check for the bone and air conduction of sounds in ear Audiometry is helpful to locate and identify the type of hearing impairment. The presence of foreign body in ear canal has to be ruled out
	Balance	Rhomberg's Test—by asking the client to stand erect firstly with eyes closed and then with eyes open. With eyes close if the balance is lost or the sway significantly increase, this may reveal the balance impairment, however the presence of the sensation in the lower extremity has to be ensured to avoid the false positive findings of lost balance

Contd...

Contd...

Name	*Function*	*Test*
Glossopharyngeal	Sensations	Check the taste sensation in the posterior 1/3rd of the tongue
	Secretomotor	Ask the client for presence of dry-mouth secondary to the reduced supply of the parotid gland
	Gag reflex	Contraction of the pharynx elicited by touching the posterior pharyngeal wall
	Swallowing and	Check for the swallowing function and see the movement of pharyngeal wall while the client says "AH"
	Voice quality	The voice may be partially hoarse or abnormal due to the paralysis of the sylopharyngeus muscle
Vagus	Motor	See the function of the palate or pharynx by using tongue depressor, and observe the position of soft palate while the client phonates. Check for the symmetry of the soft palate on both the sides
		Observe the position of vocal cords at rest, during inspiration and during expiration
		Test the pharyngeal and laryngeal wall by test the client's ability to cough
	Gag reflex	Check gag reflex same as for glossopharyngeal nerve
		Presence of regurgitation reveals the impairment of the vagus nerve
Spinal accessory	Neck motion and shrugging	Check the strength of the shoulder shrugging and neck movement muscles
		Check the atrophy of sternocleidomastoid muscle (SCM)
Hypoglossal	Motor, check for the tongue strength and movement	Ask the client to protrude the tongue and note whether tongue is protruding in midline or deviated on one side
		Observe any wasting of the tongue (most early seen in the lateral margins of the tongue)
		In the advanced cases of the nerve injury the wrinkling of the tongue occurs along-with the presence of fasciculation and atrophy
		Ask the client to protrude the tongue against resistance with a tongue depressor

The mnemonic to remember the nature of the nerve function can be learned as:

"*S*ome *s*ay *m*oney *m*atters, *b*ut *m*y *b*rother *s*ays *b*ig *b*rains *m*atter *m*ore. [S=Sensory; M= Motor; B=Both Motor as well as Sensory]

In case of the unilateral loss of hypoglossal function, the mild difficulties with speaking may occur but swallowing is not impaired. However in case of bilateral impairment, the speech difficulty along with severe difficulty in swallowing (Keane JR, 1996). In the cases of severe difficulty in swallowing, the feeding training may need the tipping of head necessarily for swallowing (Feldman et al, 2005).

BELL'S PALSY

Bell's palsy is the sudden onset, unilateral, idiopathic form of peripheral facial paresis (weakness) or paralysis having no known cause. It is the most common neurological disorder of the cranial nerve, and especially the incidence increases during the winters. In majority of cases the unilateral involvement occurs however very rarely bilateral involvements can occur.

Onset and Presentation

The onset of the Bell's palsy is sudden and mostly is confused with the stroke.

The presenting features may be similar to the facial nerve entrapments and may include the following presentation during the facial muscle paresis:

- Pain in the mastoid region behind the ears.
- The excessive tear and running eyes due to the poor functioning of the orbicularis oculi muscle.
- Hyperacusis—the sudden perception of even the very less loud sound.

The physical appearance of the facial expressions is as follows (Fig 9.13.1):

- The weakness of the facial muscles is easily observable
- The weakness or paresis or paralysis of all the upper and lower face muscles is apparent
- Eye closure is not complete and while attempting the eye closure the eyes roll upward (Bells'a phenomenon)
- Dropping of the face
- Dropping of the lower corner of mouth

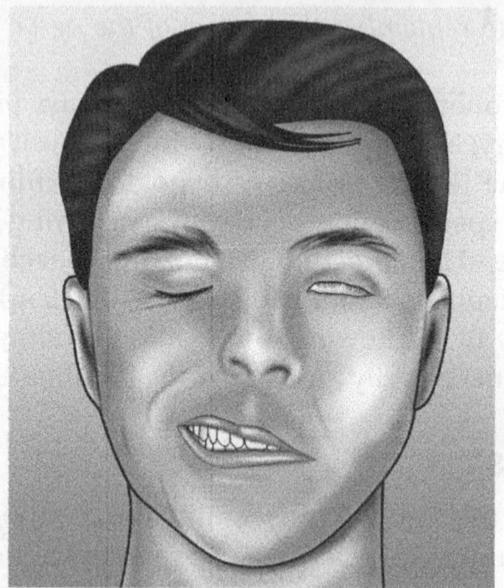

Fig. 9.13.1: The facial muscle weakness

- Closing the eye is difficult and incomplete
- Speaking, whistling is difficult because the air cannot remain inside mouth and leaks out form the unclosed corner of mouth
- The non-verbal gestures are lost (laughing, pleasure, facial expression, surprise, interest, worries).

Diagnosis

The exact cause of the Bell's palsy is not known however the idiopathic involvement (McCormick , 1972) is established and the temporary dysfunction of the facial nerve (7th cranial nerve) has been reported (May et al, 1983). Due to the involvement of the facial nerve the symptoms and presentation may be similar to the facial nerve palsy except few differences (discussed later).

In fact, during the sudden onset facial muscle paralysis the other causative factors have to be ruled out to lay down the idiopathic origin. Therefore, the Bell's palsy is the disease of the exclusion.

Sequel

The sudden onset of the facial muscle paresis in case of the Bell's palsy may be frightening for the patients due to the fear of the stroke, tumor, neuropathy, etc.

In majority of the cases of Bell's palsy the recovery occurs completely and spontaneously over 4-6 weeks (Peitersen, 1982), however rare number of cases continue to present with the following problems for extended time or permanently:

- Partial residual paralysis or paresis
- Some involuntary movements while performing the voluntary movement of the face (facio-motor synkinesis)
- Involuntary lacrimation after the voluntary movement of facial muscles (autonomic synkinesis).

Causes

The exact cause of the Bell's palsy is not known however the following conditions may put the facial nerve to undergo temporary and irreversible inflammation of the Bell's palsy and therefore have to be ruled out:

- Otitis media (acute as well as chronic)
- Rupture of the ear drum
- The infection in the ear canal
- Viral infections such as rubella, mumps, herpes simplex, cytomegalovirus
- The surgery in the ear or throat region
- Polyneuritis
- Parotid tumors
- Herpes zoster—the small blisters and vesicles are seen on the body
- Cardiofacial syndrome (lower lip palsy).

Management

The true Bell's palsy has very good prognosis due to its self limiting nature. The management of the Bell's palsy starts immediately after its onset and continues even when the results of the investigative procedures are awaited. The goals of the management (Rowlands et al, 2001) consist of the preventing the neuronal damage; the enhancement of the recovery process; preserving the strength of the involved muscle till the recovery does not occur.

The first line of management consists of the:

- Relaxation of the client to reduce the anxiety
- The supportive therapy
- Protection of the eyes from getting dried

- Initiating appropriate means to start anti-inflammatory interventions
- The American academy of the neurology recommends the use of the acyclovir and the prednisone for the faster reduction of the probable nerve inflammation and the faster recovery of the client (Grogan and Gronseth, 2001).

During the flaccid state of the muscles the orthotic intervention may be given in form of the "S" shaped clip to support the corner of mouth for preventing the dropping of the corner of mouth

Non-pharmacological approaches consist of the physical therapy (McCormick, 1972), gentle massaging, acupuncture and the orthotic supports.

The proper eye care:

- Avoiding the excessive drying of the eyes
- Use saline eye drops each half hourly
- Wash faces and eye frequently without applying the excessive stretch or the pressure over the weak muscles
- During sleep the eyes must be covered with a wet cloth to avoid the excessive dryness and the fall of foreign object in to the eye
- During sleep the eye lubricants are advised
- The artificial tears are used to avoid the dryness of eye and prevent corneal ulceration.

Exercises for the facial muscles:

- Perform the exercise for the facial muscles (including the muscles of the facial expression)
- Look surprise
- Look frowning
- Close tight and open wide eyes
- Fill air in mouth
- Smile and do grinning
- Say words like "Oh", "we", "aaiee", "you"
- Hold straw in mouth to perform the sucking of juices
- Hold straw in mouth and blow air out to make bubbles in water
- Whistle
- Blow off the candle
- Fill the balloons with mouth
- Fill air in mouth
- Suck in large volume of air in mouth, and then shift the air inside closed mouth from one part of mouth to other.

Electrical stimulation:

- While the recovery process is still underway, the artificial electric stimulation is advised to preserve the contractibility of the muscles and the excitability of the nerve
- The intermittent galvanic stimulation with the small periods of frequent stimulation may be recommended
- The prolonged stimulation of localized region should be avoided as it may lead to the chemical or electric burns.

Facial massage with gentle effleurage strokes is helpful to prevent the edema of the facial muscles.

In the rare cases of the Bell's palsy where the recovery remains absent or irreversibly incomplete, the electrodiagnostic findings may be recommended. If found unfavorable, the surgical interventions may be recommended for causing the decompression of the compression region of the nerve (Dellon, 1992).

FACIAL PARALYSIS

Facial palsy is the supra-nuclear (Upper motor neuron) lesion characterized by the weakness and the movement loss of the lower part of the face or the more severely than those of the upper face muscles. The weakness is presented in all those muscle which are supplied by the facial nerve. This is the upper motor neuron lesion type condition unlike the Bell's palsy which is a lower motor neuron type (due to the infra-nuclear involvement) paralysis of the facial nerve supplied muscles.

This supra-nuclear lesion involves the weakness of the muscles of the emotional presentation of the face, and mimics paralysis.

Features of the Facial Palsy

- Difficulty in closing the eyes completely and forcefully
- The continuous drooling of the saliva from mouth
- Speech difficulty is faced and the voice does not remain clear
- The emotional expression and the facial expressions are lost including the loss of the expression of the joy, sadness, sorrow, surprise
- The face appears to be the totally blank and expression less.

Anatomy of the Facial Nerve

Facial nerve is the 7th cranial nerve and originates from the facial nucleus of the lower pontine area. The facial nucleus is under the control of the frontal lobe of the cerebral cortex by the corticobulbar fibers.

The upper portion of the facial nucleus has the corticobulbar fibers from the bilateral cerebral cortex, while the lower part of the facial nucleus has the fibers which cross to the contralateral side to supply the lower facial muscles of the opposite side. The upper portion has the bilateral innervation and supplies the upper part of face including the forehead. Therefore in order to observe the complete paralysis of the forehead region the corticobulbar projections from both the frontal lobes must have been impaired. The lower portion of the facial nucleus supplies the contralateral side of the lower face muscles including buccinator, platysma, stylohyoid and the posterior belly of digastric muscle.

The facial nerve divides into three branches near the angle of mandible. These three branches are the ophthalmic (upper branch), mandibular and the maxillary.

The upper branch innervated frontalis (frowning muscle), orbicularis oculi (for closure of the upper eyelid), corrugators supercilli.

The zygomatic branch supplies the zygomatic major and minor (smiling muscle), levator labi superioris (the elevation of the upper lip), the dilator nasalis (for the dilatation of the nostrils).

The buccal branch innervates the buccinators (the puffing muscle of mouth) and the orbicularis oris (opening of the mouth).

The mandibular division innervates the risorius (smiling muscle), depressor labii inferioris (for the depression of the lower lip), mentalis, and lower parts of the orbicularis oris muscle.

The injury to the facial nerve may be incomplete (neuroprexia) when the portion of the nerve is involved; or the complete (when the whole nerve is involved).

Causes of the Facial Palsy

- Skull base fracture
- The fracture of the mastoid process or the adjoining region
- The excessive pressure within ear canal such as during deep water diving
- Infection of the middle and inner ear—otitis media, otitis interna, mastoiditis
- Metabolic pathologies such as diabetes, hypertension
- Tumor of the parotid gland
- Facial nerve tumor

- The surgery of the parotid gland
- The osteomyelitis or the osteopetrosis of the mastoid process or the internal auditory meatus.

Clinical Presentation

The onset of the features of the facial nerve involvement may occur either sudden onset or the gradual onset.

The location of the involved site, the possible etiology and the prognosis of the facial nerve paralysis is important to be documented.

- Careful history about the possible causes of the facial nerve involvement must be noted. These may include the chronic or acute ottitis media; the herpex zoster infection; the cytomegalovirus or the history of the surgery to the middle or the inner ear. The other causes such as the parotid gland tumor; long standing ear pain or post-auricular pain may be other causative factors.
- A complete and detailed examination of the head and neck region is important.
- The careful note about the salivation, tearing, taste, sound perception is important.
- The strengthening of the muscles supplied by different branches of the facial nerve.
- The muscles of the facial expressions must be checked for the strength and the functioning.

INVESTIGATIVE PROCESS

- The investigative procedures are recommended for identification of the causative factor of the facial palsy.
- CT and MRI scans are useful to locate the intracranial lesions or fractures. Also these are helpful for the visualization of the facial nerve across its course, its discontinuity or the swelling.
- Electrodiagnostic methods to determine the extent of the nerve disruption.
- Laboratory investigation to diagnose any infection or the tumor.

Management

For the management of the synkinesis and hyperkinesis the botulinum toxin injection.

In the cases of the cases where the nerve recovery fails and the prognosis of recovery is absent, the surgical interventions are advised.

The unpredictable prognosis of the surgical outcomes and the poor possibility of regaining the facial symmetry and balance must be explained to the client before surgical interventions.

The surgical options available for the facial paralysis include the nerve grafting, the nerve reconstruction, tendon transfer surgeries are advised (Skirven and Callahan, 2002).

9.14: NEURITIS AND NEURALGIA-BRACHIAL, SCIATICA

Neuritis is the inflammation of the nerve.

CAUSES

The inflammation of the nerve can occur due to the various possible causes some of them are as follows:

- Mechanical factors could be involved in the inflammatory processes within nerve
- The excessive pressure over the nerve due to the surrounding tissue irritation, the pressure due to the bony prominences (osteophytes, extra ribs, the fracture, the ulnar nerve irritation due to excessive cubitus valgus), the pressure due to the ends of the fractured bones and the healing callus of the fracture site (the Tardy ulnar nerve palsy after the friction due to the healing callus of the medial humeral epicondylar fracture).
- The excessive pressure due to the POP cast (used for stabilization of fractures), or the splints or crutches or the tight plaster casts
- Direct mechanical pressure over the nerve due to tumor
- Trauma such as contusion, the irritation secondary to the bruises
- The systemic pathologies such as diabetes mellitus, rheumatic arthritis, Reiter's syndrome
- The toxic pathologies such as arsenic, lead toxicopathy
- The metabolic causes such as diabetes mellitus, vitamin B_{12} deficiency, Beriberi, hypothyroidism, alcoholic neuropathy, porphyria
- *Infective causes*: Herpes simplex, leprosy, GBS, herpes zoster shingels

- *Chemical injury*—The contact with acids
- Radiation exposure
- Autoimmune diseases such as Multiple Sclerosis

Signs and Symptoms

The presenting feature of the neuritis varies with the number and type of nerve(s) involved, the cause of the nerve inflammation, the severity of the nerve involvement.

The common presentation of the neuritis is initially associated with the pain in the affected nerve distribution, the pain, the muscles (myalgia) supplied by the affected nerve, altered sensation and the pain hypersensitivity in the sensory region supplied by the affected nerve.

As the extent of the nerve pathology progresses the more prominent symptoms such as numbness, tingling, pins and needle sensations, muscles cramps, weakness tremors may occur. In more prominent cases the complete nerve may get damaged or the neurotmesis may occur resulting in the complete loss of function, the complete paralysis of the muscles supplied by the affected nerve, and the complete loss of deep tendon reflex (DTR). The autonomic changes may occur such as loss of blood flow regulation, the skin nutrition; the dry, wrinkled and the scaly appearance of the skin supplied by the affected nerve. In prolonged cases of the severe neuritis the complete nerve damage may occur leading to the signs of the complete denervation such as the fasciculations, the tremors.

The neuritis affects the peripheral nerves therefore the features are presented in the distribution region of the affected nerve. The increased pain sensitivity occurs, due to which the client may complain of the excessive pain with the sensations such as touch. Even the touch of the cloth or hair or the cold air may elicit pain. For the purpose of assessment, pathology identification and the management the difference between neuritis and similarly representing neuralgia, have to be laid down (Table 9.14.1).

Treatment

The most optimal treatment of the neuritis or the neuralgia depends on the cause of symptoms and it aims at the pain relief and preservation of symptoms. The causative factors are dealt with the medical or surgical interventions, while the associated symptoms, complications and pain are dealt with physiotherapy interventions.

TABLE 9.14.1 Differences between neuritis and neuralgia

Neuritis	*Neuralgia*
Includes the inflammation of the nerve or its covering (epineurium, perineurium, endoneurium)	Does not involve the inflammatory process in the nerve or its sheath
The causes of the neuritis may involve the metabolic, nutrition, systemic pathologies	The most common cause of the neuralgia is the pressure or the poor nutrition or the nerve root avulsion
The pain occurs as acute, dull or aching type pain	The nature of the pain includes intense pain, sharp shooting, throbbing
The pain is more continuous unless analgesics or the anti-inflammatory medicines taken	The pain is more intermittent compared to the neuritis
The reflexes are normal in case of interstitial neuritis	There may be muscle twitches or tremors due to the irritation of the motor fibers, however the paralysis does not occur due to the neuralgia itself

Physiotherapy Treatment

Cryotherapy—helps to reduce the inflammation and allows the recovery of the nerve.

Massage is generally not tolerated by majority of the neuritis patients, due to increased sensitivity of pain towards the touch or pressure. However in cases where the sensitivity is not high, the gentle strokes of effleurage helps to reduce the spasm and alleviation of pain to acceptable extent.

In cases of the neuritis affecting the parenchyma of nerve the management needs to be similar to that of the complete peripheral nerve injury. The prevention of pressure sore, the heat burn and the cut injuries are important. The prevention of contractures and joint deformity is highly important; however the causative pathology has to be simultaneously dealt with.

The passive ROM exercises may be desirable in cases of the significant nerve inflammation, however it must be kept in mind that in no way the interventions must aggravate inflammatory processes. Therefore, during Passive Rom or active-assisted ROM exercises the traction or the stretching or the friction of the affected nerve has to be avoided.

The complete rest of the affected nerve is important to avoid the aggravation of the inflammation. For this purpose the slab, splint and the sling may be useful. The active movement of the bony lever and muscles may cause the traction over the nerve or the gliding of nerve, therefore the complete rest of the affected extremity may be necessary depending on the extent of nerve involvement.

TENS (Transcutaneous Electrical Nerve Stimulation) is found to be highly useful and a safe modality for the management of the pain associated with the neuralgia and neuropathy. The placement of the electrodes and the number of the channels used for the management of the pain, depends on the extent and size of the painful region. Depending on the pain location and distribution the placement of the electrodes of a channel may be as follows:

- One electrode proximal and one electrode distal to the painful region
- The placement of the electrodes over the course of the nerve
- The placement of the electrodes over the same dermatomal region, as involved in the painful region
- The placement of the electrodes over the nerve roots or the spinal segments supplying the region of the pain
- The placement of the electrodes over the same region of the contra-lateral extremity.

Generally depending on the severity of pain, the TENS therapy may be given from one hour to several hours per day for each patient. The maximum pain relief in neuralgic conditions may occur up to 4-6 weeks (Jin et al, 2010) however the pain relief beyond this duration is generally not very significant.

However one must keep in mind that the TENS is not the treatment modality rather a supportive modality. Therefore, if the causative factors are not treated while using the TENS for pain relief, the pain relief does not sustain beyond a month after the pain relief by TENS (Peiber et al, 2010).

In chronic cases the nerve tissue mobility exercises (the neural tissue tension techniques) are helpful to break the adhesion of the nerve sheath with the surrounding nerve sheath. This is important to increase the nerve excursion and to avoid the nerve traction.

Brachial Neuralgia

Anatomy

Brachium is the region located between shoulder and the elbow, pain of this region is commonly considered to be the brachial neuralgia, however the accurate pathology of the brachial neuralgia must include the region of the upper extremity innervated by the nerves from the brachial plexus. The pain of the brachial neuralgia may be manifested in the region of shoulder, upper arm, forearm and/or hand region. This pain may occur either of the upper, middle or the lower cord of the brachial plexus.

Introduction

Brachial neuralgia is a rare condition which affects the brachial plexus, and is characterized by severe, burning pain in the shoulder and upper arm accompanied with pronounced upper arm weakness in any of the muscle or region innervated by the brachial plexus. The symptoms exist in form of combinations of symptoms therefore indicated involvement of the multifocal lesions.

Brachial neuralgia (BN) may involve any muscle or any region innervated by the brachial plexus, in any way and combination of symptoms, indicating involvement of multifocal lesions.

Incidence

- The true brachial neuralgia is a rare type of condition.
- Previous reports found the incidence of about 2-3 cases per 100000 (MacDonald et al, 2000) however the incidence reports on Indian population is lacking.
- The incidence of brachial neuralgia is seen among those who have sedentary occupations such as prolonged use of the computers, prolonged TV watching, the drivers, etc.

Clinical Features

Matric, et al (2010) described the following presentation of the brachial neuralgia:

- Pain is the most dominant feature
- Pain is most severe in acute phase
- Pain appears suddenly and unprovoked as burning pain
- Pain aggravates if arm is firmly pressed against body during sleep, therefore it causes sleep disturbance

- Pain is very intense and most of patients do report unbearable and most intense pain ever felt (usually the reported pain scores 7 or higher on 10 point VAS scale)
- The clinical picture may present as motor or sensory presentation depending on the type of nerve involved
- Sometimes the pain may appears in the distributions of the nerves, which do not belong to brachial plexus therefore diagnosis may be difficult to be made
- In most of patients (upto 89%) the pain aggravates during night, especially between midnight and 7 a.m. It therefore disturbs sleep and causes severe exhaustion due to lack of rest.

Beside these manifestations, the pain is usually of the sharp-shooting type, stabbing, burning, radiating in nature. The pain is definitely disabling and may come in form of light flashes. The client is mostly afraid of having the relapse of similar pain.

The pain stays for relatively longer duration among males while compared to the female counterpart.

Causes

The pathology of the brachial neuralgia may involve anything which could cause the:

- Irritation of the brachial plexus or the associated nerves
- Inflammation of the brachial plexus or the associated nerves
- Compression or the pinching of the brachial plexus or the associated nerves.

Diagnosis

Diagnosis is difficult to be made due to variety of factors and highly variable presentation.

During early stage most of the cases cannot be distinguished from the other diseases of the cervical spine and arm (Matric et al, 2010).

Majority of patients are misdiagnosed and cervical radiculopathy or problem of the shoulder joint.

The brachial neuralgia pain on left side of body may be confused with the referred pain related to the heart attack.

One important distinguish between brachial neuralgia and cervical radiculopathy can be made by local palpation and the nerve tension tests. In case of the cervical radiculopathy these tests are positive, while in most of the brachial neuralgia these tests are negative.

Muscle weakness in the brachial neuralgia my develop within 13 days in males and 8 days in females (Matric et al, 2010).

Differential Diagnosis

- Cervical radiculopathy
- Multifocal neuropathy
- Joint pathology of shoulder, elbow or cervical region
- Tumor.

Physiotherapy Management

The physiotherapy management of the brachial neuralgia is similar to that of the neuritis or the sciatica. Due to the irritation of the nerve or the brachial plexus portion, the rest in the soft collar is important in certain cases. The cause of the the brachial plexus or the associated nerves irritation has to be ruled out.

Sciatica

Sciatica is the condition characterized with the pain in lower back region along with the route of the sciatic nerve and its distribution. Sciatic nerve is the largest and thickest nerve in body therefore the route of pain includes the lower lumbar or the lumbo-sacral region, the buttock region, posterior aspect of thigh, posterior aspect calf and the foot region. Pain radiation may be in one or both of the lower extremity.

Features

Pain is generally the sharp-shooting in nature.

The aggravated with the increased intra-abdominal pressure or by the mechanisms that increase the stretch over the sciatic nerve.

The clients complain the pain starting from the lower lumbar region (either one or both paravertebral region; the lumbo-sacral junction) and travelling upto the whole route of the sciatic nerve. In cases of the significant compression over the nerve the numbness may be felt in the course of nerve or over the foot region due to the complete impede of the nerve impulses through nerve.

The ankle jerk is diminished or completely absent.

Pain increase with the sneezing, coughing, trunk flexion.

Causes

Sciatica is caused due to the compression and/or irritation of the sciatic nerve.

The patients in majority of cases report the complaint of sudden onset pain after lifting the heavy weight or while assuming the flexion posture or while returning to neutral spine position from the trunk flexed position. In the first few hours or days the pain may remain localized to the lower back region and then it progresses down quickly.

The common causes related to the sciatica can be as follows:

- The prolapsed inter-vertebral disc in the spine
- The osteophytes formed in the vertebral bodies can impinge upon the adjacent nerve roots
- The degenerative changes in the vertebral bodies of the spine related to the lumbar spondylosis or fracture or the spondylolisthesis
- The formation of the tumor or the malignant growth in the vertebral region.

Symptoms

The most common complaint of the sciatica is the pain and the numbness or the tingling like sensation in the route of the sciatic nerve.

The pain and the tingling can appear after the period of the prolonged sitting or after lifting the heavy weight, after sneezing/coughing or the trunk flexion.

Diagnosis

Diagnosis of the sciatica is generally based on the history, presenting features and the clinical testing of the client. The confirmation may be done with the help of MRI to determine the exact extent of the disc herniation, the nerve root obstruction and the status of the spine.

The investigative procedures may be used for ruling out the other medical or more serious causes of the sciatica.

The straight leg raising test (SLR) is mostly positive (Fig. 9.14.1) with the reproduction of the pain between the 30 to 70 degree hip flexion with knee straight in the supine lying position.

Pain may appear in peripheral fashion or the centralization manner. In the peripheral form of sciatica the pain starts in the spine and extends or progresses downward towards the calf or ankle. In the centrally directed fashion the pain starts in the calf and leg, and progresses proximally towards the spine.

The deep tendon reflex is diminished or absent in the ankle jerk.

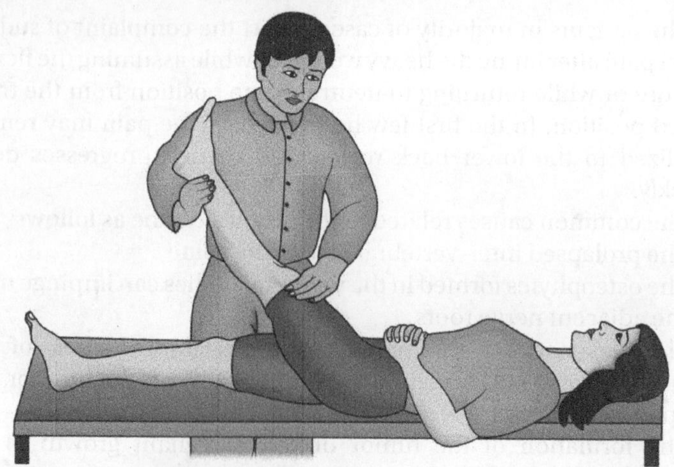

Fig. 9.14.1: The straight leg raise (SLR) assessment of the sciatica. In sciatica the pain is present in range of the 35 to 70 degree of passive hip flexion with knee extended

The motor weakness may be seen in the myotome corresponding to the affected nerve root. The client may assume the limp or the antalgic gait during ambulation.

Treatment

Self-care at Home

- The client must be instructed to avoid the postures which aggravate the traction over the nerves. In case of sciatic nerve inflammation (sciatica), the client must avoid certain postures such as:- excessive bending, the jerky movements of spine and lower extremity, the forceful kicking movement of simultaneous hip flexion with knee extension, the heavy weight lifting, sitting on lower chair, use of the Indian style low height lavatory.
- In case of the ulnar neuritis, the client must avoid the repeated elbow flexion and extension as it would aggravate the traction over the ulnar nerve.
- *The resting position of nerve:* The rest of the nerve in comfortable and the relaxed position is important. In sciatica, the bed rest in comfortable position, with gentle hip and knee flexed posture in

side lying position (the position is also called as Fetal position). The crook lying position with a pillow under the knees help to flatten the lordosis and helps to reduce the traction over the nerve.

Physiotherapy Interventions

The gentle massage of the gluteal region muscles (if touch sensitivity is not high) helps to improve the circulation while simultaneously activating the mechanoreceptors for causing pain relief

The gentle breathing exercises and deep breathing exercises in cases where bed rest is recommended due to significant sciatic nerve inflammation. There is little evidence to support the use of bed rest for acute pain (Van tudler, et al. 1997).

Gentle active contractions of the gluteal muscles, the prone lying passive trunk extension are advised so as to slack the sciatic nerve. As the condition of the client improves, the further progression may be recommended. The exercises of the spine would be recommended as per the cause of the sciatic nerve involvement. If the cause of the sciatica includes the prolapsed intervertebral disc posterior herniation, the spinal extension exercises are helpful (Fig. 9.14.2). If the cause of the nerve inflammation lies anterior to the nerve root in the spinal canal, the flexion exercises would be helpful.

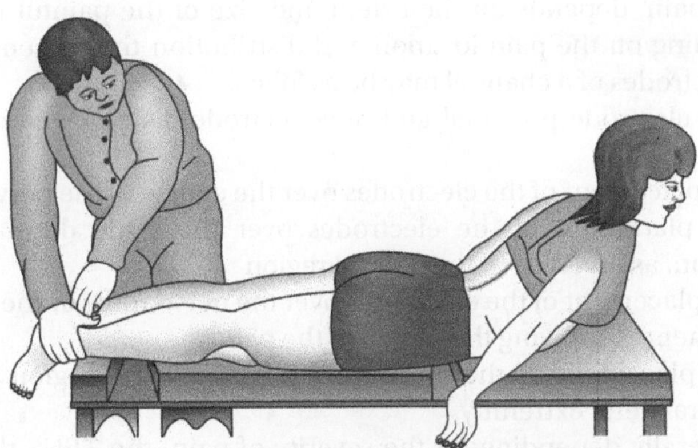

Fig. 9.14.2: The active spinal extension exercise in case of low back pain

The reduction of the inflammation is also achieved with the help of the cryotherapy application. The cryotherapy may be given in form of the ice packs, the direct application of ice in a towel, the ice massage. The site of the cryotherapy application includes the area presenting with the soreness, inflammation and the pain.

The sciatica related pain is minimal in the position of the crook supine lying with a pillow under knees, the prone lying, the side lying fetal position, or the reclining chair position.

The lumbosacral support orthosis (the lumbar belt) may be recommended in the clients having acute pain, however the prolonged and unjudicial use of these orthosis may worsen the sciatica due to the weakness or the altered proprioception of the spinal muscles and the related proprioceptors.

Similarly the rest or bed rest is advisable during acute phases of the pain, however the bed rest beyond two days is discouraged as it would lead to the weakness of the muscles. The client is advised to stay active within the limits of the pain, and must avoid the pain aggravating postures and tasks.

Relaxation exercises help the client to develop better awareness of own's body and helps to relieve the muscular spasm.

TENS (transcutaneous electrical nerve stimulation) is found to be highly useful and a safe modality for the management of the pain associated with the neuralgia and neuropathy. The placement of the electrodes and the number of the channels used for the management of the pain, depends on the extent and size of the painful region. depending on the pain location and distribution the placement of the electrodes of a channel may be as follos:

- One electrode proximal and one electrode distal to the painful region
- The placement of the electrodes over the course of the nerve
- The placement of the electrodes over the same dermatomal region, as involved in the painful region
- The placement of the electrodes over the nerve roots or the spinal segments supplying the region of the pain
- The placement of the electrodes over the same region of the contralateral extremity.

Generally depending on the severity of pain, the TENS therapy may be given from one hour to several hours per day for each patient. The maximum pain relief in neuralgic conditions may occur up to 4-6 weeks (Jin, et al. 2010) however, the pain relief beyond this duration is generally not very significant.

However, one must keep in mind that the TENS is not the treatment modality rather a supportive modality. Therefore if the causative factors are not treated while using the TENS for pain relief, the pain relief does not sustain beyond a month after the pain relief by TENS (Peiber, et al. 2010).

In cases of the significant sciatic nerve impairment, the weakness of the lower extremity muscles (may affect quadriceps, hamstrings or the ankle dorsi or plantar flexors) occurs. For speeding up the recovery process, the faradic nerve stimulation (faradism) is recommended to improve the function and strength of the weak muscles.

In recovery phases and the chronic phases of the sciatica, the stretching and flexibility exercises of the lower extremity muscles (hamstring and posterior calf muscle) are advised. Similarly the spinal muscle strengthening exercises, spinal endurance exercises and the core stabilization exercises (special emphasis on the multifidus and transverses abdominis muscle) are recommended. The core stabilization exercises are found to be useful for the prevention of the low back pain and for the functional enhancement (such as balance performance) in case of those (Aggarwal, et al. 2010) who are at higher risk of developing low back pain (Table 9.14.2).

In cases where radicular signs are present, the pain fails to centralize with movement, or may present the lateral shift/list, the mechanical traction or auto-traction is used to help the client for centralizing the features (Fritz, et al. 2003).

Patients, who exhibit the centralization of pain during lumbar spine ROM testing, are treated with specific exercises (flexion or extension) which help to promote the centralization of symptoms (Fritz, et al. 2003; Werneke and Hart, 2001). The patients, who present the history of the previous episodes of "instability catches" are believed to have clinical instability in the spine (Fritz, et al. 2003; Ogon, et al. 1997). The trunk strengthening exercises and trunk stabilization exercises are found to be effective (Kumar, et al. 2009).

TABLE 9.14.2 Protocol for core stability training for prevention of low back pain and balance enhancement (Aggarwal, et al. 2010)

Week 1	
Abdominal muscle: Contraction in crook supine lying position	3 x 15 repetitions
Abdominal muscle: Contraction in prone lying position	3 x 15 repetitions
Abdominal muscle: Contraction in quadruped position	3 x 15 repetitions
Abdominal muscle: Contraction while standing on single limb	1 x 10 repetitions on each leg
Abdominal muscle: Contraction in crook supine lying position	3 x 15 repetitions
Week 2 (Session 4–6)	
Abdominal muscle: Contraction in crook lying (base position)	1 x 20 repetitions
Base position + foot lift	2 x 10
Bird dog extension	15 repetitions each leg
Seated medicine ball rotation	3 x 15
Week 3 (Session 7–9)	
Abdominal muscle: Contraction	1 x 20
Seated on Swiss ball	3 x 15 repetitions
Squat with Swiss ball	3 x 10 repetitions
Superman	2 x 10 repetitions
Week 4 (session 10–12)	
Abdominal muscle: Contraction	1 x 20 contractions
Multi-direction lunges	2 x 10 repetitions each extremity
Oblique pulley with side shuffle	15 repetitions each side rotation
Standing wall cross toss	15 repetitions on each side
Week 5 (session 13–15)	
Abdominal contraction	1 x 20 contractions
Diagonal Curls on Swiss ball	10 repetitions each side
Twist on Swiss ball	10 repetitions each side
Week 6 (session 16–18)	
Front plank stability ball	2 x 10 repetitions.
Back bridge on stability ball	2 x 10 repetitions
Stability ball pitcher squat	10 repetitions each lower extremity
Front plank stability ball	2 x 10 repetitions.

9.15: POLIOMYELITIS

It is also known as polio or infective paralysis.

Polio, or poliomyelitis, is a highly contagious viral infection that can lead to paralysis, breathing problems, or even death. The term poliomyelitis is from the Greek poliós meaning grey, myelós referencing the spinal cord, and -itis meaning inflammation.

- Inflammation of "grey matter of the spinal cord"
- Three types of virus:
  - Type I (Brunhilde)
  - Type II (Lansing)
  - Type III (Leon).

PATHOPHYSIOLOGY

Poliovirus is an RNA virus that is transmitted through the oral-fecal route or by ingestion of contaminated water. Three serotypes are able to cause human infection. The incubation period for poliovirus is 5–35 days. The viral particles initially replicate in the nasopharynx and gastrointestinal (GI) tract and then invade lymphoid tissues, with subsequent hematologic spread. After a period of viremia, the virus becomes neurotropic and produces destruction of the motor neurons in the anterior horn and brainstem. The destruction of motor neurons leads to the development of flaccid paralysis, which may be bulbar or spinal in distribution.

Mortality/Morbidity

Mortality is more frequently in cases of paralytic poliomyelitis with complications such as respiratory failure.

In certain cases of mild to moderate respiratory involvement, the respiratory failure may not be always be manifested. Such possibility may be suspected in the patients presenting with the headache, sleep problems, morning headache, sleep apnea, disorientation, chronic hypoventilation. Therefore upon finding these features, the appropriate referral to the respiratory specialist may be needed for proper investigation and intervention (Bach and Tilton, 1997).

Fatigue, morning headache, sleep disturbance, difficult arousal, daytime somnolence, impaired concentration, memory and irritability, chronic alveolar hypoventilation and sleep apnea should be suspected and patients referred to respiratory specialists.

Sex

Males and females of pediatric age are affected with equal frequency.

Age

Poliovirus affects mainly children. However, individuals of any age (especially those who are immunocompromised) may also develop the disease.

Signs and Symptoms

There are four recognized stages:

1. Acute paralysis and/or weakness
2. Recovery and rehabilitation
3. Neurological stability
4. Post-polio syndrome/sequelae.

The spectrum of disease varies from inapparent infection to paralytic disease.

- In mild cases, the following non-specific signs and symptoms are observed and usually resolve within a few days:
  - Fever
  - Headache
  - Nausea
  - Vomiting
  - Abdominal pain
  - Oropharyngeal hyperemia
- Non-paralytic poliomyelitis is characterized by the symptoms described above in addition to the following:
  - Nuchal rigidity
  - More severe headache
  - Back and lower extremity pain
  - Meningitis with lymphocytic pleocytosis (usually)
- Paralytic poliomyelitis occurs in fewer than 5% of affected patients and is characterized by the following:
  - Compromise of the motor neurons may be localized or widespread
  - More frequently, asymmetric loss of muscle function is observed with involvement of major muscle groups
  - Muscle atrophy is generally observed several weeks after the beginning of symptoms
  - Recovery may be complete, partial, or absent.

SUBCLINICAL INFECTION

- No symptoms, or symptoms lasting 72 hours or less
- Slight fever
- Headache
- General discomfort or uneasiness (malaise)

- Sore throat
- Red throat
- Vomiting.

NON-PARALYTIC POLIOMYELITIS

- Symptoms last 1 to 2 weeks
- Moderate fever
- Headache
- Vomiting
- Diarrhea
- Excessive tiredness, fatigue
- Irritability
- Pain or stiffness of the back, arms, legs, abdomen
- Muscle tenderness and spasm in any area of the body
- Neck pain and stiffness
- Pain front part of neck.

TABLE 9.15.1 The precautions to be followed during acute stage of poliomyelitis

Do's for the acute stage	*Don'ts for the acute stage*
The hospital admission is needed if the child develops breathing problems, difficulty swallowing	No injection has to be given
Complete rest is important	No exercise or massage is to be done
The proper care must be taken to prevent the spread of the polio, therefore the hands should be properly washed with antiseptic solutions	The client is not allowed to sit or stand or move to avoid the loading on joint and muscles
The client's cloth has to be washed separately	Don't let the joint segment or the muscle to assume a gravity dependent or unsupported position
Relaxed position of the limbs is advisable however the proper changes must be made in the positions regulary to avoid the development of the muscle contractures	No surgery can be performed during the acute stage
The water bedding or air bed or water filled gloves are to be placed over the bony prominences to prevent the formation of ulcers	

- Back pain or backache
- Leg pain (calf muscles)
- Skin rash or lesion with pain
- Muscle stiffness.

PARALYTIC POLIOMYELITIS

- Fever, occurring 5 to 7 days before other symptoms
- Headache
- Stiff neck and back
- Muscle weakness, asymmetrical (only on one side or worse on one side)
- Rapid onset
- Progresses to paralysis
- Location depends on where the spinal cord is affected.

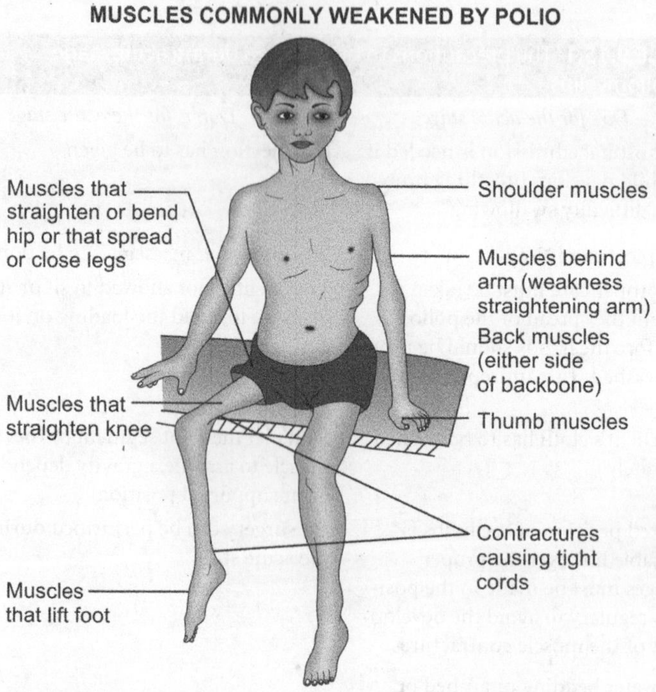

MUSCLES COMMONLY WEAKENED BY POLIO

Fig. 9.15.1: Various muscles which are commonly weakened/atrophied in polio and those which undergo contracture in polio

- Abnormal sensations (but not loss of sensation) of an area
- Sensitivity to touch, mild touch may be painful
- Difficulty beginning to urinate
- Constipation
- Bloated feeling of abdomen
- Swallowing difficulty
- Muscle pain
- Muscle contractions or muscle spasms, particularly in the calf, neck, or back
- Drooling
- Breathing difficulty.

During acute stage of polio, certain precautions (Table 9.15.1) have to be followed to avoid the progression of the disease and to minimize the associated complications.

Typical characteristics of post-polio residual paralysis

- The symptoms include weakness, fatigue, pain and loss of function
- It is stage four of the polio virus and occurs after a time of disease stability
- The spontaneous recovery of present weakness, contracture and deformity is not possible. Therefore, whatever paralysis is present in this stage is permanent in nature. Certain muscles are commonly affected in terms of weakness and contracture development in the polio patients (Fig. 9.15.1).

Causes

- Polioviruses are enteroviruses within the Picornaviridae family. These viruses are resistant to ether and chloroform but can be inactivated by formaldehyde. They multiply in the GI tract but are particularly neurotropic.
- Documentation suggests that infections with polioviruses can be potentiated by factors such as exercise and tonsillectomy. Additionally, patients who are immunocompromised, such as those with human immunodeficiency virus (HIV) infection, B-cell disfunction, immunoglobulin A (IgA) deficiency, or severe combined immunodeficiency, are particularly at high risk of developing poliomyelitis when exposed to both wild-type polioviruses and vaccine-attenuated viruses present in the oral poliovirus vaccine.

Classification

Polio can be classified as either symptomatic or asymptomatic. About 95% of all cases display no symptoms (asymptomatic polio), and between 4 and 8% of cases display symptoms (symptomatic polio). Symptomatic polio can be broken down further into a mild form called non-paralytic or abortive polio and a severe form called paralytic polio (occurring in 0.1 to 2% of cases).

Paralytic polio also may be classified as:

- Spinal polio—attacks motor neurons in the spinal cord and causes paralysis in arms and legs and breathing problems
- Bulbar polio—affects neurons responsible for sight, vision, taste, swallowing, and breathing
- Bulbospinal polio—both spinal and bulbar polio.

Many people with non-paralytic polio are able to make a full recovery, while those with paralytic polio generally end up with permanent paralysis.

MANAGEMENT ON THE BASIS OF THE CONDITION OF THE PATIENT

In acute stage (pre-paralytic stage):

- The exertion and excessive exercises must be avoided as it will aggravate the condition
- Complete physiological rest is needed
- Relief of the pain is important to be achieved, as the continuous pain may lead to the arthrogenic inhibition of the muscles and may lead to the weakness of these muscles on long-term basis. For the pain relief, the therapeutic agents such as heat (Willen and Grimby, 1998), TENS, stretching, relaxation exercises, appropriate walking aid, orthosis (Warring, et al. 1989), etc. are helpful
- Relaxation of the painful spasm is done by the relaxation exercises, gentle hydro-collateral packs with mild warmth (the excessive heating is to be strictly contraindicated)
- Proper positioning of the whole body and the body part is important for avoiding the overstretching of the weak muscles and the prevention of the joint deformity
- The positioning must be modified to provide the complete support to the limbs and to avoid the development of the pressure sores
- The complete support with the pillows and sandbags will offload the possible overloading of the joints.

- In case of the involvement of the brain-stem nuclei, the bulbar muscles (in case of the bulbar polio) are weak or paralyzed, leading to the difficulty in swallowing the food and saliva; the frequent choking of the pharyngeal region; and the difficulty in maintaining the breathing occurs due to respiratory muscle paralysis (Dean and Ross, 1991). These are to be coped accordingly. The ventilator support is needed to preserve the respiration and improving the vital capacity of lungs. The postural drainage may be done to improve the secretion clearance
- Incentive spirometry helps to train the ventilator muscles.

During recovery phase:

- During this phase, the manual muscle charting (MMT) of the whole muscle groups of the involved extremity is to be done to formulate the short and long-term goals. Such muscle charting is to be performed periodically over period of time to determine the progression or the improvement of the weakness (Bohannon, 2005)
- Some critics do argue that the MMT cannot document the actual amount of strength available in the muscles and may be subjected to the higher degree of subjectivity (Bohannon, 2005). Therefore, the other objective strength assessment tools are available for making the objective documentation of the muscle strength. Such tools may include the dynamometer or isokinetic device
- The weakened group muscles are identified and the strengthening of these muscles may be started with adequate rest in between
- During early stages, the low grade active, active assisted exercises and the hydro-pool therapy (Prins, et al. 1994) may be helpful to minimally loading the joint and applying the overloading stimulus in a controlled and accepted manner
- Focus on the minimal resistance exercise with the special attention to prevent the trick or the compensatory movements
- The proprioceptive neuromuscular facilitation (PNF) techniques can be utilized to improve the neural firing within the motor circuit
- Assistive devices may be given (such as tricycle, axillary crutches) may be needed to improve the functional status of the client by supporting the important joints such as knee, foot, pelvis in the functional position and reducing the undue stresses of the extremity joints

- The lower extremity weakness (Perry, et al. 1993) and/or development of joint deformity or contractures (Lord, et al. 2002) may lead to the diminished functional performance. Therefore for improving/maintaining the ambulatory performance, it is important to minimize the lower extremity weakness and joint deformity.
- Splints must be check for avoiding the harm to the body part due to the sharp edges or the unnecessary assembly of the supporting orthosis
- The client him/herself must be motivated to walk so as to get the maximum cooperation from the client. The externally imposed tasks on the client without self-motivation fails to get the maximum cooperation and the results of improvement remain unsatisfactory
- The strengthening exercise program must be implemented in a graded fashion and with the adequate rest period in between so as to allow the improvement to occur in positive direction. The inadequate recovery period and the sudden progression in the applied overloading may cause the further damage to the muscles. The objective documentation of the available strength and the progression of resistance for strengthening can be made with the help of equipments such as isokinetic or dynamometers. The isokinetic equipments, Cybex device could be used safely for the variety of isometric and isotonic exercises for polio patients (Einarsson, 1991)
- These patients are more prone to develop multiple joint pain and the myofascial pain syndromes. The patients with higher activity report more pain than the sedentary patients (Klein, et al. 2004). The management of these pain is important to save the patient compliance towards the rehabilitation regime and to preserve the functional status
- Aerobic exercise such as upper extremity ergometry, the supported swimming, fast walking may be recommended. The participation in the recreational sports and the group sports may be more beneficial. The aerobic conditioning exercises also help to improve the generalized blood flow in the body and muscles; to tackle the myofascial pain
- Due to the influence of the polio, there are chances of limb length discrepancy, and this must be meticulously and appropriately compensated for, before starting the ambulatory and the other exercise program. The uncompensated limb length discrepancy

are at higher risk of leading to the development of the scoliosis and the pelvic misalignment
- The scoliotic and kyphoscoliotic deformities of spine lead to the impaired functioning of the spinal cord and the pulmonary system
- Due to the spinal deformities, and the increased obesity secondary to diminished physical exertion, the polio patients have higher risk of developing breathing problems (Bach, 1995).

The residual paralysis phase (chronic phase):
- The muscle weakness and the deformity remaining in this phases are permanent and irreversible in nature therefore the aim of this phase does not focus on the strengthening program, rather they believe in the functional rehabilitation of the client
- The residual deformity may be compensated with appropriate assistive and orthotic device to stabilize the limb during functional tasks and to prevent the progression of the deformity
- Correct use of brace and calipers is important to avoid the pain in the lower extremity; similarly the correct use of crutches, wheelchair and other orthosis is important to avoid the pain in the joints of the upper extremity (Gawne and Halsteal, 1995)
- The prevention of the further development of the contractures and deformities is important
- The polio patients have higher joint and bone loading due to the abnormal functioning of the muscles, therefore they are more prone to develop the arthritic changes in joints as well as joints derangements. The early stage management of these complications help to delay the progression of the deformity or dysfunction to the debility level (Gawne and Halstead, 1995)
- The vocational rehabilitation of the client may be needed
- The occupational changes or the work station modification may be recommended
- When the recovery phase is over, the residual deformities may impose the compensatory movement pattern in the client which may be unacceptable and therefore need the surgical interventions for the correction of deformities and the contracture releases
- The progressive resistance exercises may be recommended for preserving the strength of the residual muscles
- During functional tasks and the training, the fatigue and overexertion has to be strictly avoided as this would cause the deterioration of the client's status

- The fatigue may not be apparent at rest, therefore the fatigue assessment for the polio patients must also be done during different level of exercises (Dean and Ross, 1991; Weinberg, et al. 1999) and the tasks
- The common used surgical interventions include the:
  - Joint arthrodesis of the unstable joints—splayed joints, the genu recurvatum, the unstable flail ankle, etc.
  - The muscle lengthening procedures to release the contractures (most commonly for the hamstring, hip flexors, plantar flexors)
  - The tendon transfer surgeries
  - The soft tissue contracture
  - The arthrotomy or the osteotomy to realign the bones (wedge osteotomy to realign the vertebral bones)
  - The correction of the limb length discrepancies—either by the shortening of the long bone (by osteotomy) or by the lengthening of the small bones (by Ilizarov's technique).

Complication of the surgical interventions

- Nerve problem—the traction injury to nerve; the numbness in the distal part of nerve; iatrogenic paralysis of the supplied nerves
- Vascular complication—the sudden entrapment of the blood vessels; the vascular spasm
- Deformity may aggravate when the surgical implant dislocates
- The pin tract infection or the infection of the metallic implant may occur
- The excessive lengthening may lead to the unstable joint
- The arthrodesis may lead to the arthritis in the proximal and the distal joints
- Due to the use of ambulatory aids, or the inefficient movement patterns the patients of polio and residual paralysis, have higher energy consumption (Brehm, et al. 2006) for even the basic activities such as walking, cycling, daily routine tasks. The reduction in fatigue, the improvement in movement efficiency can result from the aerobic exercises for six weeks, at low to moderate intensity appropriate as per the individual requirements (Dean and Ross, 1991).

POST-SURGICAL PHYSIOTHERAPY

The aims of the post-surgical physiotherapy include:

- To avoid the recurrence of the contractures
- To avoid the infection of the surgical site and wound

- To strengthen the muscles in the gained range
- To re-educate the muscle for the new action after the tendon transfer
- To train the client to get the maximum benefit out of the surgical interventions
- To maximize the functional outcome. The progression of weakness or muscle atrophy may be the result of the decreased muscle use, decreased mobility, reduced endurance and function. The clients who have presented significant functional recovery despite weakness, present the higher scope of recovery (Gawne and Halstead, 1995). Therefore one important aim while dealing with the patients of the polio, is to minimize the weakness and maintain the functional performance as long as possible.

For the Soft tissue release surgery:
- The preoperative physiotherapy aims to gain the maximum mobility and the flexibility of the 'to be operated' muscles
- Postoperatively the mobility is to be maintained in the proximal and distal joints of the operated joints
- Positioning of the client are important for prevent the again development of the contractures
- The prone-lying position is advised for preventing the development of the hip flexor contractures.
- The AFO (ankle foot orthosis) may be advised to maintain the neutral position of the ankle after tendo-achlis lengthening
- Graded mobility exercises are important to gain the movement and to preserve the soft tissue mobility after the motion at the operated site is permitted
- Beside hospital or the clinical based program the home exercise program are also important
- The muscle strengthening and endurance exercises are to be done to regain the active maintenance of the concerned joint and muscles
- Re-education of the joint to have weight bearing and the joint loading to avoid the recurrence of the soft tissue contracture.

For tendon transfer surgery:
- Preoperative management consists of gaining the mobility at the proximal and distal portion of the 'to receive transfer' muscles. The strengthening of the donor tendon are advised. The synergist groups of the donor muscle must be trained for the strength to

avoid the weakening of the group action once its component has been transferred.

- Re-education of the transferred muscle for its new action
- The electrical stimulation may be used for assisting the learning of new action and this may be synchronized with the patient's efforts
- The passive ROM exercises, followed by the assisted to resisted exercise
- The biofeedback to improve the patient's cooperation
- The static orthosis in the early stage followed by the dynamic splints.

For the Arthrodesis:

- Preoperative management consists of the non-weight bearing (NWB) exercise and the NWB ambulation is taught, the muscle needed for the crutch ambulation are strengthened, the mobilization and the strengthening of the muscles at the 'to be operated joint' and the joints in the vicinity of this joint
- After operation the limb is immobilized in the POP (plaster of Paris) cast therefore the NWB ambulation is recommended.

9.16: MENINGITIS

Meningitis involves the inflammation of the meningeal lining of the brain and spinal cord (Saez, 2003) secondary to the infective pathological state, in the person of any gender or any age.

■ CAUSES

- Most common cause of the meningitis is infection
- The infections can be due to bacterial, viral (Ginsberg, 2004) or the fungal origin
- Bacterial origin is the most common cause of meningitis and the most life-threatening too. These have to be dealt at emergency and may cause death within hours
- The *Neisseria meningitides*, pnumococcal bacteria are the mostly involved in the bacterial meningitis in adults. In children, the *Haemophilus influenza* are most commonly involved for the bacterial meningitis
- The viral meningitis is less common and is caused by enteroviruses, herpes simplex virus

- The fungal causes of the meningitis include the *Cryptococcus* fungal infections
- The non-infectious causes of the meningitis include malignancy (Chamberlain, 2005), antibiotics overdoses, intravenous immuno-globulins (Moris, 1999)
- The bacterial form of the meningitis is most dangerous and has to be dealt at emergency. The viral form is relatively less serious and the recovery is faster and complete.

Presentation of the Meningitis

The meningitis infection is more common during winter. The infection is more common in the people with diminished immunity such as in young children, geriatric patients, immunocompromised responses. Meningitis can affect people anywhere, at any age and at any time. The initial features of the meningitis resembles like any other infections, therefore the early stage is difficult to be diagnosed. Therefore the initial features include following:

- Fever, severe headache, drowsiness
- Nausea, vomiting, neck stiffness, drowsiness
- Lethargy, weakness, disorientation
- Photophobia (difficulty in tolerating the light)
- In some cases where the Intracranial pressure (ICP) rises the inability to tolerate sounds occurs
- The Kernig's sign is positive, i.e. in the supine lying position the hip and knee are placed in the 90° flexed position, when the knee is extended, the pain increases and the client resists the extension of the knee. Also the neck flexion causes the knee extension in order to reduce the tension within the dural sheath surrounding the spinal cord.
- In case of bacterial meningitis, the rigidity is present in the neck muscles, the nuchal region, and the muscle tone of the neck muscles increases, therefore the passive neck flexion is difficult (Van de Beek, 2004) and painful
- The tone of the neck muscle increases secondary to spasm and the protective response to avoid the pain during neck movement
- In extreme cases, the swelling occurs within matter of the brain, and causes rise in the intracranial pressure, the disorientation and coma

Other signs of meningism include the presence of positive Kernig's sign or Brudzinski's sign. Kernig's sign is assessed with the patient lying supine, with the hip and knee flexed to 90 degrees. In a patient with a positive Kernig's sign, pain limits passive extension of the knee. A positive Brudzinski's sign occurs when flexion of the neck causes involuntary flexion of the knee and hip. Although Kernig's and Brudzinski's signs are both commonly used to screen for meningitis, the sensitivity of these tests is limited. (Attia J, 1999)

Meningitis can lead to brain swelling and cause further disability, including coma and even death.

Treatment

- Physiotherapist has the supporting role to deal with the complication of the meningitis, and to preserve the integrity of the vital organs of the body
- Physiotherapist help to cope with the acute phase complications and management
- The acute phase management consists of the
  - Passive ROM exercises of the major joints of the body to prevent the development of the muscle contractures and the joint deformity. The special care has to be taken to avoid the overstretching in the combined movement of the hip and knee simultaneous flexion, as this position would tend to irritate the dura more
  - The prevention of the pressure sores is done by the frequent turning of the patient, the frequent inspection of the pressure tolerant regions to see any feature of the excessive erythema, superficial skin breaching or the pressure ulcers
  - The regions having higher risk of developing ulcers (such as sacral region, scapular region, the heels, the olecranon process) must be carefully inspected and must be supported with the pressure dissipating mechanisms such as water bed, air bed, water filled gloves, etc.
- During the phase of the unconsciousness and the drowsiness, the physiotherapist is responsible for the prevention of the pulmonary congestion and for the preservation of the integrity of the body functional system
- The postural drainage positions may be used for facilitating the drainage of the secretions, however, the care must be taken to avoid the undue rise in the intracranial pressure as this would aggravate the condition of the client by further pressurizing the brain tissue.

- The deep breathing exercises and the coughing or huffing mechanisms are not of much use due to the noncompliance form the patient side secondary to the unconsciousness and the altered sensorium
- The percussion, vibration and the shaking can be used to dislodge the accumulated secretions and to direct them towards the main bronchus. The care must be taken not to raise the ICP as these maneuvers have been found to raise the ICP
- Furthermore the removal of secretions from the pharyngeal region is not possible, therefore for the secretion removal the suctioning may be used, again the timing of the suctioning must be very small to avoid the rise in the ICP and the brain hypoxia
- The residual weakness and the paralysis are managed by the physiotherapist who helps to regain the strength and the functional movement
- Therapist is also responsible for making them able to cope with the residual weakness and the disabilities, and to maximize the functional independence
- For the irreversible residual deformities and the disabilities the ambulatory aids or the assistive devices may be recommended to promote the quality of life and the functional independence
- The aims of the therapeutic rehabilitation can be framed after the complete assessment, and the re-assessment
- Physiotherapy is also important to train the activity of daily living.

ENCEPHALITIS

Encephalitis is the pathological state characterized by the localized or the diffused inflammation of the brain tissue leading to the presentation of the malfunctioning of the involved portion of the brain.

Symptoms of the encephalitis are the mixed features of the infection, the increased intracranial pressure (ICP) and the malfunctioning of the involved portion of the brain.

Causes

- Viral infections—when the viruses directly attach the brain and the spinal cord leading to the inflammation
- The most common viruses leading to the encephalitis are enterovirus, herpes simplex, arboviruses

- The sequel of the previous viral infections when the presentation of the encephalitis appears after the 2–3 week after some other previous infection
- The involvement of the brain tissue may be in form of the localized manner (when only the portion of the brain tissue is involved) or the diffused manner when the large portion of the brain tissue is involved.

Symptoms

- Sudden fever (in the direct viral infection) or the fever after the 2–3 weeks of some other previous infections
- Loss of appetite
- Headache, and
- Vomiting
- Increased sensitivity to the light and the sound
- Irritability
- The difficulty in maintaining balance while walking
- In severe cases, the client presents with the loss of consciousness.

Signs

- Presentation of the mild to moderate increased ICP:
  - Headache,
  - Photophobia
  - Drowsiness
  - Irritability
  - Sonophobia
  - Low grade confusion
  - The impairment of the judgment
  - The features of the meningeal irritation occurs such as neck stiffness, the Kernig sign, neck muscles rigidity or tone increase
- Features of the significant increase in the ICP:
  - Altered sensorium
  - The seizures and the severe compromise of the physical functions occurs
  - The signs of the increased ICP may be seen as altered pupillary reaction
  - In severe cases the brain death may occur
  - The vegetative posturing such as decerebrate rigidity or the decorticate posturing.

Diagnosis

- The clinical features of the encephalitis come into picture
- The detailed neurological examination is to be conducted
- The basic mental status examination (MMSE—mini mental state examination) reveals the confused or the drowsiness of the patient
- The CSF pressure analysis indicates the amount of the pressure of CSF with in brain ventricles or the CSF channels
- The CSF cerebrospinal) fluid examination for the content analysis reveals the presence of the specific features such as protein content, the protein compositions, white blood cells, the amount of glucose, the nature of the infective organism
- The MRI imaging would help to localize the extent of the brain tissue involvement and the degree of the involvement
- The specific analysis of the CSF for the specific infective agent can be done by the advanced technology such as ELISA (Enzyme-linked immunosorbent assay) and the PCR (polymerase chain reaction).

Treatment

- Medical management of the encephalitis is symptomatic. The steroid and the methylprednisolone are given to reduce the brain swelling and the inflammation. The medical management also deals with the convulsions and the seizures
- The bed rest is given to stabilize the vitals signs
- The fluids, antibiotics and the electrolytes are given intravenously for meeting the demands of the body and maintaining the homeostasis
- Antibiotic management is to be given as per the identified infective organisms and special viral agents
- In the clients who are very sick and in the state of the unconsciousness, the mechanical ventilation is needed to maintain the respiratory status
- The long-term care might be needed depending on the severity of the involvement, therefore in such cases the education of the family members about the home management, of the client has to be given.

Physiotherapy Management

Acute Phase Management

- The acute phase management consists of the:

- Joint ROM (range of motion) exercises of the major joints of the body to prevent the development of the muscle contractures and the joint deformity. This is important to avoid the overstretching as this may lead to the irreversible damage and the fibrosis of the muscles
- The prevention of the pressure sores is done by the frequent turning of the patient, the frequent inspection of the pressure tolerant regions to see any feature of the excessive erythema, superficial skin breaching or the pressure ulcers.
- The regions having higher risk of developing ulcers (such as sacral region, scapular region, the heels, the olecranon process) must be carefully inspected and must be supported with the pressure dissipating mechanisms such as water bed, air bed, water filled gloves, etc.

- During the phase of the unconsciousness and the drowsiness, the physiotherapist is responsible for the prevention of the pulmonary congestion and for the preservation of the integrity of the body functional system.
- The postural drainage positions may be used for facilitating the drainage of the secretions, however the care must be taken to avoid the undue rise in the intracranial pressure as this would aggravate the condition of the client by further pressurizing the brain tissue.
- The deep breathing exercises and the coughing or huffing mechanisms are not of much use due to the noncompliance from the patient side secondary to the unconsciousness and the altered sensorium.
- Generally, the encephalitic patients are disoriented and the frightened therefore they may not be able to understand the happenings of his/her surroundings and may resist the efforts of the nursing staff, medical practitioner and the physiotherapists. In such circumstances, it is important to have the presence of the family member nearby so that the patient does not get anxious or afraid
- The percussion, vibration and the shaking can be used to dislodge the accumulated secretions and to direct them towards the main bronchus. The care must be taken not to raise the ICP as these maneuvers have been found to raise the ICP.
- Furthermore the removal of secretions from the pharyngeal region is not possible, therefore for the secretion removal the

suctioning may be used, again the timing of the suctioning must be very small to avoid the rise in the ICP and the brain hypoxia.

In the Recovery and the Chronic Phases

- The detailed physiotherapy assessment is reconducted to assess the recovery potential and the residual impairments. This is important for framing the new goals for long-term and short-term basis
- The strength, balance, movement patterns, walking abilities, the functional performance, the social interaction and the cognitive abilities have to be carefully and adequately assessed
- The pain management is an important role of the physiotherapist. Generally because of the altered conscious or the altered sensorium, it is not easy and always possible to identify the pain status of the client therefore the facial expressions, the body part movement, and the sounds made by the client can be used as indicator of the pain. The alleviation of the pain or atleast 'no aggravation of pain during intervention' is an important aspect of the ethical physiotherapy management of the encephalitic patient
- The physiotherapy interventions in the long-term rests to target the:
  - Improvement of the functional skills
  - The enhancement of the quality of life (QOL)
  - To improve the social, mental and physical well being
  - The training to better deal with the residual impairments
  - The specific training needed for the occupational demands
  - The vocational rehabilitation of the client.

The problems of the speech difficulty can be dealt by the qualified speech therapist.

The long-term support of the family members and the social groups is important. This can be integrated and coordinated with the help of multidisciplinary specializations such as social workers, speech therapist, physiotherapist, social support groups, the encephalitic supports organizations, neuropsychologist.

POLYNEURITIS

Polyneuritis is the condition characterized by the simultaneous inflammation of the multiple nerves cells of the body at different sites.

Cause

- The multiple pathological conditions may be responsible for the development of the polyneuritis
- The causes of the polyneuritis or the polyneuropathy involve the systemic diseases or the conditions which affect the multiple systems in the body or produce the generalized presentations
- The GBS (Guillain Barre Syndrome) is a common form of polyneuritis which is a demyelinating type of nerve affection and is characterized by the damage to the myelin sheath of the nerve.
- The multiple nerve inflammation may occur in the persons with very high or very low immune responses
- In the patients of the weak immune mechanisms the inflammation of the nerves go unnoticed, however once the symptoms of nerve impairment start appearing, the polyneuritis is suspected.
- Vitamin B_{12} deficiency
- The diabetes
- Alcoholism
- Poison or the arsenic neuropathy
- Fluoroquinolone overdoses (Cohen, 2001)
- The prolonged chemotherapy (Wilkes, 2007) used for the management of the cancer.

Pattern of the Nerve Involvement

In case of the polyneuritis either the whole nerve (less commonly) or the small portion of nerve (more commonly) is involved. The portion affected in the partially involved nerves may be either the nerve cell body, the axon, surrounding its myelin sheath. Not necessarily all the nerves of the particular region of body are affected.

The common pattern of the nerve involvement is as follows:

- Distal axonopathy—the cell bodies remain intact and the axons are affected. Example is diabetic neuropathy
- Demyelinating polyneuropathies—the myelin sheath surrounding the nerves are damaged leading to the impairment of the impulse conduction across the axons
- The neuronopathy or the ganglionopathy—where the proximal portion of the nerve such as cell body or the ganglion, are affected. This is the less common pattern and may affect either the sensory cell bodies (in sensory neuronopathy) or the motor cell body (anterior horn cell involvement or the motor neuron disease)

Features

- The presenting features of the polyneuritis depend on the number, type and the severity of the nerve involvement
- The neurological symptoms such as pain, sensory alteration (hypersensitivity or the hyposensitivity), the motor weakness, tingling or numbness, the muscle atrophy are the common features of the nerve involvement. The autonomic manifestations include the poor blood pressure control, the erectile dysfunction, the postural hypotension
- In cases of the early stages of the diabetic neuropathy or nerve involvement, the sensory alterations, numbness, pain, tingling sensations can occur in feet and hand even before the diabetes is diagnosed. Such cases have higher tendency of developing the diabetic neuropathy advanced form later on, therefore these patients require the early stage interventions and attention, as these client can recover in early stages with the diet, exercises, blood sugar monitoring and the weight control programs (Jim ete, al. 2010).

Differential Diagnosis of the Polyneuropathy

- Vasculitis
- Multiple neuralgias
- The amyloidosis
- GBS—Gullian Barre's syndrome
- Infections such as Herpes simplex, Shingles, leprosy.

This is a comprehensive process and needs involvement of multispeciality expertise team. Physiotherapists are required to work as team member, and design the intervention program after carefully understanding the objective of intervention and minimizing the associated risks/harm to the client.

Management of the Polyneuropathy

The early stage interventions focus on the:

- Identification and the elimination of the causative factor
- Preventing the progression of the deterioration
- Maintaining the strength, endurance, sensory integrity and the functional capacity of the client
- Improving the strength and the functional capacity of the client

- Manage the complications or the associated impairments such as neuropathic pain, sensory loss, the muscle weakness or paresis
- In the cases with the extensive nerve problem and the irreversible impairment, the supportive intervention is needed and the vocational rehabilitation might be an important aim.

The detailed neurological assessment is carried out to determine the extent of the nerve damage, the prognosis of the condition, the identification of the causative mechanism. Once the causative mechanism is identified, the interventions are done to remove this cause, and to prevent the progression of the symptoms. The electrodiagnostic and the other investigative procedures help to differentiate among the different causes of the possible neuropathy and various conditions having the similar presentation.

The detailed physiotherapy assessment helps in framing the short and long-term goals.

The recovery stage physiotherapy helps to regain the function and motor control.

The loss of balance can be compensated to certain extent with the help of the means to improve the sensory response of the limbs, and with the help of the balancing exercises.

The precautions are explained to avoid the possibility of suffering injuries secondary to the sensory and motor loss.

For the neuropathic pain, the symptomatic treatment and the prolonged application of the TENS (transcutaneous electric nerve stimulation) is needed (Pieber, 2010).

Tilt-bed exercises are helpful for the conditioning of the patients suffering from the postural hypotension.

The bladder training and the management instructions are explained to the client to deal with the bladder dysfunction.

9.17: TRAUMATIC HEAD INJURIES

Head injury includes the either closed (when integrity of skull bones maintained) or opened (when the integrity of the bony skull is disrupted) trauma to the skull portion of body with or without involving the injury to the brain tissue.

Head injury is an insult to the brain caused by an external physical force that may produce altered or diminished level of consciousness which results in impairment of cognitive, physical, emotional or behavioral functioning. These may be either temporary or permanent and cause partial or complete physical disabilities or psychological malfunctioning. In common practice, the term 'head injury' and the 'traumatic head injury' are used interchangeably.

Three things which can affect the pressure within the intracranial cavity are:

- Brain
- Blood
- Cerebrospinal fluid.

The classification of the head injury may be based on:

Type of injury (Table 9.17.1)

- Concussion
- Contusion—The bruise to the brain
- Laceration

Location of accumulation of blood

- Extradural hematoma
- Subdural hematoma
- Subarachnoid hematoma
- Intraparenchymal hematoma.

Depending on the integrity of the overlying bones of the skull

- *Closed injury*: When the overlying skull bones are intact and their continuity is not breached
- *Open injury*: When the overlying skull bones are injured or fractured.

Depending on the nature of the tissue involvement

- Diffused injury
- Localized injury.

Consequences of Head Injury

The presentation of the head injury varies with the type of injury, mechanism of injury and the time elapsed after the injury.

The consequences of the direct impact of the injury causing forces could include:

- *Due to concussion*: The transient disorientation, loss of balance and the headache. These are transient in nature and complete recovery occurs rapidly
- *Contusion*: No organic or permanent damage occurs to the brain tissue. Local swelling of the parenchyma of brain may occur, however in majority of cases the recovery occurs completely. The recovery time may be more than that of the concussion

TABLE 9.17.1 Classification of head injury on the basis of type of injury

	Concussion	*Contusion*	*Laceration*
Definition	Concussion is the most common and mildest form (Satz, et al. 1997) of head injury which is characterized by the temporary loss of brain function	Contusion is the bruise to the brain with or without the accumulation of blood in the brain tissue and the damage to the blood vessels of the brain. The pia-archnoid membranes are not damaged The part of brain is squeezed against the skull bone	This is the severe form of head injury where the pia-arachnoid membranes are damaged therefore the portion of brain is torn (Hardman, et al. 2002)
Causes	The head on collision and the direct strike of head with some stationery or moving objects	May be a kind of accelerating (moving object hits static person) or the decelerating injury (moving person strikes the static object)	The cause is mostly the penetrating injury or severe diffused injury to the brain. High velocity trauma causing the rapid movement of brain with in skull also tears blood vessels due to shearing forces
Signs and symptoms	Concussion present with the variety of physical, cognitive and the emotional symptoms The physical symptoms include headache, dizziness, nausea, vomiting, balance and coordination problem	Features of contusion depend on the part of brain that has received bruise Coup-countercoup pattern is present Most common site of contusion is the frontal and temporal lobe	This is a emergency condition and needs the medical or surgical interventions depending on the findings of the MRI, CT scan and other investigative procedures

Contd...

Contd...

	Concussion	*Contusion*	*Laceration*
Treatment	Almost all concussions resolve without any medical interventions, however 12–24 hour observation is need The headache, or dizziness may need medical interventions The repeated concussion may need surgery for scarring or ischemia	Aims to prevent the rise in ICP thus strictly avoid the hypotension, the hyponatremia, hypercapnia	The surgical decompression of the affected area The decompression helps to prevent the increase in the ICP The supporting management for the ventilation, neurological and medical support
Prognosis	Concussion resolves spontaneously without interventions. No brain tissue damage is involved The presenting features are strictly physiological and non-structural	Majority of contusion recover spontaneously without medical interventions Cause the increase in ICP and pressurize the delicate brain tissue	Prognosis is variable depending on the severity of the injury

- *Laceration*: It occurs when the damage to the brain tissue has occurred, and the recovery may be either absent or the incomplete. It is a severe form of head injury and in large number of cases the surgical interventions are needed. Moreover the residual disability or impairment is permanent in nature
- The direct impact force of the high velocity nature may lead to the skull fracture
- The movement of the brain within the skull due to inertial forces may lead to the tear of the brain tissue and the supplying blood vessels
- Head injury may result in subarachnoid hemorrhage, depressed skull fracture, widespread diffused axonal injury, the extravagation of blood into the cavities with in brain, the injury to the vital nuclei located in the brain (various cranial nerve nuclei, the respiratory/satiety/thermostat center, etc. located in the brain stem portion). Depending on the region involved, the presentation of the client may vary
- Diffuse axonal injury may occur when the white matter of the brain is affected due to shearing forces causes different tissues to slide over others.

The **consequences** which are secondary in nature could involve:
- Hemorrhage
- Infections
- Herniation of the brain tissue or the brain stem
- Edema of the brain tissue
- Ischemia or the hypoxia of the brain tissue due to the impaired blood supply to the brain region secondary to the blood vessel injury followed by tissue fibrosis.

Effect of Neurological Impairment on the Gas Exchange

Beside these direct and indirect consequences the presentation may also vary according to the associated injuries sustained by the client. These injuries may include the rib fracture, flail chest, hemo-pneumothorax, multiple fractures, and lung contusion.

Damage to the respiratory centers causes: Hypercapnia, hypocapnia, Cheyne-Stoke breathing; ataxic breathing.

Regurgitation of fluid and meal in the pharynx region; the loss of the protective pharyngeal reflexes may lead to the acute form of aspiration pneumonia.

The coughing mechanism may be impaired leading to the inability to clear off the secretions from the lungs and respiratory passages.

Effect of Head Injury on Brain

Brain injury leads to the increased cerebral edema, which increases ICP (intracranial pressure). This in turn leads to the capillary compression with in brain and the cerebral hypoperfusion.

Following head injury the intracranial pressure (ICP) increases. The ICP further increases due to following factors:

- Head down posture. Therefore the postural drainage positions which use head down position, are contraindicated
- Turning the head—it increases the pressure in the one side of head thus leading to the compression, hypoxia, ischemia, and the increased ICP
- The physiotherapy interventions such as vibrations, percussions, suctioning, postural drainage positions also increase the ICP
- ICP also increases by the stress, coughing, noise, hypertension, anxiety, hyperglycemia, fever, etc.
- Fever leads to the increased ICP secondary to the increased metabolism of the cerebral tissue. Each degree increase in the body temperature increased the cerebral metabolism by about 10%.

The management of the increased ICP is by:

- Elevation of head (about 15–30 degrees from horizontal) to increase the CSF outflow and decrease the ICP.
- Use of the steroids to reduce the development of cerebral edema
- Additional means to counteract the causative mechanism also needs to be implemented.
- Relaxation exercises to reduce anxiety and stress
- Avoid the neck flexion and prone lying as it obstructs the CSF outflow
- The postural drainage can be carried out if ICP < 15 mm Hg and CPP (central perfusion pressure) > 50 mm Hg.

PHYSIOTHERAPY ASSESSMENT OF THE HEAD INJURY PATIENT

Respiratory Status

- Is the breathing spontaneous or the mechanical ventilator derived?

- Is the mechanical ventilation being given by the mouth piece, or by the tracheostomy? The ventilation through tracheostomy indicates the prolonged duration for which the ventilator support is needed. Moreover in case of the tracheostomy intubated patient the coughing mechanism is impaired and the sputum production is high secondary to the irritation of the airways by the mechanical tube of ventilator
- What is the pattern of respiration? Is there any evidence of the paradoxical breathing? Is the rib cage expansion uniform and adequate?
- Is the depth and frequency of breathing normal or altered? Is the tissue oxygen saturation level within normal range or not?

Neurological Status

- This assessment may not be possible in initial sessions due to the unconsciousness, sedation medicines, anesthesia or paralysis.
- The Glasgow Coma Scale (GCS) can be used for the assessment of the patient.
- The pupillary reflex, the attitude of the limb, respiratory status and GCS score are of high important in the assessment of the unconscious patients.
- Cognitive assessment of the client—this is done as per the standard RLS (Rancho Los Amigos) scale (Table 9.17.2).

TABLE 9.17.2 RLA (Rancho Los Amigos) scale for cognitive functioning of the head injury assessment (RLA NRC, 1990)

Level I	No response to sound, light, touch or movement
Level II	Generalized response Person begins to respond to sounds, touch, movement Response is slow, inconsistent. Response may include the chewing, sweating, breathing faster, moving, moaning.
Level III	Localized response The response is more than the previous level Patient may be awake on and off during day React slowly and inconsistently Follow simple instruction such as "squeeze my hand", "look here".

Contd...

Contd...

Level IV	Confused and agitated The client is confused and frightened Does not understand what is happening around him Overreacts to what he hears, feels or sees by hitting, screaming, abusive language due to the confusion May not able to understand that people are trying to help.
Level V	Confused and inappropriate (no meaningful interaction) Client is confused and has difficulty in making sense of things around him. Not be able to understand or do the daily routine activities (such as brushing teeth) even though the physical strength is available Feels uncomfortable when many people are present in his/her room Confabulation (filling the memory gaps by making things up) is present The memory recalling is difficult for the events happening after the injury, however the events prior to the injury may be recalled.
Level VI	Confused appropriate Patient remembers the main points of the conversation but forgets the details about that Follows a schedule with assistance but gets confused if the changes are made in routine Has difficulty in concentrating on the task which involves multiple steps, such as watching the red light while driving; walk and talk at the same time.
Level VII	Automatic and appropriate Can follow a set schedule without assistance Can do routine self care work without help if physically able Has a problem in planning, starting, and following the activities. Needs supervision due to decreased safety awareness and judgment. Is slow thinker and difficulty in concentrating on work in noisy or distracting environment Has rigid and stubborn thinking.
Level VIII	Purposeful and appropriate Realizes that he has problem I thinking and memory Is more flexible in thinking Shows poor judgment in new situation and may need some assistance.

Evaluation of the Impairments

- The impairment is important to be identified so as to start their earlier management and to prevent the aggravation of these impairments
- The strength and tone of all important muscles has to be assessed at all joints of body
- The flexibility assessment to check the tightness or contracture of the muscles
- The range of motion and the deformity assessment at the joints
- The accurate documentation of the muscle tone as per standard tone assessment scale (Modified version of Ashworth scale). The factors leading to the increased or decreased in the muscle tone also need to be documented
- The quality timing of the Deep tendon reflexes (DTRs) and the superficial reflexes has to be documented. The abnormal reflexes such as flexor withdrawal, tonic labyrinthine reflex (TLR), asymmetrical tonic neck reflex (ATNR), symmetrical tonic neck reflex (STNR) also need to be carefully evaluated and documented if present
- Evaluation of sensory impairments
- Evaluation of motor impairment
- Evaluation of the ambulation, mobility, hand skills, transferring abilities
- To check whether the abnormal synergy pattern of movement are present or not.
- Evaluating the complex task level of performance.

Evaluation of the BADL (basic activity of daily living) and IADL (instrumental activity of daily living). The common used tool of assessment is the functional independence measure scale (FIMS).

Evaluation of the balancing performance.

REHABILITATION OF THE TRAUMATIC BRAIN INJURY

The role of physiotherapist extends right from the acute phase of the trauma up to the complete rehabilitation of the patient. The aims of the physiotherapy interventions for traumatic brain injury are as follows:

- Maintain the functional integrity of the patient
- In acute phase
  - Preserve the functional capabilities of the patient
  - Optimize the breathing and the pulmonary status

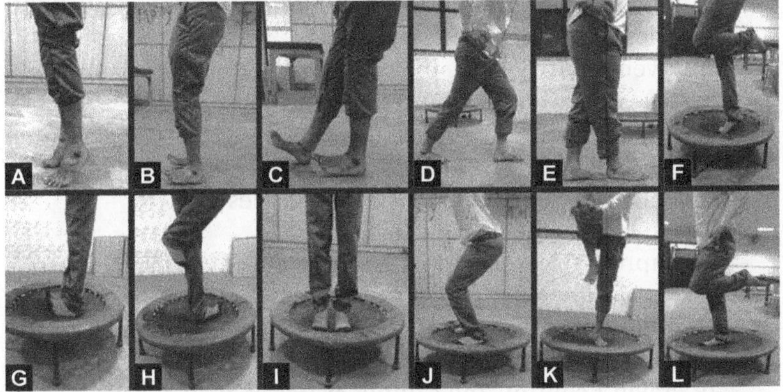

Figs 9.17.1A to L: Balance training exercise program: (A) Heel raise; (B) Toe raise; (C) Bilateral toe raise; (D) Bilateral heel raise; (E) Single leg support with heel raise; (F) Side lunges; (G) One leg standing with high thigh raise; (H) Single leg standing with toe raise; (I) Single leg standing; (J) Trampoline training toe raises; (K) Trampoline training heel raise; (L) Single leg standing with heel raise on trampoline, m-single leg standing with partial squat on trampoline, o-single leg standing with toe raise on trampoline, o-bilateral mini squats on trampoline.

  - Prevention of the secretion accumulation
  - If pulmonary secretions are present, then physiotherapist helps to clear off the secretions from lungs
  - To position the patient in appropriate posture to minimize the pressure ulcers, to prevent development of the abnormal postural reflexes, to optimize the ventilation-perfusion ratio in the vital organs of the body
  - To minimize the development of muscle tightness, joint deformity and contractures
  - To preserve the mobility and ranges at the joints
  - To preserve the sensory awareness of the body and the surroundings
  - To prevent the development of the spasticity in the muscles
  - To prevent the development of the abnormal postural reflexes (flexor withdrawal, ATNR, STNR, etc.).
- During subacute phase
  - To help the client to gain the sensory inputs and able to utilize them for the regaining the control of the body
  - To gradually counteract the factors which could have increased the risk of functional impairment

- Interventions to prevent the development of the spasticity (if spasticity not already present)
- Interventions to reduce the spasticity (if spasticity has already set in)
- To implement the method to negate the influence of abnormal postural reflexes
- To help the strengthening of weak muscles
- To stretch out the tight muscles
- To improve the exercise tolerance and the muscular endurance
- To regain the balance (Figs 9.17.1A to L) in sitting, standing positions. The various exercises can be implemented for the balance training, according to the principle of the COG (center of gravity) control. The sample exercises may consist of heel raise, toe raise, alternate heel and or raise, heel walking, toe walking, single leg standing, single leg standing with partial squat or deep squat, etc.
- To regain the control of the spine
- To provide appropriate bracing or orthotic support to gain the stability at joints, and the improved functional performance
- To improve the ability to carry out the voluntary movement at the joints through functional or complete ranges, in an efficient, coordinated and the functional manner
- To educate the family members about their expected cooperation with the client, and to gain their maximum support in favor of the client

- During chronic phases
  - To make the client to perform maximum capacity while living with the irreversible residual deformity
  - To train the client for advanced balancing tasks
  - To train the client for advanced functional tasks and the activities helpful to improve the performance at the occupational level
- Regain the maximum functioning of the client with in feasible limits
- Attempt to improve or gain the new functional skills.

Early Positioning in Bed

- Appropriate positioning in supine, prone or side lying position
- The proper and periodic changes in the posture to avoid the development of the excessive secretion accumulation in lungs,

stagnation of the blood, to prevent development of the pressure sores

- Sustained supine position leads to the increased risk of developing the ulcers in sacral, scapular and spinous process region
- The appropriate positioning of the body is important to prevent the development of the abnormal muscle tone in the muscles of the body and to prevent the development of the abnormal reflexes (such as TLR, ATNR, flexor withdrawal, etc.)
- Positioning may increase the ICP, however if the head alignment is maintained to prevent the venous obstruction, the rise of ICP is within acceptable limits (Chudley, 1994).

Emphasize the Respiratory Function

The highly important aim of the physiotherapy intervention in head injury patient is to prevent the reduction of the blood perfusion to vital organs and simultaneously assisting the management of the other associated trauma. The importance must be given to the respiratory status of the patient. The improvement of the respiratory status and the protection of airways is the very important goal of early physiotherapy interventions.

Specifically the aims must be to prevent hypoxemia (PaO_2 <8 kPa), hypotension (Systolic BP < 90 mm Hg), increased intracranial hypertension (ICP> 20 mm Hg), and the prevention of hypercapnia ($PaCO_2$ > 6kPa) (Roberts, 2002).

Ensure the adequate oxygenation of the tissues.

Protection of the airways by removal of secretions—the mechanical suctioning, gentle airways clearance techniques.

The reduction of ICP (intracranial pressure) is important to maintain the adequate cerebral perfusion pressure and to prevent the secondary brain damage.

MHI (manual hyperinflation) is advised for the prevention of atelectasis and the lung collapse, however the period of MHI must be kept brief to avoid the abrupt rise in ICP. The airway pressure up to 40 cm H_2O and the double tidal volume is needed to re-expand the atelectatic lung (Rothen, et al. 1993; Robert, 2002).

To stimulate the cough response the rib-springing technique is useful.

- Maintain the musculoskeletal integrity
  - The prevention of the secondary effects of immobility
  - Prevention of ulcers and joint deformities

- Improving the sensory awareness and the arousal through sensory stimulus
  - Increase the sensory input via tactile, auditory, visual stimuli. Provide the sensory stimuli in controlled stimulation, and check for the response with each stimulus.

MANAGEMENT OF TONE AND SPASTICITY

- Proper positioning of the patient
- Discourage the position which leads to the development of the abnormal reflexes. The supine position leads to the increased tonic labrynthine reaction (TLR)
- Cryotherapy leads to the temporary inhibition of the spasticity
- The orthotic support is helpful for allowing the prolonged weight bearing which in turn leads to the reduction in the spasticity
- The management of the factors which aggravate the spasticity such as stress, pain, noise, etc.

Improving the motivation of the patient:
- Goal formation should be appropriate
- Attention span
- Treatment of all basic level components.

Complex level treatment: This is the task on whole task practice through:
- Electromyogram (EMG) biofeedback
- Functional electrical stimulation (FES) to strengthen or activate the weak muscles
- Practice of goal oriented tasks
- Modification of environment according to the requirement and the encouragement of the client.

PHYSICAL MEDICINE AND REHABILITATION OF THE HEAD AND TRAUMATIC BRAIN INJURY

Following traumatic brain injury, the individual needs to progress through a four-stage process of acute care, rehabilitation, resettlement and long-term adjustment (Tyerman, 1991; Campbell, 2002).

The pre-injury status, the nutrition status, family support, social status, psychiatric illness and the medical history is important to consider as these may play pivotal role in determining the extent of possible recovery.

The GCS (Glasgow coma scale) low score may indicate the significant injury to the brainstem, subarachnoid hemorrhage and this may delay the recovery process (Eames and Wood, 1989).

The strengthening exercises of the weaker group muscles.

The stretching exercise of the tight muscles.

The use of splint, braces, orthosis may be recommended as per the physical evaluation and the strength available in the muscle groups.

Positioning may be done to minimize the muscle tightness and the contracture formation.

The patients generally will present with the hypotension and the dizziness while attempting to get up from the bed, therefore the gradual progressive inclination may be used for the adaptation of the vestibular apparatus, the spinal proprioceptors, and the gradually progressive conditioning of the autonomic nervous system (ANS) to maintain adequate blood pressure in the vascular channels of the body. For this purpose, the tilt-table may be used.

Heterotrophic ossification is a common problem encountered in the head injury patients who have been bed-ridden for a long time, and have reduced tone in the muscles. When this ectopic bone has been formed, the extra caution must be taken while overloading the weak muscles during strengthening and ambulatory tasks. The passive vigorous mobilization and the jerky movements have to be avoided.

For gaining the maximum possible functional rehabilitation, the gradually progressing functionally oriented task skills must be implemented. Appropriate feedback about the performance and about the achievements made in the direction of target goals must be fed back to the patient as an indicator of the success of his/her efforts made.

For the management of head injury patients, the recommendations have been made according to their cognitive abilities score as per RLA scoring method (Table 9.17.3).

The training for the stair use (Figs 9.17.2A to F). The client training must also include the training for the effective and safe usage of the stairs during ascending or descending. The stair training must incorporate the training for the forward steppage, backward steppage, and sideways steppage. In case, the client has to use the walking aid for the ambulation, it is important to training him/her the safe and effective use of this aid.

TABLE 9.17.3 Management according to the RLA (Rancho Los Amigos) scale score, (RLA NRC, 1990 patient information)

Level I Level II Level III	Improve the arousal through sensory inputs Explain the client what you are going to do. Example: "I am going to move your hand". Give brief and simple instructions. "Look at me" instead of "can your turn your head towards me?" Keep room calm and quiet Show the patient the pictures of the closed relative, dear friend, favorite site seeing, etc. After each command, give adequate time for responding.
Level IV Confused and agitated	Explain the patient where he is Assure him he is safe Make him feel home and comfortable Do not force him to do activities, but listen what he wants to do and follow his lead with in safety limits Avoid the distractions, and excessive noise in the room Limit the number of visitors to 2–3 days so that patient feels comfortable and is able to avoid being agitated on watching strangers.
Level V (Confused and inappropriate)	Repeat the things frequently to make him remember Remind him the day, date, name and location of his home or hospital Command must be short and simple, and the repetition must be made with same words instead of using synonyms or other words Give adequate rest while having difficult in paying attention Gradually reduce the rest period.
Level VI (Confused and inappropriate)	Repeat things as to improve the memory Assist him in starting and continuing the activities Encourage the individual to participate in all therapies Give positive feedback when doing the desired activity.
Level VII (Automatic and appropriate) Level VIII (Purposeful and appropriate)	Treat the patient as an important member of the decision making team His opinion must be respected Discuss with him the problems without criticizing Strongly courage to participate in therapy regime Encourage to keep a small diary for making notes of the tasks or activities as a mean of dealing with memory problems Encourage to be as independent as possible however be cautious about the driving, smoking, working, etc. Social worker and psychologist may help to improve the response.

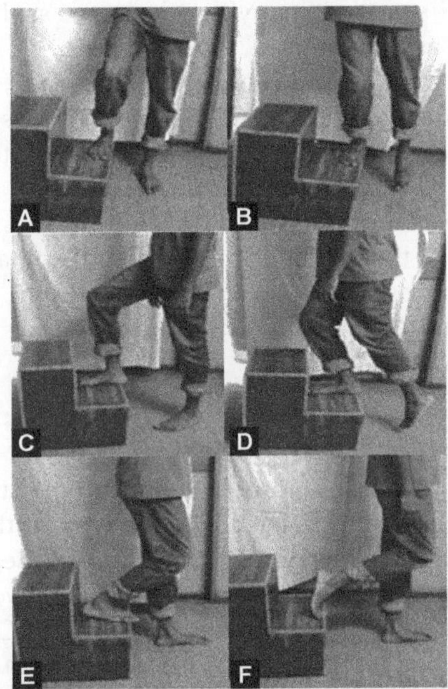

Figs 9.17.2A to F: Training for the effective and safe use of stairs: (A) Side step up starting position; (B) Side step up final position; (C) Front step up starting position; (D) Front step up final position; (E) Stair descend initial position; (F) Stair descend final position

9.18: SPINAL CORD INJURY

Spinal cord injury may involve the impairment of the highly important spinal cord and/or various ascending or descending tracts which carry signals towards brain or from the brain. Depending on the level of spinal cord injury, the extent of damage and the associated pathological states, the injury may involve the whole or a part of spinal cord section at some specific level or at multiple levels. Also the various nerve roots emerging from the spinal cord may also get injured leading to sensory, motor, autonomic or mixed presentation.

CAUSES OF SPINAL CORD INJURIES

The spinal cord injury may occur due to a number of conditions which may include following (the causes are not restricted to following):

- Pathological space occupying lesions such as tumors, meningioma, astrocytoma
- Trauma—fall from height, vehicle accidents, war, diving injury,
- The injury to the blood vessels supplying the spinal cord due to osteophytes, emboli, arterial aneurysm, arterial traumatic rupture, arterial occlusion/narrowing
- The infections of the spinal cord- myelitis
- The infection of the myeline sheath around spinal cord—in case of multiple sclerosis
- The increased pressure within spinal cord or the herniation of the spinal cord in spina bifida.

LEVEL OF LESION

The location of the level of injury is important to establish as this is critical in determining the prognosis, the type of the intervention needed, etc. While considering the vertebral body segments and the spinal cord segments, the discrepancy occurs between the both in terms of the levels. All cervical nerves from C1 to C7 pass through the intervertebral foramen at the level of the same number vertebral body level. The C8 nerve root and the remaining lower nerve roots of the spinal cord pass below the numbered level of the vertebral body. Higher numbered nerve root is located more laterally with in spinal cord. All thoracic segments of the spinal cord lie between T1 and T9 vertebra. The all lumbar nerve roots and spinal cord lumbar segments lie between T10 to T11. All sacral nerve roots lie between T12 and L1. To label the level of spinal cord injury, the most distal normal segment is mentioned along with last segment showing the partial or complete normal functioning. Example incomplete below T1 and complete below T4 means that at T1 normal functioning is present, the T2, T3 and T4 nerve roots are functioning partially, the whole spinal cord below T4 cord segment is completely non-functional.

CLASSIFICATION OF SPINAL CORD INJURY

The classification of the spinal cord injury is done in grade A to grade E using the criteria standardized by the American Spinal Injury Association (ASIA) commonly also called as ASIA scoring (Table 9.18.1).

The Asia scoring is an important assessment tool for predicting the possible recovery of the client. Patients with complete sensorimotor

TABLE 9.18.1 American Spinal Injury Association (ASIA) impairment scale for neurological classification of spinal cord injury (Dobkin, et al. 2003)

Injury grade	*Essential criteria*
A	Complete spinal cord injury No sensation is present in S4 and S5 dermatome.
B	Incomplete injury Sensory function is preserved below the neurological level of injury Motor function is not present below the neurological level of injury The S4 and S5 region sensations are intact but motor function is compromised.
C	Incomplete injury The motor function is partially preserved below the neurological level, as below the neurological level more than half muscles have strength less than grade 3 of manual muscle testing.
D	Incomplete injury The motor function is partially preserved below the neurological level, as below the neurological level at least half muscles have strength ≥ (equal or more) than grade 3 of manual muscle testing.
E	This is the normal state where the motor and sensory scores are normal.

loss, i.e. ASIA grade A and those graded ASIA B within 1 week to 1 month of the SCI recover walking in no more than 10 to 15% of cases (Dobkin, et al. 2003). Several experimental studies in SCI suggested that BWSTT (body weight supported treadmill training) may increase the possibility of the Asia graded B, C and D patients of walking over the ground (Dobkin, 1999; Wernig, et al. 1998).

SENSORY AND MOTOR TESTING FOR SPINAL CORD INJURY

The motor and sensory grading of impairment is important to document the extent of the injury involvement, and this is done by the ASIA motor and sensory scoring. The motor testing is done by the manual muscle technique for checking the strength of the key group of muscles, which are believed to have the nerve supply by the specific nerve roots arising at the specific neurological level of the spinal cord (Table 9.18.2).

The Sensory examination in ASIA scoring is done by based on the sensation related neurological response to the touch, cold, hot

TABLE 9.18.2 The key muscles used for the motor testing in a spinal cord injury patients

Spinal cord neurological level	*Key muscle group tested for motor assessment*
C1 to C5	Neck flexors
C1 to T1	Neck extensors
C3 to C5 combined	Diaphragm
C4	Scapula elevation (shrugging)
C5	Elbow flexion
C6	Wrist extension
C7	Elbow extension
C8	Finger flexors (distal phalanx of middle finger)
T1	Intrinsic muscles of hand; finger abductors (little finger abduction)
L1, L2	Hip flexors
L3	Knee extensors
L4	Ankle dorsiflexors
L5	Great toe extension
S1	Ankle plantar flexors

and pinprick sensations in the specific dermatomes supplied by the specific levels of the spinal cord (Fig. 9.18.1).

MEASUREMENT SCALES

The ASIA score does not provide the impairment of the function and the associated disability encountered by the patient during daily living activities. For the functional activity documentation, the functional independence measure (FIM) is used.

EFFECTS CLINICAL EFFECTS OF SPINAL CORD INJURY

The injury to the spinal cord may result in the:

- Loss of motor power and the voluntary movement of the body part
- Loss of the superficial sensation or deep sensation
- Loss of autonomic regulation and vasomotor control
- Loss of the voluntary control over the bowel or/and bladder regulation.

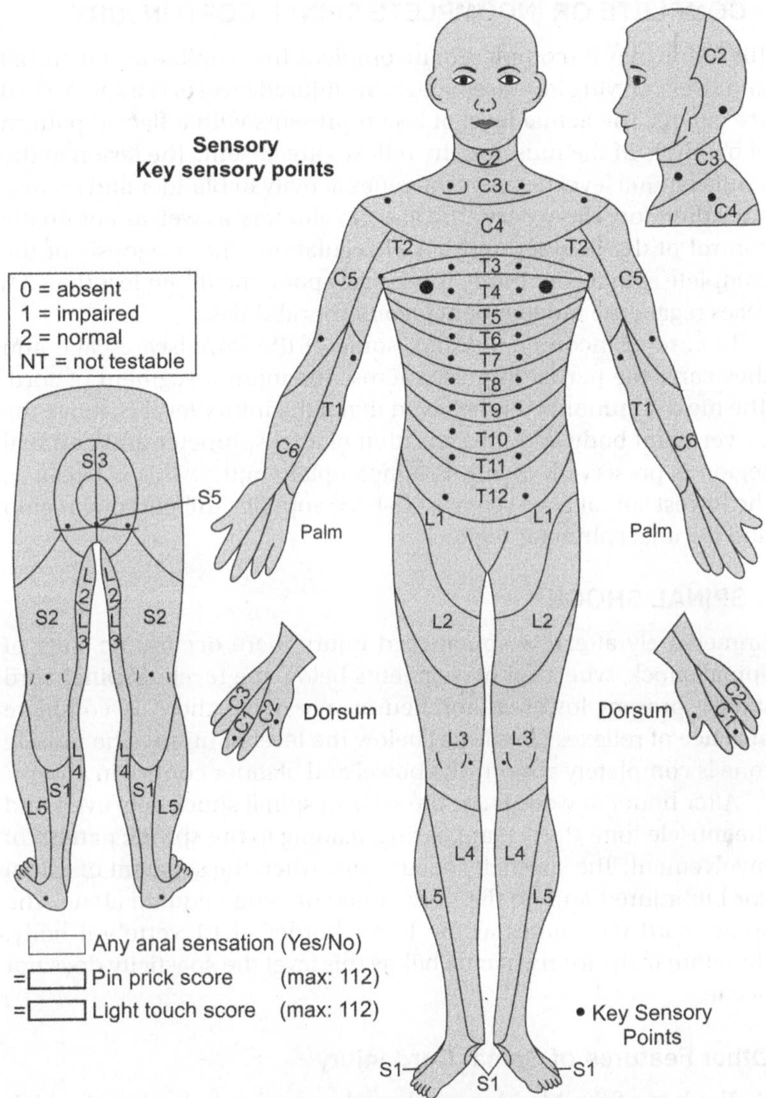

Fig. 9.18.1: The dermatomal region for sensory testing of spinal cord injury

COMPLETE OR INCOMPLETE SPINAL CORD INJURY

The lesion may be complete or incomplete. In complete lesion, the all impulses carrying impulses across the injured level of the spinal cord are cut off. The actual level of lesion presents with a flaccid pattern of paralysis in the muscles, the reflexes are absent. The lesion at the cauda equina level destroys the reflex activity in bladder and rectum anus therefore there occur the loss of voluntary as well as automatic control of the bladder and bowel regulation. The prognosis of the complete spinal cord injury is relatively poor and about less than 5% cases regain the independent locomotors abilities.

In case of incomplete lesion some of the impulses escape and they carry the partial impulses across the injured segment of cord. The most commonly it is believed that if the injury level is above the L1 vertebral body and the sensation of anal sphincter and perianal region is preserved, then it is a incomplete injury. This is because; the lowest spinal cord segment (S4-S5) supplies the perianal region and the anal sphincter region.

SPINAL SHOCK

Immediately after the spinal cord injury there occurs the state of spinal shock, where all he segments below the level of spinal cord injury, present lower motor neuron paralysis, there is complete absence of reflexes (Areflexia) below the level of injury. The muscle tone is completely absent. The bowel and bladder control in absent.

After hours to week later, the state of spinal shock gets over, and the muscle tone starts reappearing, leading to the spastic pattern of involvement. The spasticity occurs only when the segment of spinal cord in injured and no the nerve route or cauda equine alone. The spinal cord terminates at the lower border of L1 vertebral body, therefore if any injury occurs below this level the spasticity does not occur.

Other Features of Spinal Cord injury

- The loss of the bladder and bowel control may lead to the high residual volume of urine in bladder and the chronic prolonged constipation. The high residual volume of urine leads to the higher risk of urinary tract infection
- The loss of the sensations in the affected dermatomes lead to the higher risk of frictional injury, decubitus ulcer, the burns and the injury by sharp objects

- The injury in the higher cervical spinal segments leads to the impairment of breathing control. The injury at C1/C2 level leads to the diaphragm paralysis and the necessity of the mechanical ventilation
- The loss of autonomic control leads to the difficulty in regulation heart rate, respiration, vasomotor control, body thermal homeostasis, the difficulty of the visceral organ functioning
- The loss of the control from the higher centers and brain control over muscle tone leads to the increased in muscle tone in form of the spasticity
- The injury above the level of T6 level leads to autonomic dysreflexia, which is characterized by the abnormal fluctuation in blood pressure, sweating, blood vessel tone, and the autonomic changes
- The loss of the muscle active action for the prolonged period of time leads to the disuse atrophy, muscle fibrosis and the osteoporosis.

Physiotherapy Assessment

The physiotherapy interventions start as soon as the vital signs of the client are stable. On the first interaction the physiotherapist carries out the detailed assessment of the client, to identify the restrictions, the targets areas, the framing of the short and long-term goals. The detailed assessment has to be properly documented, as it provides the vital information to determine the prognosis and the mandatory changes in the intervention strategies. The documentation of the everyday incidents is also important including the urinary tract infections, the efforts performed by the client, the participation by the client, the inspection notes of the areas prone to develop decubitus ulcers, the changes in the medicine regimen, etc.

Physiotherapy has to be performed the detailed neurological examination and this must contain the details about the:

- Demographic features
  - The name, age, gender of the patient
  - The contact number or address
  - The occupational history of the patient is important to determine if the client can resume his/her previous job or not. This is also important for determining the type of vocational rehabilitation or the job modifications that might have to be needed in later stages
  - Family history of the diseases

- History of injury
  - How did the injury occur?
  - The mechanism of injury?
  - The timing of injury?
  - The onset of symptoms was acute or gradual?
  - What was the rapidity of the alterations in symptoms or signs?
  - The medical or surgical history of the patient?
  - Is there any history of similar presentation in the past time?
  - Does the patient have any significant medical pathology such as tumor, malignancy, diabetes, rheumatoid arthritis, MS, polyneuropathy, bladder incontinence, bowel incontinence, etc.?
- The overall present condition of the patient
  - Patient is conscious or unconscious?
  - Is the injury site stable or not?
  - What interventions have been done so far?
  - What is the general condition of the client?
  - Is the patient medically, neurologically or orthopedically stable?
  - What is the present status of the associated fracture or injuries?
  - What is the status of the chest, lung function, the chest expansion, oxygen saturation, the electrolyte balance in the body?
- Motor examination
  - What is the current motor level of the functioning?
  - The detailed manual muscle charting (MMT) has to be done for the key muscles of the body in both upper and lower extremities.
  - The deep tendon reflexes (DTR) has to be documented on the standard DTR grading scale.
  - Is there presence of the spasticity in any muscle or muscle group? If spasticity is present in the muscles, the degree of the spasticity has to be carefully documented for each muscle group on standard spasticity grading scale (Modified Ashworth scale or the Ashworth Scale)
- Sensory Examination
  - What is the sensory level of the involvement? What sensations are present and which are absent?
  - The sensory examination across the dermatome pattern has to be meticulously documented. Are the 'saddle region' sensations present or not?

  - The sensations for the anterior, lateral and posterior column of the spinal cord have to be tested to identify various syndromes associated with the spinal cord injury.
- The level of the lesion can be known to a good extent by the interpretation of the sensory and motor presentation so far. This is important because the prognosis of recovery, the type of the interventions needed, vary significantly depending on the level of the injury
- The bladder function:
  - What is the current status of the bladder functioning?
  - Has there been any improvement or the deterioration in the bladder function since the onset of injury?
  - Are the sensations of the bladder fullness or emptying present?
  - Can the patient control the micturition reflex or not?
  - Is there any evidence of the urine dribbling, or the continuous leakage of the urine?
  - The amount of the urine dribbling coughing, sneezing or the other valsalva maneuver has to be documented. The palpation of urinary bladder may reveal the extent of the bladder fullness.
  - Ultrasound imaging or/and cystography may be helpful to determine the residual urine volume in the bladder and the bladder capacity. This helps to determine the type of impairment in the bladder functioning and the most optimal strategies needed
- Bowel functioning
  - What is the current status of the bowel function?
  - Is the patient able to voluntarily control the bowel function and the process of defecation or not?
  - Are the saddle region sensations present or not?
  - Is the anal reflex and/or bulbocavernous reflex present or not?
  - What is the frequency of the defecation?
- Chest examination and respiratory function
  - The examination of the chest region is important
  - The volume and values of various Spirometric variables are useful to highlight upon the pulmonary functioning
  - Is there any evidence of the rib fracture (s)?
  - Is there any evidence of the paradoxical breathing?
  - Is the chest expansion adequate?
  - Does the auscultation with stethoscope reveals the presence of normal or/and abnormal breathing sounds?
  - Is the air flow across various segments of lungs adequate?

- Functional activity evaluation
  - This involves the evaluation of the functional ability in bed, in sitting and standing positions
  - The ability to perform the various transfers to be tested while examining the spinal cord injury patients include
    a. Transfers between beds,
    b. Transfers in beds,
    c. Transfers between bed and chair, and returning back
    d. Transfer from bed and wheel chair, and return back
  - The ability to execute the transitions between various positions (such as prone lying, side-lying, sitting, standing, supine lying, etc.) needs to be carefully documented
  - The ability to perform various tasks such as ability to use hands, ability to bring glass towards mouth, ability to use pen or pencil for writing, etc. also need to be documented. This functional testing is performed in the limbs depending upon the level of the injury and the number of the limbs involved.
  - The functional activity evaluation includes the examination of the BADL (basic activities of daily living) as well as the IADL (instrumental activities of daily living)
- Walking abilities
- Multiple challenges faced by the SCI patients during functional ambulation include:- reduced muscle strength; increased energy demands; inefficient gait patterns; asymmetry in limb functioning; inefficient weight transfers between limbs; increased need of orthotic interventions; decreased step length; increased spasticity in the limbs; reduced step height; excessive plantar flexion during swing phase. These impose the great challenges and put the risk of reduced safety and efficiency of the client during ambulation (Edelle, et al. 2001)
- The important aim of the physical rehabilitation of the spinal cord injury is to re-establish the independent walking abilities.
- The most common scale used for the evaluation of the walking ability is WISCI (walking index for the spinal cord injury). This scale appears to be more sensitive and detailed about the walking recovery than other scales (Morganti, et al. 2005). The WISCI (Table 9.18.3) is a 21-level hierarchical scale which includes the gradations of physical assistance and devices required for walking. Improvement in walking is based on the change of scores from admission to discharge (Morganti, et al. 2005)

TABLE 9.18.3 The walking index for the spinal cord injury (WISCI) (Morganti, et al. 2005)

Level	*Description*
00	Patient is cannot stand and/or participate in assisted walking.
01	Ambulates in parallel bars, with braces and support of two persons, less than 10 m.
02	Ambulates in parallel bars, with braces and physical assistance of two persons, 10 m.
03	Ambulates in parallel bars, with braces and physical assistance of one person, 10 m.
04	Ambulates in parallel bars, no braces and physical assistance of one person, 10 m.
05	Ambulates in parallel bars, with braces and no physical assistance, 10 m.
06	Ambulates with walker, with braces and physical assistance of one person, 10 m.
07	Ambulates with two crutches, with braces and physical assistance of one person, 10 m.
08	Ambulates with walker, no braces and physical assistance of one person, 10 m.
09	Ambulates with walker, with braces and no physical assistance, 10 m.
10	Ambulates with one cane/crutch, with braces and physical assistance of one person, 10 m.
11	Ambulates with two crutches, no braces and physical assistance of one person, 10 m.
12	Ambulates with two crutches, with braces and no physical assistance, 10 m.
13	Ambulates with walker, no braces and no physical assistance, 10 m.
14	Ambulates with one cane/crutch, no braces and physical assistance of one person, 10 m.
15	Ambulates with one cane/crutch, with braces and no physical assistance, 10 m.
16	Ambulates with two crutches, no braces and no physical assistance, 10 m.
17	Ambulates with no devices, no braces and physical assistance of one person, 10 m.
18	Ambulates with no devices, with braces and no physical assistance, 10 m.
19	Ambulates with one cane/crutch, no braces and no physical assistance, 10 m.
20	Ambulates with no devices, no braces and physical assistance, 10 m.

- Recovery of locomotion, therefore, has become a primary goal of both pharmacological and rehabilitative treatment (Wernig, et al. 1992)
- Beside the WISCI, the other suggested method to assess the walking ability in the SCI patients includes the SCIFAI (spinal cord injury functional ambulation inventory). The SCIFAI (Table 9.18.4) is found to be reliable, sensitive and valid tool for assessing walking function in the individuals with SCI who possess some ambulatory function. This is a straightforward method and includes the all domains that are critical to walking performance (Edelle, et al. 2001)
- Assessment of the wheel chair handling abilities
  - The strength testing is to be done for the muscles which are needed for the use of wheel chair
  - The specific activity which is to be tested varies with the type of lesion and the extent of the involvement of the injury.
  - The important activities which are to be evaluated for the wheel chair usage include:
    a. Ability of the client to maintain sitting balance in the wheel chair
    b. Ability of the client to manipulate the brakes of the wheel chair
    c. Ability of the client to pick the objects from floor
    d. Ability of the client to reach down to the foot plates
  - For the documentation of the wheel chair usage ability, WST (Wheelchair skill test) version 4.1 (Table 9.18.5) is a commonly used test, and it offers a practical, safe, well tolerated, exhibits good to excellent reliability, excellent content validity, fair construct and concurrent validity, and moderate usefulness (Kirby, et al. 2002).

The client is believed to have passed the skill if he can perform these mentions skills independently and safely. The total score of the WTS represents his wheelchair ability performance score. Higher value of the WTS score means better performance.

REPAIRING THE SPINAL CORD

The repair of the injured spinal cord is very delicate and skillful procedure. Also this is highly unpredictable even because the regeneration of the injured neurons/axons in central nervous system (CNS) does not necessarily occur.

TABLE 9.18.4 The SCIFAI inventory for the walking assessment in the spinal cord injury patients (Edelle, et al. 2001)

Parameter	*Activity*	*Scoring Left*	*Scoring right*
Weight shift	Shifts weight to stance limb Weight shift absent or only onto assistive device	1 0	1 0
Step width	Swing foot clears stance foot on limb advancement Stance foot obstructs swing foot on limb advancement Final foot placement does not obstruct swing limb Final foot placement obstructs swing limb	1 0 1 0	1 0 1 0
Step rhythm	At heel strike of stance limb, the swing limb: • Begins to advance < 1 second • Needs 1–3 seconds to begin advancing • Requires > 3 seconds to begin advancing	 2 1 0	 2 1 0
Step height	Toes clear foot throughout swing phase Toe drags at initiation of swing phase only Toe drags throughout swing phase	2 1 0	2 1 0
Foot contact	Heel contacts floor before forefoot Forefoot or foot flat first contacts with floor	1 0	1 0
Step length	Swing heel placed forward of stance toe Swing toe placed forward of stance toe Swing toe placed rearward of stance toe	2 1 0	2 1 0
Assistive devices			
Upper extremity balance or weight-bearing devices	None Cane (s) Quad cane (s), forearm or axillary crutch (es) Walker Parallel bar	4 3 2 2 0	4 3 2 2 0
Lower extremity assistive devices	None AFO KAFO RGO	3 2 1 0	3 2 1 0

Contd...

Contd...

Parameter	*Activity*	*Scoring Left*	*Scoring right*
Temporal or distance measures			
Walking mobility	Walks regularly in community (rarely or never uses W/c) Walks regularly in home/occasion in community Walks occasionally in home and rarely in community Walks rarely in home and never in community Walks for exercises only Does not walk	5 4 3 2 1 0	5 4 3 2 1 0
Two minute walk test	Total distance walked in two minutes (in number of feet per minute)		

TABLE 9.18.5 Wheelchair skill testing (WTS) version 4.1

Skills of WTS testing	
1.	Rolls forward 10 m
2.	Rolls forward 10 m in 30s
3.	Rolls backward 5 m
4.	Turns 90° while moving forward—left and right
5.	Turns 90° while moving backward—left and right
6.	Turns 180° in place—left and right
7.	Maneuvers sideways—left and right
8.	Gets through hinged door in both directions
9.	Reaches 1.5 m high object
10.	Picks object from floor
11.	Relieves weight from buttocks
12.	Transfers from WC to bench and back
13.	Folds and unfolds wheelchair
14.	Rolls 100 m
15.	Avoids moving obstacles—left and right
16.	Ascends 5° incline
17.	Descends 5° incline

Contd...

Contd...

18.	Ascends 10° incline
19.	Descends 10° incline
20.	Rolls 2 m across 5° side-slope—left and right
21.	Rolls 2 m on soft surface
22.	Gets over 15 cm pot-hole
23.	Gets over 2 cm threshold
24.	Ascends 5 cm level change
25.	Descends 5 cm level change
26.	Ascends 15 cm curb
27.	Descends 15 cm curb
28.	Performs 30s stationary wheelie
29.	Turns 180° in place in wheelie position—left and right
30.	Gets from ground into wheelchair
31.	Ascends stairs
32.	Descends stairs

During the very early stage of spinal cord injury, the steroids, methylprednisolone are given to prevent the progression of edema. The researches regarding the process of speeding up the process of regeneration are still under laboratory set ups. The promising effects of the stem cell therapy, neurotropic factor injections and the nerve cell grafting are yet to be established.

Rehabilitation of the spinal cord injury patient (Table 9.18.6).

The presenting features vary with the type, severity and level of the injury. Physiotherapy has important role to perform at all levels (Pillastrini, et al. 2008) for the rehabilitation of the spinal cord injury (SCI).

The important immediate and the long-term goals of the physiotherapy and occupational therapy programs focus at:

- Minimize the deterioration of the function
- The preservation of the functions of the body parts
- The maintenance of the integrity of the function
- To bring the client back to the normal life in best possible way
- Restoring the function of the client (Wikipedia, 2010)
- Enable the client to participate in the activities of basic and advanced daily routine tasks in best possible extent

TABLE 9.18.6 The management and rehabilitation of the spinal cord injury patient
Acute phase care and management of the stable patient
Focuses support and prevention
Appropriate positioning
Positioning to prevent the development of the spasticity
The static or supporting splints to support the resting position of joints to prevent overstretching
Range of motion exercise to prevent deformity and contracture
The active-assisted exercises to maintain the strength and the contractibility of the muscles
Regular turning in bed and wheel chair to prevent contractures
The preservation of the motivation and the dignity of the client
The bowel and bladder management
The preservation of the pulmonary status with deep breathing exercises, the airway clearance techniques
The guidance to perform the self care skills with the available strength and the capacity
Education about positioning, turning, regular movements, and the nutrition to the patient and the family members
Special care for the anesthetic skin or the poor nutrition skin
The education to prevent the urinary tract infections
Maintain the sensation of the client with respect to the proprioception and the kinesthetic awareness by regular passive ROM exercise and active-assisted exercises.
Subacute Phase (Rehabilitation Phase)
Reframing the short-term and long-term targets
Consider the activities important to perform the coping with home environment, occupational demands, community set up
To improve the independence status of the client
Replace the static splints with the dynamic or functional splints which enhance the activity demands by the client while simultaneously assisting the movement
Positioning and the activities which prevent the development of the spasticity or help to cope with the spasticity (if spasticity has already set in)

Contd...

Contd...

To train the client to use the available movement or strength to carry out the functional tasks. The client having wrist muscle strength and the absent strength of hand intrinsic muscles, may be trained to execute the tenodesis effect to bring about finger/hand closure and opening to grasp and release the objects.
Strength, endurance and coordination activities to train towards meeting the occupational demands
Transfer training:
The basic transfer and advance mobility training for within bed mobility; bed to chair; chair to bed; bed to wheelchair; wheelchair to bed; wheelchair to floor; floor to wheelchair; wheelchair to toilet seat and back are important for improving the mobility and independence
The sliding board and the parallel bars also help to improve the mobility
Wheel chair training
Selection of the most suitable wheelchair as per the client's demands, financial status and the comfort
Power wheelchair may be better for those who have reduced strength or the endurance in the upper extremity muscles. This is also appropriate to increase mobility on uneven terrains
Prevention of the pressure sores
If the pressure sore has already developed then the prophylactic measures and the therapeutic modalities are important to speed up the healing process
Maintain the motivation of the client and the compliance with the exercise regime
Management of the spastic or flaccid bladder
Home environment modifications
If needed the building of ramp and the lifts may be useful
Widened doors and the corridors
The use of adaptive equipments may improve the functional independence in the kitchen, washrooms
Occupational therapist helps in the training of skills in a wheelchair accessible kitchen
Adaptive aids and equipments help to improve the independence
The adaptive strategies can be trained for carrying out the domestic activities (laundry, kitchen, parenting, bathing)
Self care training

Contd...

Contd...

Training for the independence in the bathing, grooming, feeding, and bladder/bowel management
Adaptive device may include—hand held shower, wheelchair accessible commode, shower commode shower,
Training for managing the transport and driving
The transfer from wheelchair to driving seat
Under "return to driving program" the training is done to enhance the return to the driving status
The training to use the public transportation such as buses, taxi, parking accessibility
Return to the pre-injury level of the leisure and recreation
The return to the work and study skills
In cases the client need the special attention, the special schools may be recommended
Community living skills
Driving and the wheelchair mobility skills are important to regain the community level of the mobility
The sexual health also needs to be paid attention however this is the area which remains almost undiscussed.
Chronic Phase (Reintegration into the Community)
Continue with the subacute interventions with appropriate progressions
The process of community integration and the community participation to improve the quality of life
Focus on restoring the client's role in terms of personal, family, social and community roles
Maintain the motivation of the client and the compliance with the exercise regime
Vocational rehabilitation
The better adaption with the residual disabilities to efficiently perform the tasks and activities.

- Enhance the physical, mental and social well being of the client
- To make them able to perform the self care (bathing, hygiene, feeding, dressing), productivity (paid work, volunteering, care giving, parenting) and the leisure tasks (the activity done during

spare time) (Krupa, et al. 2009; Wikipedia, 2010) in efficient and dignified manner

- To make them able to perform the mobility tasks (transfers, wheel chair mobility, ambulation and the basic ADL activities) independently or with at least the minimal support
- Establishing and promoting the early biomechanical stability of the injured segment, and preserving the stabilization till the injured tissue is under healing process.
- Prevent the progression in the area of injury and prevent neurological degradation
- Speed up the process of neurological recovery
- Simultaneous management of the spinal cord injury, the management of the multi-system impairment
- The long-term prevention and the management of the associated complications such as pressure ulcers, septicemia, and the ischemia of the neural tissues
- As the time after the injury progresses without stabilization, there occurs the increase in the edema with in spinal cord which further reduces the chances of neural recovery.

ADL TRAINING

- Depending on the level of injury, the execution of the daily activity is difficult for patients with spinal cord injury, however the meticulous training can guide them through the rehabilitation approaches to become independent or atleast the minimally dependent
- For training the ADL activities the detailed ADL assessment is important to identify the limitations and capacity to perform the target tasks; to identify the challenges; to frame the short-term and long-term goals
- After the assessment and the target identification, the target task is further break down in to smaller components and the individual components are trained with appropriate feedback and the practice. When these components are learned and practiced adequately, the all components are integrated together to perform the target tasks
- The specific muscle groups useful for performing functional tasks, may be trained for the strengthening or the endurance performance

- When the accurate execution of the target task lies beyond the possible capacity of the client (restriction imposed due to the SCI) the environment modification may be done and the assistive devices may be prescribed for the better functional performance.

Management of the Bladder

The Acute Lesion

The problems associated with the impairment of the bladder control depend on the length of the time after injury, level of injury, extent of the injury. During stage of the spinal shock, the bladder is completely flaccid, devoid of micturition reflex, absent muscle action therefore it shows the failure to voluntarily void the urine. This in turn leads to the accumulation of the urine in bladder which is followed by overflow incontinence of the distended bladder.

METHODS TO DEAL WITH FLACCID BLADDER

- Emptying the maximum volume of urine while attempting voiding. This provides relatively a large duration for which the overflow incontinence may be deferred
- Preventing the development of the urine infection.

Urethral catheterization. It has advantage that after catheterization the more volume may be accommodated in the bladder for the bladder distension, which in turn gives stimulus for the micturition, therefore attempts to optimize the impulses to the bladder regulating center of spinal cord. The following are the common methods used for catheterization:

- Intermittent
- Indwelling
- Suprapubic drainage (Green, 2004)—used in cases where the recovery of the bladder muscle tone is delayed by weeks. This makes a bore in the suprapubic region for allowing the drainage of the urine from bladder.

Other option for controlling the bladder emptying may include the sacral nerve root stimulators to stimulate the anterior S2, S3 and S4 nerve roots for promoting the bladder emptying at will.

Maintenance of the bladder diary for documenting the amount of fluid intake or excreted. Depending on the amount of intake the catheterization may be done after regular time intervals so as to

7. Shumway-Cook A, Anson D, Haller S. Postural sway biofeedback: its effect on re-establishing stance stability in hemiplegic patients. Arch Phys Med Rehabil. 1988;69:395-400.
8. Sullivan PE, Markos PD, Minor MD. An Integrated Approach to Therapeutic exercise: Theory and Clinical Application. Reston, Va: Reston Ltd. 1982.
9. Wall JC, Turnbull GI. Gait asymmetries in residual hemiplegia. Arch Phys Med Rehabil. 1986;67:550-3.
10. Wang R-Y. Effect of proprioceptive neuromuscular facilitation on the gait of patients with hemiplegia of short and long duration. Phys Ther. 1994;74:1008-1115.

9.3

1. Anke AGW, Stenchjem AE, Kvalvik Stanghelle J. Pain and life quality within two years of spinal cord injury. Paraplegia. 1995;33:555-59.
2. Aung TS, Masry WS. Audit of a British centre for spinal injury. Spinal Cord. 1997;35:147-50.
3. Azouvi P, Mare M Thiebaut JB. Intra-thecal baclofen administered for control of severe spasticity: functional improvement and long term follow-up. Archives of Physical Medicine and Rehabilitation. 1996;77:35-9.
4. Bagley JC, Cochran TP, Sledge CB. The impingement syndrome in paraplegia. Journal of Bone and Joint Surgery America. 1987;69:676-8.
5. Cariga P, Ahmed S, Mathias CJ, Gardiner BP. The prevalence and association of neck (coat-hanger) pain and orthostatic (postural) hypotension in human spinal cord injury. Spinal Cord. 2002;40:77-82.
6. Curtis KA, Roach KE, Brooks Applegate E. Development of the wheelchair users pain index (WUSPI). Paraplegia. 1995;33:290-3.
7. Eltorai I, Montroy R. Muscle release in the management of spasticity in spinal cord injury. Paraplegia. 1990;28(7):433-40.
8. Frey-Rindova P, de Bruin ED, Stussi E. Bone mineral density in upper and lower extremities during 12 months after spinal cord injury measured by peripheral quantitative tomography. Spinal Cord. 2000;38: 26-32.
9. Soni BM, Mani RM, Vaidyanathan S. Treatment of spasticity in a spinal cord-injured patient with intrathecal morphine due to intrathecal baclofen intolerance - a case report and review of literature. Spinal Cord. 2003;41:586-9.
10. Szollar SM, Martin EME, Parthemore JG. Demineralisation in tetraplegic and paraplegic man over time. Spinal Cord. 1997;4:223-8.

9.4

1. Bannister R. Brain's Clinical Neurology. Oxford, England: Oxford University Press. 1979.
2. Langford CA, Gilliland BC. Arthritis associated with systemic disease and other arthritides. In: Fauci AS, Braunwald E, Kasper DL, Hauser SL, Longo DL, Jameson JL, Loscalzo J, eds. Harrison's Principles of Internal Medicine. 17th ed. New York, NY: McGraw-Hill Professional. 2008:2177-83.
3. Long WJ, Scuderi GR. Porous tantalum cones for large metaphyseal tibial defects in revision total knee arthroplasty a minimum 2-year follow-up [published online ahead of print]. J Arthroplasty. 2008.
4. Morris ME, Summers JJ, Matym TA, Lansek R. Current status of the motor program. Physical therapy. 1994;74:738-52.
5. Troyer J, Levin BR. Proximal Tibia Reconstruction with a Porous Tantalum Cone in a Patient with Charcot Arthropathy. Knee Orthopedics. 2009;32(5):358.

9.5

1. Brockelhurst G. Clinics in Developmental Medicine, Spina Bifida for the Clinician. No. 57. Philadelphia, PA, JB Lippincott Co. 1976.p.29.
2. Caroline T, Smith BA, Kubo M, Chang CL, Moerchen V, Murazko K, et al. Stepping Responses of Infants With Myelomeningocele When Supported on a Motorized Treadmill. Phys Therapy. 2009;89:60-72.
3. Cherian A, Seena S, Bullock RK, Antony AC. Incidence of neural tube defects in the least-developed area of India: a populationbased study. Lancet. 2005;366:930-1.
4. DeSouza LJ, Carroll N. Ambulation of the braced myelomeningocele patient. J Bone Joint Surg [Am]. 1976;58:1112-8.
5. Duffy CM, Hill AE, Cosgrove AP. Three dimensional analysis in spina bifida. J Pediatr Orthop. 1996;16:786-91.
6. Sousa JC, Telzrow RW, Holm RA, McCartin R, Shurtleff DB. Developmental Guidelines for Children with Myelodysplasia. Physical Therapy. 1983;63(1):21-9.

9.6

1. Barry MJ. Physical Therapy Interventions for Patients With Movement Disorders due to Cerebral Palsy. J Child Neurol. 1996;11(1):S51-S60.
2. Basford JR. Therapeutic Heat, Microwaves and Cold. Encyclopedia of Pain. 2007;20:2461-4.

3. Bobath K, Bobath B. The neurodevelopmental treatment In: Scrotton D, ed. Management of the motor disorders of children with cerebral palsy. Oxford: Blackwell Scientific Publications Ltd. 1984.
4. Butler C, Campbell S. Evidence of the effects of intrathecal baclofen for spastic and dystonic cerebral palsy. Developmental Medicine & Child Neurology. 2000;42:634-64.
5. Butler C, Darrah J. AACPDM Evidence Report: Effects of neuro-developmental Treatment (NDT) for Cerebral Palsy. Developmental Medicine and Child Neurology. 2001;43:778-90.
6. Cook AS, Horak FB. Assessing the Influence of Sensory Interaction on Balance. Phys Ther. 1986;66:1548-1550.
7. Gerszten PC, Albright LA, Graham F, Johnstone. Intrathecal baclofen infusion and subsequent orthopedic surgery in patients with spastic cerebral palsy. Journal of Neurosurgery. 1998;88(6):1009-13.
8. Gregson JM, Leathley M, Moore AP, Sharma AK, Smith TL, Watkins CL. Reliability of the tone assessment scale and the modified ashworth scale as clinical tools for assessing poststroke spasticity. Archives of Physical medicine and rehabilitation. 1999;80(9):1013-6.
9. Hagberg B, Hagberg G, Beckung E, Uvebrant P. Changing panorama of cerebral palsy in Sweden. VIII. Prevalence and origin in the birth year period 1991–94. Acta Pædiatrica. 2001;90(3):271–7.
10. Jahnsen R, Villien L, Egeland T, Stanghelle JK, Holm I. Locomotion skills in persons with cerebral palsy.Clin Rehabil. 2004;18:309-16.
11. Knott M. "Neuromuscular Facilitation in the Child with Central Nervous System Deficit." JAmer Phv Ther Assoc. 1966;46:721-4.
12. Knox V, Evans LA. Evaluation of the functional effects of a course of Bobath therapy in children with cerebral palsy: a preliminary study. Dev Med Child Neurol. 2002;44:447-60.
13. Koman A, Paterson Smith B, Shilt J. Cerebral palsy. Lancet. 2004;363: 1619-31.
14. Kothari R, Singh R, Singh S, Jain M, Bokariya P, Khatoon M. Neurophysiologic findings in children with spastic cerebral palsy. Journal of Pediatric neurosciences. 2010;5(1):12-7.
15. Kuban KCK, Allred EN, Michael O'Shea, Paneth N, Pagano M, Leviton A. ELGAN Study Cerebral Palsy-Algorithm Group: An algorithm for identifying and classifying cerebral palsy in young children. J Pediatr. 2008;153(4):466-72.
16. Levine MG, Kabat H, Knott M, Voss DE. Relaxation of Spasticity by Physiological Technics. Arch Phys Med Rehab. 1954;35:214-23.
17. Lister MJ. Contemporary Management of Motor Control Problems: Proceedings of the II Step Conference. Alexandria: The Foundation for Physical Therapy. 1991;137-9.

18. Martin B, Tydeman C, Flodmark O. Clinical and MRI Correlates of Cerebral Palsy. JAMA. 2006;296:1602-8.
19. Morris C. Definition and classification of cerebral palsy: A historical perspective. Dev Med Child Neurol Suppl. 2007;109:3-7.
20. Odding E, Roebroeck ME, Stam HJ. The epidemiology of cerebral palsy: Incidence, impairments and risk factors. Disability & Rehabilitation. 2006;28(4):183-91.
21. Sahrmann SA, Norton BJ. The relationship of voluntary movement to spasticity in the upper motor neuron syndrome. Annals of Neurology. 1977;2:460-5.
22. Weindling AM, Cunningham CC, Glenn SM. Additional therapy for young children with spastic cerebral palsy: a randomized controlled trial. Health Technol Assess. 2007;11:16.

9.7

1. Hughes RA, Raphael JC, Swan AV, van Doorn PA. Intravenous immunoglobulin for Guillain-Barre syndrome. Cochrane Database Syst Rev. 2009;1:CD002063.
2. Hughes RA, Wijdicks EF, Barohn R. Practice parameter: immunotherapy for Guillain-Barre syndrome: report of the Quality Standards Subcommittee of the American Academy of Neurology. Neurology. 2003;61(6):736-40.
3. Meythaler, Miller RG, Sladky JT, Stevens JC, Hughes RAC, Wijdicks EFM, et al. Practice parameter: Immunotherapy for Guillain Barré syndrome: Quality Standards Subcommittee of the American Academy of Neurology. Neurology. 2003;61:736-40.
4. Shy ME. Peripheral neuropathies. In: Goldman L, Ausiello D, eds. Cecil Medicine. 23rd edn. Philadelphia, Pa: Saunders Elsevier: chap. 2007;446.
5. Tardy SV. Guillain-Barré syndrome and influenza virus infection. Clinical Infectious Diseases (The University of Chicago Press). 2009;48(1):48-56.
6. Yuki N. Campylobacter genes responsible for the development and determinant of clinical features of Guillain-Barré syndrome. Nippon Rinsho. Japanese Journal of Clinical Medicine. 2008;66(6):1205-10.

9.8

1. Baatile JBS, Langbein WE, Weaver F, Maloney Ms, Jost MB. Effect of exercise on perceived quality of life of individuals with Parkinson's disease. Journal of Rehabilitation Research and Development. 2000;37(5): 529-34.

2. Bloem BR, Grimbergen YA, Cramer M, Willemsen M, Zwinderman AH. Prospective assessment of falls in Parkinson's disease. J Neurol. 2001;248:950-8.
3. Garrett NA, Brasure M, Schmitz KH, Schultz MM, Huber MR. Physical inactivity: direct cost to a health plan. Am J Prev Med. 2004;27:304-9.
4. Gauthier L, Dalziel S, Gauthier S. The benefits of group occupational therapy for patients with Parkinson's disease. Am J Occup Ther. 1987;41: 360-5.
5. Goetz CG, Thelen JA, Macleod CM, Carvey PM, Bartley EA, Stebbins GT. Blood levodopa levels and Unified Parkinson's disease rating scale functions: with or without exercise. Neurology. 1993;43:1040-2.
6. Hirsch MA, Toole T, Maitland CG, Rider RA. The effects of balance training and high-intensity resistance training on persons with idiopathic Parkinson's disease. Arch Phys Med Rehabilitation. 2003;84:1109-17.
7. Keus SHJ, Bastiaan RB, Erik JMH, Alexandra BB, Munneke M. Evidence-Based Analysis of Physical Therapy in Parkinson's disease with Recommendations for Practice and Research. Movement Disorders. Physical therapy. 2007;22(4):451-60.
8. Pahwa R, Lyons KE, Koller WC. Handbook of Parkinson's Disease (3rd edition). Chapter 25: Therapy with botulinum toxin. Marcel Dekker Inc. New York. 2003.
9. Marchese R, Diverio M, Zucchi F, Lentino C, Abbruzzese G. The role of sensory cues in the rehabilitation of Parkinsonian patients: a comparison of two physical therapy protocols. Movement Disorder. 2000;15:879-83.
10. Morris ME, Iansek R, Matyas TA, Summers JJ. Stride length regulation in Parkinson's disease. Normalization strategies and underlying mechanisms. Brain. 1996;119(2):551-68.
11. Muller V, Mohr B, Rosin R, Pulvermuller F, Muller F, Birbaumer N. Short-term effects of behavioral treatment on movement initiation and postural control in Parkinson's disease: a controlled clinical study. Movement Disorder. 1997;12:306-14.
12. Nieuwboer A, De Weerdt W, Dom R, Truyen M, Janssens L, Kamsma Y. The effect of a home physiotherapy program for persons with Parkinson's disease. J Rehabil Med. 2001;33:266-72.
13. Rubinstein TC, Giladi N, Hausdorff JM. The power of cueing to circumvent dopamine deficits: a review of physical therapy treatment of gait disturbances in Parkinson's disease. Movement Disorder. 2002;17:1148-60.
14. Sasco AJ, Paffernbarger RS, Gemdre I, Wing AL. The role of physical exercise in the occurrence of Parkinson's disease. Archive of neurology. 1992;49:360-5.

15. Scandalis TA, Bosak A, Berliner JC, Helman LL, Wells MR. Resistance training and gait function in patients with Parkinson's disease. Am J Phys Med Rehabilitation. 2001;80(1):38-43.
16. Schrag A, Jahanshahi M, Quinn N. How does Parkinson's disease affect quality of life? A comparison with quality of life in the general population. Movement Disorder. 2000;15:1112-8.
17. Toole T, Hirsch MA, Forkink A, Lehman DA, Maitland CG. The effects of a balance and strength training program on equilibrium in Parkinsonism: a preliminary study. Neuro Rehabilitation. 2000;14:165-74.

9.9

1. Bohannon RW, Smith MB. Interrater reliability of a modified Ashworth scale of muscle spasticity. Phys Ther. 1977;67:206-7.
2. Compston A, Coles A. Multiple sclerosis. Lancet. 2002;359(9313):1221-31.
3. DeBolt LS, McCubbin JA. The effects of home-based resistance exercise on balance, power, and mobility in adults with multiple sclerosis. Arch Phys Med Rehabil. 2004;85:290-7.
4. DeBolt LS, McCubbin JA. The effects of home-based resistance exercise on balance, power, and mobility in adults with multiple sclerosis. Arch Phys Med Rehabil. 2004;85:290-7.
5. Ericsson RP, Lie MR, Wineinger MA. Rehabilitation in multiple sclerosis. Mayo Clin Proc. 1989;64:81and 828.
6. Freal JE, Kraft GH, Coryell JK. Symptomatic fatigue in multiple sclerosis. Arch Phys Med Rehabil. 1984;65:135-7.
7. Gehlsen GM, Grigsby SA, Winant DM. Effects of an aquatic fitness program on the muscular strength and endurance of patients with multiple sclerosis. Phys Ther. 1984;64:653-7.
8. Hough A. Physiotherapy in respiratory care: a problem-solving approach to respiratory and cardiac management. 2nd edn. London: Chapman & Hall. 1996.p.1-163.
9. Kasser SL, McCubbin JA. Effects of progressive resistance exercise on muscular strength in adults with multiple sclerosis. Med Sci Sports Exerc. 1996;28:S143.
10. Klefbeck B, Nedjad HJ. Effect of inspiratory muscle training in patients with multiple sclerosis. Arch Phys Med Rehabilitation. 2003;84:994-9.
11. Kraft GH, Freal JE, Coryell JK. Disability, disease duration, and rehabilitation service needs in multiple sclerosis: patient perspectives. Arch Phys Med Rehabilitation. 1986;67:164-8.
12. Mc Alphine D, Course, Diagnosis in Multiple Sclerosis: A Reappraisal. London, England. Churchill Livingstone. 1972;197-223.

13. Podsiadlo D, Richardson S. The timed "Up & Go": a test of basic functional mobility for frail elderly persons. J Am Geriatr Soc. 1991;39:142-8.
14. Reingold SC. Defining the clinical course of multiple sclerosis: results of an international survey. National Multiple Sclerosis Society (USA) Advisory Committee on Clinical Trials of New Agents in Multiple Sclerosis. Neurology. 1996;46(4):907-11.
15. Sadovnick AD,, Eisen K, Ebers GC, Paty DW. Cause of death in patients attending multiple sclerosis clinics. Neurology. 1991;41:1193-6.
16. Sharma KR, Kent-Braun JA, Mynhier MA, Weiner MW, Miller RG. Evidence of an abnormal intramuscular component of fatigue in multiple sclerosis. Muscle Nerve. 1995;18:1403-11.
17. Skelton DA, Greig CA, Davies JM, Young A. Strength, power, and related functional ability of healthy people aged 65-89 years. Age Ageing. 1994;23:371-7.
18. Smeltzer SC, Utell MJ, Rudick RA, Herndon RM. Pulmonary function and dysfunction in multiple sclerosis. Arch Neurol. 1988;45:1245-9.
19. Swensson B, Gerdle B, Elert J. Endurance training in patients with multiple sclerosis: five case studies. Phys Ther. 1994;74:1017-26.
20. Troyer DA, Pride NB. The respiratory system in neuromuscular disorders. In: Roussos C, Macklem PT, editors. The thorax: lung biology in health and disease. New York: Marcel Dekker. 1985.p.2135-40.

9.10

1. Arora NS, Rochester DE. Respiratory muscle strength and maximal voluntary ventilation in undernourished patients. Am Rev Respir Dis. 1982;126:5-8.
2. Ashworth NL, Satkunam LE, Deforge D. Treatment for spasticity in amyotrophic lateral sclerosis/motor neuron disease. Cochrane Database systematic review. 2006;25(1):CD004156.
3. Caroscio JT, Mulvihill MN, Sterling R, Abrams B. Amyotrophic lateral sclerosis: Its natural history. Neurol Clin. 1987;5:1-8.
4. Dworkin JE, Hartrnann DE. Progressive speech deterioration and dysphagia in amyotrophic lateral sclerosis: case report. Arch Phys Med Rehabil. 1979;60:423-5.
5. Francis K, Bach JR, Delisa DL. Evaluation and rehabilitation of patients with adult motor neuron disease. Archives of physical medicine and rehabilitation. 1999;80:951-63.
6. Gubbay SS, Kahana E, Zilher N, Cooper G, Pintov S, Leibowitz Y. Amyotrophic lateral sclerosis: a study of its presentation and prognosis. J Neurol. 1985;232:295-300.
7. Hillel AD, Miller R. Bulbar amyotrophic lateral sclerosis: patterns of progression and clinical management. Head Neck. 1989;11:51-9.

8. Kasarskis EJ, Neville HE. Management of ALS: nutritional care. Neurology. 1998;47(2):S118-20.
9. Radunovic A, Annane D, Jewitt K, Mustfa N. Mechanical ventilation for amyotrophic lateral sclerosis/motor neuron disease. Cochrane database systematic review. 2009;7(4): CD004427.
10. Robbins J. Swallowing in ALS and motor neuron disorders. Neurol Clin. 1987;5:213-29.
11. Slowie LA, Paige MS, Antel JR. Nutritional considerations in the management of patients with amyotrophic lateral sclerosis (ALS). J Am Diet Assoc. 1983;83:44-7.
12. Wijesekera LC, Mathers S, Talman P, Galtrey C, Parkinson MH, Ganesalingam J, et al. Natural history and clinical features of the flail arm and flail leg ALS variants. Neurology. 2009;72(12):1087-94.
13. Wikipedia, 2010. Accessed on 24th august-2010, !2:00 PM. http://en.wikipedia.org/wiki/Motor_ neurone_disease.
14. Yorkston KM, Strand E, Miller R, Hillel A, Smith K. Speech deterioration in amyotrophic lateral sclerosis: implications for the timing of intervention. J Med Speech-Language Pathol. 1993;1:35-46.

9.11

1. Gardner WJ. Hydrodynamic mechanism of syringomyelia: its relationship to myelocel. J. Neurol Neurosurg Psychiat. 1965;28:247.
2. Johnston L. Human spinal cord injury: new and emerging approaches to treatment. Spinal Cord. 2001;39:609-13.
3. Rossier AB, Foo D, Shillito J, Dyro FM. Post-traumatic cervical syringomyelia. Brain. 1985;108:439-61.
4. Schurch B, Wichmann W, Rossier AB. Post-traumatic syringomyelia (cystic myelopathy):a prospective study of 449 patients with spinal cord injury. J Neurol Neurosurg Psychiatr. 1996;60(1):61-7.
5. Williams B. On the pathogenesis of syringomyelia: a review. Journal of the Royal Society of Medicine. 1980;73:798-806.
6. Williams B. On the pathogenesis of syringomyelia: a review. Journal of the Royal Society of Medicine. 1980;73:799.

9.12

1. Francis K, Bach JR, Delisa DL. Evaluation and rehabilitation of patients with adult motor neuron disease. Archives of physical medicine and rehabilitation. 1999;80:951-63.
2. Wijesekera LC, Mathers S, Talman P, Galtrey C, Parkinson MH, Ganesalingam J, et al. Natural history and clinical features of the flail arm and flail leg ALS variants. Neurology. 2009;72(12):1087-94.
3. Wikipedia. Accessed on 24th august-2010, !2:00 PM. http://en.wikipedia.org/wiki/Motor_neurone_disease.

9.13

1. Colditz JC. Splinting for radial nerve palsy. J Hand Ther. 1987;1:18-23.
2. Dellon AL. Client evaluation and management considerations in nerve compression. In Rayan GM, editor: Hand clinics: nerve compression syndromes, Philadelphia. 1992, WB Saunders.
3. Feldman EL, Grisold W, Russell JW, Zifko UA. Atlas of Neuromuscular Diseases: A Practical Guideline. Springer Wien New York publisher. 2005;77.
4. Grogan PM, Gronseth GS. Practice parameter: Steroids, acyclovir, and surgery for Bell's palsy (an evidence-based review): report of the Quality Standards Subcommittee of the American Academy of Neurology. Neurology. 2001;56(7):830-6.
5. Gutman S. Quick reference neuroscience for rehabilitation professionals, Thorofare, NJ. 2001, SLACK.
6. Keane JR. Twelfth nerve palsy: analysis. Arch Neurol. 1996;53:561.
7. Lundborg G. Peripheral nerve injuries: patho-physiology and strategies for treatment. J Hand Ther. 1993;6(3):179-88.
8. Lundy-Ekman E. Neuroscience: fundamentals for rehabilitation, Philadelphia, 1998, WB Saunders.
9. May M, Blumenthal F, Klein SR. Acute Bell's palsy: prognostic value of evoked electromyography, maximal stimulation, and other electrical tests. Am J Otol. 1983;5(1):1-7.
10. McCormick DP. Herpes-simplex virus as a cause of Bell's palsy. Lancet. 1972;1(7757):937-9.
11. Peitersen E. The natural history of Bell's palsy. Am J Otol. 1982;4:107-11.
12. Rowlands S, Hooper R, Hughes E. The epidemiology and treatment of Bell's palsy in the UK. Eur Neurol. 2001;9:63-7.
13. Skirven TM, Callahan AD. Therapist's management of peripheral-nerve injuries. In: Mackin EJ, Callahan AD, Skirven TM, et al. (Eds). Rehabilitation of the Hand and Upper Extremity, 5th edn. St Louis, 2002, Mosby.

9.14

1. Aggarwal A, Zutshi K, Munjal J, Kumar S, Sharma V. Comparing stabilization training with balance training in recreationally active individuals. International Journal of Therapy and Rehabilitation. 2010;17(5): 244-253.
2. Fritz JM, Delitto A, Erhard RE. Comparison of Classification-Based Physical Therapy With Therapy Based on Clinical Practice Guidelines for Patients with Acute Low Back Pain: A Randomized Clinical Trial. Spine. 2003;28:1363-72.

3. Jin DM, Xu Y, Geng DF, Yan TB. Effect of transcutaneous electrical nerve stimulation on symptomatic diabetic peripheral neuropathy: a meta-analysis of randomized controlled trials. Diabetes Res. Clin. Pract. 2010;89(1):10-5.
4. MacDonald BK, Cockerell OC, Sander AS, Shorvon SD. The incidence and lifetime prevalence of neurological disorders in a prospective community-based study in the UK. Brain. 2000;123:665-76.
5. Marti V, Podnar S, Jovin Z. Clinical Manifestations of Brachial Neuralgia. Curr Top Neurol Psychiatr Relat Discip. 2010;18(1):49-56.
6. Ogon M, Bender BR, Hooper DM. A dynamic approach to spinal instability: Part II. Hesitation and giving way during interspinal motion. Spine. 1997;22:2859-66.
7. Pieber K, Herceg M, Paternostro-Sluga T. Electrotherapy for the treatment of painful diabetic peripheral neuropathy: a review. J Rehabil Med 2010;42(4):289-95.
8. Kumars, Sharma VP, Shukla R, Dev R, Aggarwal A. Efficacy of dynamic muscular stabilization techniques (DMST) in the management of lumbar disc disorders. Nigerian Journal of medical rehabilitation. 2009;14(22):14-9.
9. Van Tulder MW, Koes BW, Bouter LM. Conservative treatment of acute and chronic nonspecific low back pain: a systematic review of randomized controlled trials of the most common interventions. Spine. 1997;22:2128-56.
10. Werneke M, Hart DL. Centralization phenomenon as a prognostic factor for chronic low back pain and disability. Spine. 2001;26:758-65.

9.15

1. Bach JR. Management of post-polio respiratory sequelae. Ann. N Y Acad Sci. 1995;25:753:96-102.
2. Bach JR, Tilton M. Pulmonary function and its management in post-polio patients. Neurorehabilitation. 1997;8(2):139-53.
3. Bohannon RW. Manual muscle testing: does it meet the standards of an adequate screening test? Clin. Rehabil. 2005;19(6):662-7.
4. Brehm MA, Nollet F, Harlaar J. Energy demands of walking in persons with post-poliomyelitis syndrome: relationship with muscle strength and reproducibility. Arch Phys Med Rehabil. 2006;87(1):136-40.
5. Dean E, Ross J. Effect of modified aerobic training on movement energetics in polio survivors. Orthopaedics. 1991;14(11):1243-6.
6. Einarsson G. Muscle conditioning in late Poliomyelitis. Arch. Phys. Med. Rehabil. 1991;72(1):11-4.
7. Gawne AC, Halstead LS. Post-Polio Syndrome; Patho-physiology and Clinical Management. Critical Reviews in Physical and Rehabilitation Medicine. 1995;7(2):147-88.

8. Klein MG, Keenan MA, Esquenazi A, Costello R, Polansky M. Musculoskeletal pain in polio survivors and strength-matched controls. Arch. Phys. Med. Rehabil. 2004;85(10):1679-83.
9. Lord SR, Allen GM, Williams P, Gandevia SC. Risk of falling: predictors based on reduced strength in persons previously affected by polio. Arch Phys Med Rehabil. 2002;83(6):757-63.
10. Perry J, Mulroy SJ, Renwick SE. The relationship of lower extremity strength and gait parameters in patients with post-polio syndrome. Arch. Phys. Med. Rehabil. 1993;74:165-9.
11. Prins JH, Hartung H, Merritt DJ, Blancq RJ, Goebert DA. Effect of aquatic exercise training in persons with poliomyelitis disability. Sports Medicine, Training & Rehabilitation. 1994;5:29-39.
12. Waring WP, Maynard F, Grady W, Grady R, Boyles C. Influence of appropriate lower extremity orthotic management on ambulation, pain and fatigue in post-polio population. Arch Phys Med Rehabil. 1989;70(5): 371-5.
13. Weinberg J, Borg J, Bevegard S, Sinderby C. Respiratory response to exercise in post-polio patients with severe inspiratory muscle dysfunction. Arch. Phys. Med. Rehabil. 1999;80(9):1095-100.
14. Willen C, Grimby G. Pain, physical activity, and disability in individuals with late effects of polio. Arch Phys Med Rehabil. 1998;79(8):915-9.

9.16

1. Attia J, Hatala R, Cook DJ, Wong JG. The rational clinical examination. Does this adult patient have acute meningitis? JAMA. 1999;282 (2): 175-81.
2. Chamberlain MC. Neoplastic meningitis. Journal of Clinical Oncology. 2005;23(15):3605-13.
3. Cohen JS. Peripheral Neuropathy Associated with Fluoroquinolones (PDF). Ann Pharmacother. 2001;35(12):1540-7.
4. Ginsberg L. Difficult and recurrent meningitis. Neurol, Neurosurg, Psychia 2004;75(Suppl 1):16-21.
5. Jin DM, Xu Y, Geng DF, Yan TB. Effect of transcutaneous electrical nerve stimulation on symptomatic diabetic peripheral neuropathy: a meta-analysis of randomized controlled trials. Diabetes Res Clin Prac. 2010;89(1):10-5.
6. Moris G, Garcia-Monco JC. The Challenge of Drug-Induced Aseptic Meningitis. Archives of Internal Medicine. 1999;159(11):1185-94.
7. Pieber K, Herceg M, Paternostro-Sluga T. Electrotherapy for the treatment of painful diabetic peripheral neuropathy: a review. J Rehabil Med. 2010;42(4):289-95.
8. Sáez-Llorens X, McCracken GH. Bacterial meningitis in children. Lancet. 2003;361(9375):2139-48.

9. Van de Beek D, de Gans J, Spanjaard L, Weisfelt M, Reitsma JB, Vermeulen M. Clinical features and prognostic factors in adults with bacterial meningitis. The New England Journal of Medicine. 2004;351(18):1849-59.
10. Wilkes G. Peripheral neuropathy related to chemotherapy. Seminars in oncology nursing. 2007;23(3):162-73.

9.17

1. Campbell M. Cecily Partridge (editor). Physical Management and Rehabilitation of Patients with Traumatic Head Injury. Neurological Physiotherapy: Bases of evidence for practice. Whurr Publishers, London and Philadelphia. 2002;83.
2. Chudley. The effect of nursing activities on intracranial pressure. British Journal of Nursing. 1994;3(9):454-5.
3. Eames P, Wood R. The structure and content of a head injury rehabilitation service. In Wood RL, Eames P (Eds) Models of Brain Injury Rehabilitation. London: Chapman & Hall. 1989;pp.31-58.
4. Hardman JM, Manoukian A. Pathology of Head Trauma. Neuroimaging Clinics of North America. 2002;12(2):175-87.
5. Rancho Los Amigos National Rehabilitation Center (RLA NRC), patient information, Communication Disorders Department, 7601 E. Imperial Highway, Downey, CA 90242. Los Amigos Research and Educational Institute (LAREI), 1990.
6. Roberts S. Cecily Partridge (editor), Neurological Physiotherapy: Bases of evidence for practice. Whurr Publishers, London and Philadelphia. 2002;63.
7. Rothen HU, Sporee B, Engberg G, Wegenius G, Hedenstierna G. Re-expansion of atelectasis during general anaesthesia: a computed tomography study. British Journal of Anaesthesiology. 1993;71(6):788-95.
8. Satz P, Zaucha K, McCleary C, Light R, Asarnow R, Becker D. Mild head injury in children and adolescents: A review of studies (1970–1995). Psychological Bulletin. 1997;122(2):107-31.

9.18

1. Dobkin B. Overview of treadmill locomotor training with partial body weight support: a neurophysiologically sound approach whose time has come for randomized clinical trials. Neurorehabil Neural Repair. 1999;13:157-65.
2. Dobkin BH, Apple D, Barbeau H, Basso M, Behrman A, Deforge D, et al. Methods for a Randomized Trial of Weight-Supported Treadmill Training Versus Conventional Training for Walking During Inpatient Rehabilitation after Incomplete Traumatic Spinal Cord Injury. Neurorehabil Neural Repair. 2003;17:153.

3. Edelle CF, Fluet GG , Schafer SD , Schneider EM, Smith R, Downey PA, et al. The Spinal Cord Injury Functional Ambulation Inventory (Sci-Fai). J Rehabil Med. 2001;33:177-81.
4. Hayes KC, Davies AL, Potter PJ. Restorative neurological approaches to the rehabilitation of individuals with longstanding spinal cord injury. Topics in Spinal Cord Injury Rehabilitation. 2004;10(1):51-62.
5. Johnston L. Human spinal cord injury: new and emerging approaches to treatment. Spinal Cord. 2001;39:609-13.
6. Kirby RL, Swuste J, Dupulis DJ, Macleod DA, Randi M. The Wheelchair Skills Test: A pilot study of a new outcome measure. Archives of Physical Medicine and Rehabilitation. 2002;83(1):10-8.
7. Krupa T, Fossey E, Anthony WA, Brown C. Doing daily life: how occupational therapy can inform psychiatric rehabilitation practice. Psychiatr Rehabil J. 2009;32(3):155-61.
8. Morganti B, Scivoletto G, Ditunno P, Ditunno J, Molinari M. Walking index for spinal cord injury (WISCI): criterion validation. Spinal Cord. 2005;43:27-33.
9. Pillastrini P, Mugnai R, Bonfiglioli R, Curti S, Mattioli S, Maioli MG. Evaluation of a therapy program for patients with spinal cord injury. Spinal Cord. 2008;46:78-81.
10. Wernig A, Muller S. Laufband locomotion with body weight support improved walking in persons with severe spinal cord injuries. Paraplegia. 1992;30:229-38.
11. Wernig A, Nanassy A, Miller S. Maintenance of locomotor abilities following Laufband (treadmill) therapy in para and tetraplegic persons: follow-up studies. Spinal Cord. 1998;36:744-9.
12. Wikipedia, 2010. Spinal cord Injury, accessed on 18th September, 2010, 6:00 AM http://en. wikipedia.org/wiki/Spinal_cord_injury#cite_note-Pilla-14.

INDEX

Page numbers followed by *f* refer to figure and *t* refer to table

D

E

M

N

Q

R

S

T

U

V

W

Y

Z